FOURTH EDITION

RESPIRATORY CARE PHARMACOLOGY

_____ FOURTH EDITION _____

RESPIRATORY CARE PHARMACOLOGY

Joseph L. Rau Jr., Ph.D., R.R.T.

Professor and Chair
Cardiopulmonary Care Sciences
College of Health Sciences
Georgia State University
Atlanta, Georgia

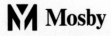 Mosby

St. Louis Baltimore Boston Chicago London Madrid Philadelphia Sydney Toronto

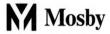

Dedicated to Publishing Excellence

Publisher: George Stamathis
Editor: James F. Shanahan
Developmental Editor: Jennifer Roche
Project Manager: Nancy C. Baker
Senior Production Editor: Jerry Schwartz
Proofroom Manager: Barbara M. Kelly
Designer: Nancy C. Baker
Manufacturing Supervisor: Karen Lewis

Copyright © 1994 by Mosby–Year Book, Inc.

Printed in the United States of America
Composition by Clarinda
Printing/binding by Donnelley-Crawfordsville

Mosby-Year Book, Inc.
11830 Westline Industrial Drive
St. Louis, Missouri 63146

Library of Congress Cataloging in Publication Data
Rau, Joseph L.
  Respiratory care pharmacology / Joseph L. Rau, Jr.—4th ed.
    p. cm.
  Includes bibliographical references and index.
  ISBN 0-8016-7184-1
  1. Respiratory therapy, 2. Respiratory agents. I. title.
  [DNLM: 1. Bronchodilator Agents—administration & dosage.
  2. Bronchodilator Agents—pharmacology. 3. Respiratory Therapy.
  WB 342 R239r 1993]
  RM161.R39   1993
  616.2'00461—dc20
  DNLM/DLC
  for Library of Congress   93-33353
                                                CIP

1 2 3 4 5 6 7 8 9 0   98 97 96 95 94

NOTICE

Every effort has been made to ensure that the drug dosage schedules herein are accurate and in accord with the standards accepted at the time of publication. However, as new research and experience broaden our knowledge, changes in treatment and drug therapy occur. Therefore, the reader is advised to check the product information sheet included in the package of each drug he plans to administer to be certain that changes have not been made in the recommended dose or in the contraindications. This is of particular importance in regard to new or infrequently used drugs.

To my son, Joe, and to all the students in respiratory care pharmacology

PREFACE TO THE FOURTH EDITION

The fourth edition of *Respiratory Care Pharmacology* marks the 15th anniversary since the first, small text, then titled *Respiratory Therapy Pharmacology*, appeared in 1978. The evolution of this text mirrors that of respiratory therapy, at least from a pharmacological perspective.

In the 1978 edition there were five classes of drugs available for aerosol inhalation: the adrenergic bronchodilators, a mucolytic, a surface-active agent (Alevaire), two steroids, and cromolyn. The second edition in 1984 more than doubled the size of the first edition, in response to demand from the profession for more information. Chapters were added on central nervous system, cardiovascular, and diuretic drugs.

In the third edition, copyrighted 1989, chapters were added on the aerosol delivery of medications and on pediatric dosing with aerosolized agents. The in-depth review of methods of aerosolizing drugs reflected the increasing diversity and knowledge of methods of aerosol delivery.

In this, the fourth edition, there are 19 chapters, compared with 14 in the first edition. The increase in chapters results from splitting some material previously combined into a single chapter. Xanthines, exogenous surfactants, aerosolized anti-infectives, and cold medications are each treated in separate chapters. Chapter 2 is further expanded to present technical descriptions of methods of aerosol delivery as well as advantages and limitations for patient use of each method.

Despite increased information and scope of responsibility in the practice of respiratory care, the fourth edition preserves the same goal of the first three: to offer a useful organization of drug knowledge for students and practitioners. It is in the hope of achieving this goal that a new edition is offered to those dedicated to respiratory care.

Every effort has been made to ensure the accuracy of information contained in this text. However, practitioners are urged to review manufacturer's detailed literature whenever administering drugs, and to keep informed of new information from research results.

Joseph L. Rau, Jr., Ph.D., R.R.T.

PREFACE TO THE FIRST EDITION

Respiratory therapy pharmacology represents one area of drug application, which can be summarized as the area of bronchoactive drugs. Respiratory therapy pharmacology is even more specific than general pharmacology, which is itself an applied field of study resting on more fundamental sciences such as chemistry and biology. Generally, the specific drugs utilized in respiratory care are delivered by aerosol, another distinguishing characteristic. The group of bronchoactive drugs is intended to provide pharmacologic care of the airway, either through control of bronchial smooth muscle, or through control of secretions. Seven categories of drugs used directly by respiratory therapy are currently included in the bronchoactive group, offering a diversely challenging field of study. In each category of drugs considered in the text, a brief review of the underlying pharmacology and physiology is first offered, and then specific drugs are identified for review. A general introductory consideration of basic pharmacologic principles and the autonomic nervous system is included, as well as drug dosage calculations, with practice problems and answers. Several drug categories (neuromuscular blockers, prostaglandins) not directly used by respiratory therapists are also discussed.

The material considered ranges from the factual and simple to the theoretical and complex, in the hope of providing useful information for all levels of personnel engaged in respiratory care. Limitations of scope to respiratory therapy drugs and drugs directly related to respiratory care is deliberate, in the belief that the field has evolved to the point of requiring in-depth treatment of well-defined subjects, rather than a comprehensive review of all topics within one text.

Joseph L. Rau, Jr., Ph.D., R.R.T.

ACKNOWLEDGMENTS

This fourth edition, as with previous editions, is possible only with the support of former teachers, colleagues, and friends in the medical professions. John Holbrook, Ph.D., has continued to offer his expertise as coauthor of Chapter 16, on central nervous system drugs. Douglas Pearce, M.D., has shared his knowledge and experience by reviewing Chapter 17, on cardiovascular agents, with helpful suggestions. As before, the greatest acknowledgment must go to students in respiratory care, whose need for knowledge remains the ultimate motivation for writing this book.

"If I have seen further, it is by standing on the shoulders of giants." (Isaac Newton, letter to Robert Hooke, February 5, 1675)

Joseph L. Rau, Jr., Ph.D., R.R.T.

CONTENTS

4   CENTRAL AND PERIPHERAL NERVOUS SYSTEMS   *97*

5   SYMPATHOMIMETIC BRONCHODILATORS   *129*

6   PARASYMPATHOLYTIC (ANTICHOLINERGIC) BRONCHODILATORS   *161*

7   XANTHINES   *179*

12   AEROSOLIZED ANTI-INFECTIVE AGENTS   *285*

13   ANTI-INFECTIVE AGENTS   *311*

14   COLD AND COUGH AGENTS   *331*

15   SKELETAL MUSCLE RELAXANTS (NEUROMUSCULAR BLOCKING AGENTS)   *349*

1

General Principles of Pharmacology

Chapter 1 presents concepts and principles of pharmacology needed for clinical practice and respiratory care. The following topics are discussed:

- Definitions of drugs and pharmacology
- Legislation regulating drug therapy
- Types of drug names
- Sources of drug information
- Sources of drugs
- Process of drug investigation and approval
- Principles of drug action from dose to effect
- The prescription and its components
- Overview of respiratory care pharmacology

The study of respiratory therapy pharmacology represents a specialized area and as such presupposes a background of general pharmacological principles, as well as more fundamental studies of chemistry, biology, biochemistry, anatomy, and human physiology. Those principles, definitions, and concepts that are most useful for general clinical practice, or especially for understanding drugs given directly by respiratory care personnel, are included as introductory material.

FUNDAMENTAL TERMS

Drugs. The many complex functions of the human organism are regulated by chemical agents such as hormones, kinins, and catecholamines. Chemicals interact with an organism to alter its function, thus illuminating the life process and at times providing methods of diagnosis, treatment, or prevention of disease. Such chemicals are called *drugs*. Most simply and universally, a drug is any chemical that alters an organism's functions or processes. Examples include oxygen, alcohol, LSD (lysergic acid diethylamide), and vitamins.

Pharmacology.   Pharmacology is the study of the interactions of drugs (chemicals) with an organism. This is the most general statement of the field. In particular, pharmacology includes specialized aspects such as dosage forms, preparation, and dispensation (pharmacy); absorption, distribution, breakdown, and elimination of drugs in the body (pharmacokinetics); and the effects and interaction of drugs within the body (pharmacodynamics). Other areas of specialized knowledge include the study of the harmful effects of drugs (toxicology), the art of treating diseases with drugs (therapeutics), and the sources of drugs (pharmacognosy).

Another specialized area of general pharmacology is pharmacogenetics, the study of the interrelationship of genetic differences and drug effects. Respiratory care personnel may often encounter a practical example of this in patients receiving succinylcholine, a neuromuscular blocking agent. Normally, this drug produces a rapid but short paralysis of skeletal muscles; in approximately 1 of 3000 patients, however, the drug causes prolonged paralysis. The drug is normally metabolized by a plasma enzyme, serum cholinesterase. The abnormal response is caused by a genetically based, abnormal or missing serum cholinesterase, and individuals with this genetic difference will require supported ventilation until the paralysis-induced apnea ends and the succinylcholine is ultimately eliminated.

LEGISLATION AFFECTING DRUGS

1906:   The first Food and Drugs Act is passed by Congress; the *United States Pharmacopeia* (USP) and the *National Formulary* (NF) are given official status.

1914:   The Harrison Narcotic Act is passed to control the importation, sale, and distribution of opium and its derivatives, as well as other narcotic analgesics.

1938:   The Food, Drug and Cosmetic Act becomes law. This is the current Federal Food, Drug and Cosmetic Act, enforced by the Food and Drug Administration (FDA), to protect the public health and to protect physicians from irresponsible drug manufacturers.

1952:   The Durham-Humphrey Amendment defines the drugs that may be sold by a pharmacist only by prescription.

1962: The Kefauver-Harris Law is passed as an amendment to the Food, Drug and Cosmetic Act of 1938. This act requires proof of safety and efficacy of all drugs introduced since 1938; drugs in use prior to 1938 have not been reviewed but are under study.

1971: On May 1 the Controlled Substances Act becomes effective. This act lists requirements for the control, sale, and dispensation of narcotics and dangerous drugs. Five schedules of controlled substances have been defined: Schedules 1 to 5 generally define drugs of decreasing potential for abuse, increasing medical use, and decreasing physical dependence. Examples of each schedule follow.

Schedule 1: heroin, marijuana, LSD, peyote, and mescaline

Schedule 2: opium, morphine, codeine, cocaine, and amphetamines

Schedule 3: glutethimide (Doriden), paregoric, and barbiturates, with some exceptions

Schedule 4: phenobarbital, barbital, chloral hydrate, meprobamate (Equanil, Miltown), and paraldehyde

Schedule 5: narcotics containing nonnarcotics in mixture form, such as cough preparations or diphenoxylate HCI (Lomotil)

NAMING DRUGS

Because a drug is a chemical, is officially regulated in the United States, and is sold as a competitive product by various manufacturers, it has a variety of labels rather than a single name.

A drug that becomes officially approved for general clinical use in the United States will have accumulated at least five different names: chemical name, code name, generic name, official name, and trade name.

Chemical Name. The chemical name indicates the drug's chemical structure.

Code Name. The code name is assigned by a manufacturer to an experimental chemical that shows potential as a drug. An example is aerosol SCH 1000, which is the code name for ipratropium bromide, a parasympatholytic bronchodilator (see Chapter 6).

Generic Name. The generic name is assigned to a chemical by the United States Adopted Name Council when the chemical appears to have therapeutic use and the manufacturer wants to market the drug. Instead of a numerical or alphanumerical code as in the code name, the generic name often is loosely based on the drug's chemical structure. For example, isoproterenol has an isopropyl group attached to the terminal nitrogen on the amino side chain, whereas metaproterenol is the same chemical structure as isoproterenol except that a dihydroxy attachment on the catechol nucleus is now in the so-called meta position (carbon-3,5 instead of carbon-3,4). The generic name is also known as the nonproprietary name, as opposed to the trade name.

Official Name.   In the event that an experimental drug becomes fully approved for general use and is admitted to the USP-NF, the generic name becomes the official name. Since an officially approved drug may be marketed by many manufacturers under different names, it is recommended that clinicians use the official name, which is nonproprietary, and not the trade name.

Trade Name.   The brand name, or proprietary name, is given by the manufacturer. For example, the generic drug isoproterenol is marketed by Winthrop as Isuprel and by Abbott as Norisodrine. Note that dosage strengths may vary with different manufacturers.

Following is an example of the different names for the same drug, beclomethasone dipropionate, an aerosolized corticosteroid used by patients with asthma:

Chemical name: 9-chloro-11β,17,21-trihydroxy-16β-methylpregna-1,4-diene-3,20-dione 17,21-dipropionate

Official name: beclomethasone dipropionate

Generic name: beclomethasone dipropionate

Trade name: Vanceril (Schering), Beclovent (Glaxo)

SOURCES OF DRUG INFORMATION

There are two official volumes that give drug standards in the United States.

The *United States Pharmacopeia* was first published in 1820 as a private medical effort, and was given official status in 1906 with the first congressional Food and Drugs Act. The USP specifies standards for such drugs as oxygen, indicated by the USP label. The USP undergoes revision every 5 years.

The *National Formulary* was first published in 1888, with the same legal status as the USP. It is published by the American Pharmaceutical Association and is continuously revised. In 1980, which was the date for revision of the USP, the USP and NF were combined into a single volume.

The *AMA Drug Evaluations* gives information and results on new drugs that are not yet officially included in the USP.

The *Physician's Desk Reference* is prepared by manufacturers of drugs and therefore is potentially lacking in the objectivity of the preceding sources. However, this annual volume does provide useful information, including descriptive color charts for drug identification, names of manufacturers, and general drug actions.

The *Hospital Formulary*, published by the American Society of Hospital Pharmacists, contains monographs and commentaries on classes of drugs (e.g., antibiotics, steroids).

Goodman and Gilman's The Pharmacological Basis of Therapeutics gives an in-depth discussion of general pharmacologic principles and modes of drug action.

Several pharmacology texts dealing more specifically with the use of drugs for the respiratory system are listed in the Bibliography.

SOURCES OF DRUGS

Although the source of drugs is not a crucial area of expertise for the respiratory care clinician, it can be one of the most interesting. Recognition of naturally occurring drugs dates to Egyptian papyrus records, to the ancient Chinese, and to the Central American civilizations, and is still seen in remote regions of the United States such as Appalachia.

The prototype of cromolyn sodium was khellin, found in the Eastern Mediterranean plant *Ammi visnaga*. This plant was used in ancient times as a muscle relaxant; today its synthetic derivative is used as an antiasthmatic agent. Similar stories can be told for curare, derived from large vines and used by South American Indians to coat arrow tips for lethal effect; for digitalis, obtained from the foxglove plant *(Digitalis purpurea)*, reputedly used by the Mayans for relief of angina, and definitely referred to by thirteenth century Welsh physicians; and for the notorious poppy, source of the opium alkaloids, immortalized in De Quincey's *Confessions of an English Opium Eater*.

Today, the most common source of drugs is chemical synthesis, but animals, plants, and minerals have often contributed the prototype of the active ingredient. Examples of each source include the following:

Animal: thyroid hormone, insulin, pancreatic dornase

Plant: khellin *(A. visnaga)*, atropine *(Atropa belladonna* alkaloid), digitalis (foxglove), reserpine *(Rauwolfia serpentina)*, volatile oils of eucalyptus, pine, anise

Mineral: copper sulfate, magnesium sulfate (epsom salts), mineral oil (liquid hydrocarbons)

PROCESS OF DRUG APPROVAL IN UNITED STATES

The process by which a chemical moves from the status of a promising potential drug to one fully approved by the FDA for general clinical use is, on average, long, costly, and complex. Although the time and cost vary for individual drugs, the process can require an average of 12 years and cost around $200 million for a single drug. Only 1 in 10,000 chemicals identified as potential drugs will reach general clinical use. The major steps in the drug approval process are discussed in the following sections and outlined in Table 1–1. These steps were reviewed by Flieger (1989) and Hassall and Fredd (1989).

TABLE 1–1.
Major Steps in the Process of Marketing a Drug in the United States

Isolation and identification of the chemical
Animal studies
General effects
Special effects on organ systems
Toxicology
Investigational New Drug approval
Phase 1 studies: small number, healthy subjects
Phase 2 studies: small number, subjects with disease
Phase 3 studies: large, multicenter studies
New Drug Application
Reporting system for first 6 months

Chemical Identification

Since a drug is a chemical, the first step in drug development is to identify a chemical with the potential for useful physiological effects. This has recently been illustrated by the plant product taxol, which was derived from the needles and bark of the Western yew tree. Taxol has demonstrated antineoplastic activity, making it attractive for investigation as an anticancer drug. The exact structure and physical and chemical characteristics of an active ingredient are established during this step of the process.

Animal Studies

Once an active chemical is isolated and identified, a series of animal studies are used to examine its general effect on an organism, as well as its effect on specific organs such as the liver or kidneys.

Toxicology studies to examine mutagenicity, teratogenicity, effect on reproductive fertility, and carcinogenicity are also performed.

Investigational New Drug Approval

At this point an Investigational New Drug application is filed with the FDA for the chemical being examined. This application includes all information previously gathered as well as plans for human studies. These studies proceed in three phases and usually require about 3 years to complete.

Phase 1.   The drug is investigated in a small group of healthy volunteers to establish its activity. This is the pharmacokinetic description of the drug (i.e., rates of absorption, distribution, metabolism, and elimination).

Phase 2.   The drug is next investigated as a treatment for a small number of patients with the disease the drug is intended to treat.

Phase 3.   The drug is investigated in large, multicenter studies to establish safety and efficacy.

New Drug Application

After a successful Investigational New Drug process, a New Drug Application is filed with the FDA, and after approval the drug is released for general clinical use. A detailed reporting system is in place for the first 6 months to track any problems that arise with the drug's use. The drug is no longer experimental (investigational) and can be prescribed by physicians for treatment of the general population.

FDA New Drug Classification System

Since some drugs are simply released in new forms or are similar to previously approved agents, the FDA has a classification system to help identify the importance of new products (Covington, 1991). An alphanumerical code is given to provide this information.

Chemical/Pharmaceutical Standing

1 = New chemical entity   4 = New combination
2 = New salt form   5 = Generic drug
3 = New dosage form   6 = New indication

Therapeutic Potential

A = Important (significant) therapeutic gain over other drugs
AA = Important therapeutic gain, indicated in acquired immunodeficiency syndrome; fast track
B = Modest therapeutic gain
C = Important options; little or no therapeutic gain

PRINCIPLES OF DRUG ACTION

The general concepts or principles of pharmacology seem on first encounter to be a confusing array of miscellaneous and poorly interrelated details. However, a conceptual framework suggested by Ariens and Simonis (1974) is useful for organizing some of these detailed concepts in a way that is more easily remembered and perhaps better understood.

Ariens and Simonis identified three basic phases of drug action, from the initial administration of a dose, through the drug's ultimate effect on the body: the *pharmaceutical phase*, the *pharmacokinetic phase*, and the *pharmacodynamic phase*. Figure 1–1 illustrates the concepts and sequential nature of

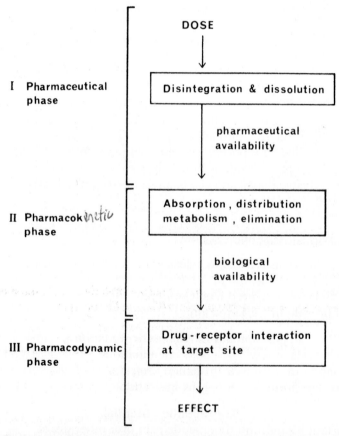

FIG 1–1. The conceptual scheme illustrating the major phases of drug action in sequence, from dosage administration to effect in the body. (Based on Ariens EJ and Simonis AM: Drug action: target tissue, dose-response relationships, and receptors. In Teorell T, Dedrick RL, and Condliffe PG, eds: Pharmacology and Pharmacokinetics, New York, 1974, Plenum Press.)

these three phases. The advantage of such a conceptualization is that it provides an organizational framework within which can be fit such details as dosage forms, routes of administration, rate of uptake, plasma half-life, and membrane transport, to mention a few.

Pharmaceutical Phase

A necessary condition for any drug action in the body is that the drug become available for absorption. The **drug dosage form** (e.g., tablet, liquid) greatly influences the disintegration and dissolution of the active substance. The **route of administration** is a second major determinant of drug availability to the body. The form in which a drug is supplied and the route of administration are related, and both are determined by other factors such as amount, susceptibility of the drug to degradation, and location of the target site in the body.

The dosage form of a drug is defined as the product or unit in which the drug is received (e.g., tablet, capsule, injectible liquid, ointment). The route of administration depends on the following factors:

1. Whether systemic or only local effect is needed
2. Desired rate of onset and duration of action of the drug
3. Stability of the drug in gastric and/or intestinal fluids
4. Whether the patient is able to swallow, retain, and absorb drugs given orally
5. Convenience vs. safety of various routes
6. Amount of drug: large amounts can be given orally or intravenously (IV), smaller doses intramuscularly or subcutaneously

Oral Route

The oral route is generally the safest, most convenient, and most economical delivery route for drugs intended to have systemic effect.

Dosage forms for the oral route include the following:

Tablet: solid dosage form prepared by molding or compressing the drug in dies

Capsule: medication contained a soluble shell of gelatin, methylcellulose, or calcium alginate

Pill: globular or ovoid dosage form prepared from a cohesive, plastic mass

Powder: mixture of dry, powdered drugs; may be used externally also (e.g., dusting powders, powders for douche solutions)

Solution: homogeneous mixture of a solvent (commonly water) and a solute

Elixir: sweetened, hydroalcoholic solution, usually flavored; other vehicles are glycerin and syrup

Syrup: nearly saturated solution of a sugar; may contain active medicinal agents

Emulsion: mixture of two immiscible liquids (usually water and an oil).

Gel: insoluble drug in a semisolid form

Parenteral Route

Parenteral literally means any route other than the intestine. The common clinical meaning, however, is the route of injection.

Types of injection include the following (Fig 1–2):

1. Intradermal
2. Subcutaneous
3. Intramuscular
4. Intravenous
5. Intraarterial: involves placing a needle into an artery for example, when drawing blood to measure blood gas levels; This route is useful for treating the specific area perfused by the artery with a drug.

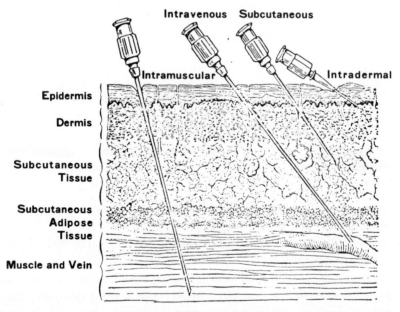

FIG 1–2.   Representation of skin layers differentiating the types of injection. (Adapted from Plein JD and Plein EM: Fundamentals of medication, ed 2, Hamilton, Ill, 1974, The Hamilton Press, Inc.)

6. Intraspinal: injection through a vertebral interspace into the spinal subarachnoid space
7. Epidural: injection through a vertebral interspace between the dura of the spinal cord and the periosteal lining of the spinal canal
8. Intraperitoneal: insertion of a needle or trocar into the peritoneal space; frequently used for peritoneal dialysis

Drugs given intravenously must be dissolved in an aqueous (water-based) solution; oil-based solutions would create emboli in the circulation. Such oil-based solutions or lipid-soluble solutions may be given intramuscularly or subcutaneously, and aspiration is performed with the syringe to detect inadvertent placement of the needle in a vein. The potency of the drug may also dictate against intravenous administration, which provides a rapid and direct effect.

Note: "Drawing up" a dose for injection is usually from either an ampule or vial.

Topical: Mucous Membranes

Topical application is often used in the rectum, vagina, or ureter as a means of systemic effect due to good absorption in these vascularized areas. Usually application to the nose or throat is intended for a localized topical effect, as with nasal spray decongestants, throat lozenges, or antiseptic sprays. Methods of topical application to the mucous membranes include the following:

Lozenges: discs or flat squares of flavored medication that dissolve in the mouth

Ophthalmic Solutions: for the eye

Nasal Solutions: for the nose

Otic Solutions: for the ear

Sublingual Tablets: for absorption under the tongue

Buccal Tablets: placed between the teeth and cheek

Suppositories: solid forms of medication prepared in a base (cocoa butter, glycerinated gelatin, or polyethylene glycols) that will soften or dissolve at body temperature. These are for rectal, vaginal, or (rarely) urethral application

Topical: Skin Application

Topical application to the skin is usually for local rather than systemic effect. There are notable exceptions to this, such as the topical use of nitroglycerin for coronary artery vasodilation. The following preparations have been used for application to the skin surface:

Powders.

Wet Preparations: dressing, soaks, and baths

Lotions: aqueous preparations that may be solutions, suspensions, or emulsions

Liniment: oily or alcoholic topical solutions, suspensions, or emulsions

Ointments: semisolid preparations that may have anhydrous bases, emulsions of oil in water, or water-washable substances such as polyethylene glycols

Creams: semisolid, less solid than ointments, with water-soluble or vanishing-cream base

Pastes: stiff, ointment-like preparations containing large quantities of powdered drugs such as zinc oxide or starch

Jellies: viscous, semisolid preparations usually made by hydrating gums; lubricant or vehicle

Inhalation

The inhalation of drugs provides a route of administration for either *systemic* effects throughout the body or *local* effects restricted to the upper (nose, throat, larynx) or lower airway. A common clinical example of an inhaled drug given for general, systemic effect is provided by gas anesthetics such as halothane. Inhaled aerosol drugs in respiratory care are intended for local effect in the airway.

Because the inhalation route of administration is relatively convenient, painless, and safe, it has been investigated for a number of agents intended for systemic effect. These agents include contraceptives (Gudmundsson et al., 1986), a diuretic (Shionoiri and Kaneko, 1986), flu vaccine (Petrescu et al., 1985), insulin (Salzman et al., 1985), and glucagon (Pontiroli et al., 1985), all administered intranasally. However, emphasis in this text is placed on drugs given by aerosol for respiratory care purposes.

A variety of devices have been or are used now to deliver drugs by inhalation whether in the gas phase or as an aerosol.

Vaporizers.   Vaporizers are heating systems that vaporize solutions such as plain water or volatile oils (anise, eucalyptol) to increase ambient humidity (Fig 1-3,A). These devices are less frequently used clinically, and the boiling liquid constitutes a serious burn hazard when used with young children. Because of this hazard and the lack of a demonstrated beneficial effect on the pulmonary system with vaporized aromatic substances (Boyd, 1970; Kaufmann et al., 1975), vaporizers should be considered obsolete.

Inhalers. Inhalers contain a relatively volatile medication embedded in some inert substance. The vapors are drawn into the nose by inhaling (Fig 1–3, **B**).

Atomizer. An atomizer uses a squeeze-bulb to force air and liquid through two separate tubes (Fig 1–3, **C**). Mixing of the air and liquid at the top of the device produces aerosolization of the liquid. There are no baffles,

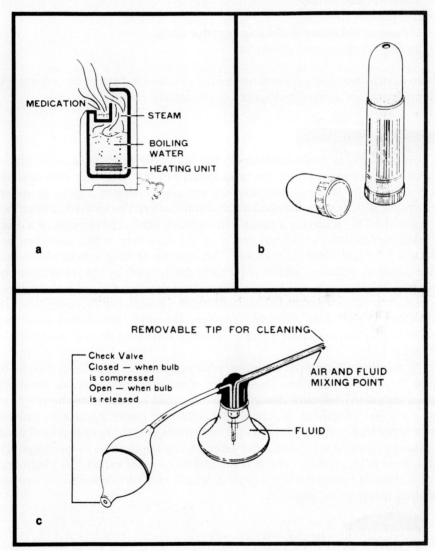

FIG 1–3. A, Vaporizer or steam inhaler. **B,** Inhaler. **C,** Atomizer.

and particle sizes may vary more than with nebulizers. These devices may be used to spray an aerosol directly into the nasal passages or the oropharyngeal region.

Other devices in common clinical use for the delivery of inhaled aerosolized drugs are the following:

- Small-volume nebulizer
- Metered-dose inhaler
- Dry-powder inhaler
- Ultrasonic nebulizer (including portable units)
- Small-particle aerosol generator

These devices are characterized more fully in Chapter 2 when discussing the administration of aerosolized agents in respiratory care.

Pharmacokinetic Phase

Once a drug is made available to the body, the pharmacokinetic phase begins. This phase describes the drug amount in the body over time and includes the major factors controlling the amount of drug at a given moment: absorption, distribution, metabolism, and elimination. The kinetics of drug levels are crucial for achieving a desired therapeutic effect. For example, if a drug is being metabolized, or broken down, at the same rate as it is absorbed, an effective dose will never be achieved. The kinetics of drug activity also influence duration of action, which is partially determined by the metabolism of the drug. For example, terbutaline sulfate is metabolized to an inactive form more slowly than isoproterenol hydrochloride, because the two drugs are not vulnerable to the same degrading enzyme. Therefore, terbutaline would be preferred over isoproterenol if longer duration is desired and all other factors are equal.

As this limited example indicates, pharmacokinetics is basic to the use of drugs for applied treatment. The kinetics of the drug (rate of onset, duration, how metabolized, effective dosage level, etc.) must be related to the needs of the particular treatment situation. The following pages attempt to outline some of the basic principles, concepts, and terms needed to understand what is meant in general by pharmacokinetics and its application to the drugs administered in respiratory care. It is not a definitive nor exhaustive treatment, and additional references are supplied, which may be needed when reviewing drug literature or research.

Absorption

To reach a given point in the body, a drug must cross a number of cellular membranes, depending on the target site and route of administration. For example, thiopental (Pentothal Sodium), an ultra–short-acting barbiturate, is intended to affect the central nervous system when used as an anesthetic. If this drug were taken orally, it would first cross the gastrointestinal epithelial lining, be absorbed into the bloodstream, circulate to the brain, and then cross the blood-brain barrier. Of course, with IV administration, common in anesthesiology, the drug bypasses the gastric mucosa, crossing only the blood-brain barrier. Thiopental is well absorbed across this barrier because of its poorly ionized state.

In general, the mechanisms for absorption of drugs include the following:
1. Passive (no energy required).
   a. Simple diffusion.
   b. Facilitated diffusion.
   c. Filtration.
2. Active (requires energy).
   a. Active transport.
   b. Pinocytosis.

Simple Diffusion. Simple diffusion across cell membranes, such as the gastric or pulmonary mucosal lining, is unfortunately not very simple. Cell membranes are composed of a double layer of lipid molecules sandwiched between two polypeptide layers. The membrane is also perforated by small pores, which allow filtration of suitably sized molecules. Simple diffusion across this membrane does not require energy but relies on a concentration gradient from one side of the membrane to the other.

In addition to a gradient, several other factors influence the ability of a drug to diffuse across cell membranes. One factor is the lipid solubility of a drug: to diffuse across a lipid layer requires that a drug be able to dissolve in a lipid substance. Another factor, which affects lipid solubility, is ionization: ions are not lipid soluble, whereas the nonionized form of a drug is lipid soluble and can diffuse across the cell membrane. Therefore, diffusion across cell membranes will be favored for poorly ionized, lipid-soluble drugs. A practical example of this is given by thiopental, a barbiturate, and tubocurarine, a paralyzing agent. Thiopental is poorly ionized in the bloodstream and will diffuse across the cell membranes into the brain, producing sedation, sleep, or anesthesia. Tubocurarine is a fully ionized compound that will not reach the brain. A patient who is paralyzed with tubocurarine for surgery cannot move at all but is fully awake because there will be no effect on the brain from the drug.

In the case of drugs that are weak acids or bases, for example, salicylic acid or quinine (a base), ionization can occur and will reduce membrane diffusion. However, the degree of ionization of such substances is determined by the surrounding pH and pKa of the drug. The pH in the body differs for various locations. For example, consider the following sites and their normal pH:

Plasma: 7.40.

Gastric Juice: 1.0.

Cerebrospinal Fluid (CSF): 7.32.

Urine: 4.5 to 8.0 (varies).

The pKa of a drug is the pH at which the drug is 50% ionized and 50% nonionized. For example:

Salicylic Acid: pKa = 3.0.

Quinine: pKa = 8.4.

Phenobarbital: pKa = 7.2.

In practical terms, this means that 50% of a drug will be ionized when the ambient pH equals the pKa of that drug. Furthermore, the direction of increasing ionization, which would *reduce* membrane diffusion, is opposite for weak acids and bases. Compare the degree of ionization for salicylic acid and quinine, given their pKa's and different pH's:

Salicylic acid; pKa = 3		Quinine (base); pKa = 8.4	
pH = 2	9% ionized	pH = 7.4	91% ionized
pH = 3	50% ionized	pH = 8.4	50% ionized
pH = 4	91% ionized	pH = 9.4	9% ionized

Aspirin (acetylsalicylic acid) is a weak acid, with a pKa of approximately 3.5, and is mostly nonionized in the stomach where the pH hovers around 1.0. Since the nonionized form is lipid soluble, aspirin is well absorbed from the gastric lining. However, by contrast quinine is almost completely ionized as the ambient pH becomes more acidic in reference to the pKa of 8.4; therefore, quinine is mainly in an *ionized* form in the stomach and is not well absorbed until it reaches the more basic intestine.

In summary, consider the pKa as a reference baseline. For a weak acid, there is less ionization in an acidic environment; for a weak base, there is more ionization in an acidic environment. The key principle is this: Cell membranes are more permeable to the nonionized form of a drug than to an ionized form.

Facilitated Diffusion.   Facilitated diffusion is similar to simple diffusion in that a concentration gradient is required for transport to occur. However, in its transport, the molecule is believed to attach to a carrier, and the transport is more rapid than in simple diffusion. This is not an active process requiring energy. An example of this type of process is given by the diffusion of glucose through the membrane of the red blood cell.

Filtration. Filtration is able to occur through cell membranes because of the presence of pores, as previously mentioned. These pores are water-filled channels approximately 40 A wide in some cells; molecules that are hydrophilic, even if lipid insoluble, can filter across the membrane if they are small enough for the pores. Such filtration can then occur in the presence of a hydrostatic or osmotic pressure gradient, as contrasted with the concentration gradient of simple diffusion. Larger channels up to 40 A occur in capillary endothelial cells and allow passage of molecules as large as albumin; water, urea, chloride, and potassium are all able to filter through membrane pores.

Active Transport. Active transport differs from the three forms of passive transport just discussed in that it requires energy and involves transfer *against* a concentration gradient. Such transport probably requires carrier mechanisms, which can become saturated when the amount of the substance transported becomes too great. An example is the pumping out of sodium ions by nerves or muscle.

Pinocytosis. Pinocytosis is a form of transport in which the cell actually engulfs extracellular fluid. Proteins and macromolecules can be slowly carried across a cell by the formation of an enclosure, or vesicle, around them. Modell et al. (1976) suggest that the resorption of liquid droplets in the alveoli may exemplify this process.

Distribution

In general, drugs will be absorbed into the bloodstream and distributed throughout the body. Accumulation may occur in the extracellular compartment (plasma, interstitial fluid, lymph); the intracellular fluid; or the special fluid systems of cerebrospinal, intraocular, peritoneal, pleural, or synovial fluids.

An area of interest and complexity for distribution is the crossing of drugs through the blood-brain barrier. Essentially the brain is enclosed in a cushion of CSF. Between the CSF and any blood vessels is the blood-brain barrier, composed of the capillary endothelium. To have an effect on the central nervous system, particularly the brain, a drug must travel from the plasma to the CSF and into brain cells. There is free diffusion between CSF and brain cells, but not between plasma and CSF. Anatomically the blood-brain barrier is created by the endothelial cells of capillaries in the brain, which are joined together by continuous, tight, intercellular junctions. In capillaries elsewhere, cells may be separated by 50–100 A. Functionally, there is active and selective control of substances in the CSF, with 7% more sodium and 30% less glucose than in extracellular fluid. The usual route of circulation from plasma to CSF and back to venous blood is as follows:

1. Plasma.
2. Choroid plexus and ventricles of brain.
3. Formation of CSF.
4. Transport to arachnoid villi.
5. Reabsorption by veins.

A classic example of drug treatment that was made difficult by the blood-brain barrier is given with parkinsonism, a disease involving poor motor coordination and regulation. A deficiency of a neurotransmitter substance called dopamine was found in the brain of patients with parkinsonism. Therefore it should be possible to give such patients dosages of dopamine to cure their tremors. Unfortunately, dopamine will not cross the blood-brain barrier, even if injected directly into the bloodstream. However, the chemical precursor of dopamine (or more correctly L-dopamine), which is levodopa (L-dopa), *is* absorbed across the blood-brain barrier by active transport, and once in the brain, it is transformed into dopamine and helps regulate motor coordination. This agent, L-dopa, has been successful in controlling the tremors of parkinsonism by being able to reach the intended site of action.

Another factor that is related to drug distribution is accumulation of drugs in fat depots. In lean persons, fat accounts for about 10% of body weight, whereas heavier individuals may have up to 30% of body weight caused by fat. Some drugs are absorbed into these lipid depots, which may cause more of the drug to be needed for therapeutic effect and a longer duration of action because of slow release of the drug from the lipid storage in people who are overweight. An example of such a drug that accumulates in lipid is phenoxybenzamine, an alpha-sympathetic blocker. Insecticides and anesthetic gases can also accumulate because they are lipid soluble.

Metabolism and Elimination

The rapidity with which a drug is biochemically altered and/or excreted is a major factor determining its duration of activity. For many drugs taken orally or by other systemic routes the liver is a major site of drug metabolism. This is true for barbiturates for instance. When taken orally a barbiturate will be metabolized by microsomal enzymes as it passes through the liver; 200 mg of pentobarbital produces drowsiness if taken by mouth but produces anesthesia if given intravenously. Sites other than the liver can contain enzymes capable of breaking down drugs. For example, the gastric mucosa contains a sulfatase enzyme that inactivates isoproterenol when taken orally. Plasma contains a cholinesterase enzyme that hydrolyzes succinylcholine (a neuromuscular blocking agent) and procaine (a local anesthetic).

Excretion of drugs from the system occurs primarily through the kidneys. Even if not chemically altered, a drug may still be eliminated in the urine after a given amount of time. However, the altered form of a chemical will often be more water soluble and less lipid soluble than the original compound and will be readily excreted by the kidneys.

There are two points of interest related to renal elimination of drugs. First, the effect of plasma and urine pH on drug ionization, given a particular pKa, affects the lipid solubility and diffusion of the drug into the urine, as previously discussed for absorption mechanisms. Second, patients in renal failure present a much more complicated drug therapy situation since the major elimination mechanism is lost. Peritoneal dialysis or hemodialysis several times a week substitutes for the normal filtration and excretion of the kidneys.

Protein Binding

In addition to absorption, distribution, metabolism, and elimination, plasma and tissue protein binding determine how much of the active drug is available for effect at a given time (biological availability). For instance, warfarin, an anticoagulant, is a commonly cited example of a drug that is 97% bound in plasma to the protein albumin. Only about 3% of the drug is free to act. Competition for the same plasma protein by other substances, such as aspirin, can radically change the biological availability of warfarin by displacing it from the albumin. Such drug interactions can significantly affect the pharmacokinetics of a drug. The amount of free, available, active warfarin could easily double to 6% in the presence of aspirin, causing hemorrhage.

The total biological availability of a drug is the net result of the interplay among the preceding pharmacokinetic factors: rate of absorption, distribution, metabolism, elimination, and protein binding.

Considered graphically, the biological availability of a drug is given by the area under a curve whose axes are the level of active drug and time or duration. The *shape* of the curve is determined by the amount of drug given, rates of absorption, metabolism and elimination, as well as any protein binding. If a drug is metabolized as rapidly as the rate of absorption for the given dose, then a somewhat flattened graph of plasma drug level over time will result. The basic pharmacokinetic concepts previously discussed are integrated and illustrated in Figure 1–4. Hypothetical time-plasma curves for 2 drugs give equal biological availability for drugs A and B. That is, the *area* under the two curves is equal. However, the *shape* of the two curves is different, and this is described as the *bioavailability profile*. In drug A, because of the overall kinetics, a threshold therapeutic plasma level is never realized. In drug B, the bioavailability profile indicates that an effect would be seen. Immediate practical results of such bioavailability profiles are the loading dose amount and the frequency of dosage administration.

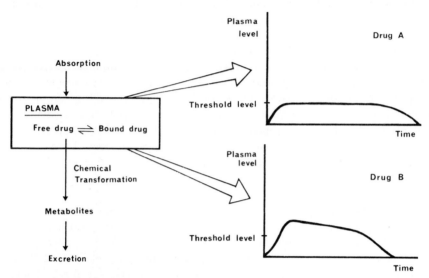

PHARMACOKINETIC FACTORS   BIOAVAILABILITY PROFILES

FIG 1–4. Diagrammatic representation of the factors determining the pharmacokinetics of a drug, with plasma-concentration curves for two hypothetical drugs (A and B), showing approximately equal biological availability but significantly different bioavailability profiles.

Application to Inhaled Drugs

The principles of pharmacokinetics also apply to inhaled aerosolized drugs. A major rationale for aerosolizing drugs used in respiratory care is to treat the lung locally as the target organ and prevent or minimize absorption and distribution throughout the body by the bloodstream. Absorption and distribution may still occur, however, causing unwanted side effects in other organs such as the heart. For example, isoproterenol, an adrenergic bronchodilator discussed in Chapter 5, is well absorbed from the mouth and lung, can increase the heart rate, and can cause vasodilation in the pulmonary circulation as the drug distributes through the bloodstream.

The principles of absorption and distribution previously presented form the basis for understanding absorption of aerosolized drugs from the lungs and distribution through the body. A good example is provided by atropine sulfate and ipratropium bromide, aerosolized anticholinergic agents discussed in Chapter 6. Both agents can block cholinergic-induced bronchoconstriction. However, atropine sulfate is less ionized than ipratropium bromide, which is fully ionized. Since cell membranes are more permeable to nonionized than to ionized forms, atropine is well absorbed from the lung when inhaled and produces numerous side effects throughout the body. These include cycloplegia, tachycardia, and central nervous system changes. Because ipratropium is fully ionized, it is not well absorbed from the lung when inhaled, and side effects are usually limited to a dry mouth. This is a local effect as the aerosolized drug is inhaled orally.

Inhalation Route of Administration.   Catecholamine agents such as isoproterenol or isoetharine are almost completely metabolized to an inactive sulfate form in the gut wall and liver when taken orally. Because of this, the oral route is not effective for achieving dilatation of the airways. If these drugs are inhaled, they do reach the airway and cause bronchial dilatation before they are metabolized to an inactive form. Inhalation is convenient and targets the organ needing treatment, making this the route of choice. Davies (1975) has described these processes for inhaled adrenergic agents and cromolyn sodium in detail.

Rate of Metabolism and Duration of Effect.   The different adrenergic agents available or under investigation also provide an illustration of how absorption, metabolism, distribution, and elimination determine the time course of a drug's activity in the body and in turn the frequency of dosing needed for efficacy. The rate of metabolism is the key factor differentiating agents in this group.

Figure 1–5 shows hypothetical curves for the measured clinical effect of

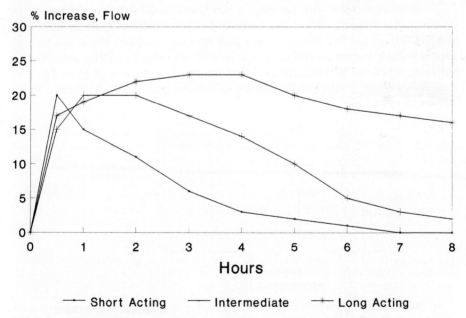

FIG 1–5.   Hypothetical time-effect curves for three different bronchodilating agents, illustrating onset, peak effect, and duration.

improved ventilatory flow rates for three types of bronchodilators: short-acting, intermediate, and long-acting agents. The short-acting curve could represent a drug such as isoetharine. Based on its time curve, this agent is too short-acting for maintenance therapy but could be useful for a before and after pulmonary function study, where a rapid peak effect and short duration are desirable. The intermediate curve, representing an agent such as albuterol with a slower peak effect but longer duration, is more suited to maintenance therapy and would require dosing 3 or 4 times a day, depending on the severity of airway obstruction. Finally, a long-acting agent, such as the investigational drug salmeterol, could provide maintenance therapy with an even less frequent dosing of twice a day and would be very useful for preserving airflow during the night.

Pharmacodynamic Phase

The final phase of drug action, the pharmacodynamic phase, refers to the interaction of the drug molecule with its target receptor site. It is this interaction of molecules that ultimately answers the question of *how* a particular drug works.

Receptor Theory

Beginning in 1878 with Langley, it has been theorized that a drug exerts its effect at a specific site in the body and is physically in contact with that site to bring about the effect. Using a lock and key analogy, the site is the receptor or lock for which the drug is a specific key (Fig 1–6). The structure of the drug is related to the corresponding structure of the receptor, and just as one key can fit one lock but not others, so one drug is specific to certain types of receptors but not others.

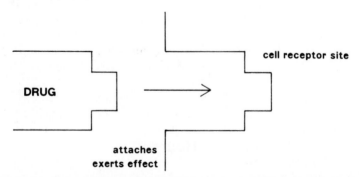

FIG 1–6. Diagrammatic representation of a drug-receptor interaction.

The essential concepts for explaining drug action are as follows:

1. The drug has to actually reach the receptor.
2. The drug is specific to its matching receptor.
3. This specificity is based on the chemical structure of the drug.

One of the basic concepts of drug-receptor interaction is that a drug must physically combine with a target receptor to produce an effect. For inhaled aerosol drugs, this means that the aerosol must enter the airways and then actually reach the site of action. If the drug is a mucus-controlling agent, it can interact with the mucous blanket. For a beta-adrenergic bronchodilator, the drug must be absorbed *through* the mucous and periciliary layers, the pulmonary epithelium, and finally into the bronchial smooth muscle where the drug can attach to the β_2 receptors causing bronchodilatation. A mast cell stabilizing agent such as cromolyn sodium probably is similarly absorbed. Use of radiolabeled drugs has shown that the absorption from airway lumen to subsurface tissue and even the bloodstream occurs rapidly (within minutes) and is probably by diffusion.

The last two concepts describe the matching of drug structure to a receptor. This is usually termed the *structure-activity relationship* of the drug, or SAR. Different effects in drug action can be caused by very minute changes in drug chemical structure, emphasizing the degree of exactitude required in drug-receptor matching. This correspondence of structure is even stereospecific, as indicated by the relative physiological inactivity of *d*-epinephrine, the right-handed stereoisomer of epinephrine. The body does respond to *l*-epinephrine, the levorotatory form.

The receptor model explains why one drug can affect certain organs or systems but not others, why small changes in chemical structure bring about significant changes in drug action, and how a drug can compete with endogenous chemicals to block the usual effect of those chemicals. The clinical usefulness of a drug is directly related to the specificity of its action. For example, acetylcholine is a poor drug for treatment because it activates far too many receptor sites. Acetylcholine is analogous to a pass key that is universal to many locks, whereas a more specific drug such as metaproterenol can fit only one.

The autoregulation of the body is based on certain chemical keys fitting matched receptor locks. By "duplicating" the endogenous chemical key with a drug, one can mimic the natural chemical's effect. This is the basis of therapeutics in pharmacology.

While the receptor concept is fundamental in explanations of drug activity, the receptors themselves are somewhat hypothetical entities inferred from the structure-activity differences of the drugs acting on the receptors. The chemical structure of the drugs is understood in detail; the molecules that are thought to comprise the target or corresponding receptor are largely unknown. Receptors are thought to be of molecular size and may be found on particular enzyme molecules, or they may be functional proteins or protein-lipid complexes on cell membranes. Drug-receptor interaction is probably analogous to an enzyme-substrate interaction. In respiratory care, these concepts may be applied to the question of the beta receptor, which responds to bronchodilators. Research (Lefkowitz, 1976; Sahyoun et al., 1977; Steer et al., 1975) indicates that this receptor is likely a protein complex on the surface of the cell membrane, rather than the enzyme adenyl cyclase as previously thought.

Several terms, based on drug-receptor interaction, are applied generally in discussing drugs and their effects.

Drug affinity: Measure of the tendency of a drug to combine with a particular receptor

Drug efficacy: Measure of the tendency of the drug-receptor complex to cause a specific response. The terms *agonist* and *antagonist* can then be defined, using the distinction between affinity and efficacy

Agonist: Drug or agent that not only has an affinity for a corresponding receptor but also possesses efficacy (i.e., creates the effect mediated by the receptor)

Antagonist: Drug that has affinity but lacks efficacy

Drug Interactions

With the increasing complexity of drug therapy, and with most critical patients encountered by respiratory care personnel on multiple drug therapies, concepts of drug interaction become very useful for understanding patient reactions. Appendix D provides further information on this topic. The terms used to describe these interactions—addition, synergism, potentiation, and antagonism—are used ambiguously, and definitions vary. The situation is made complex by the increased understanding of drug actions. Two drugs may act on the same receptors in the same way, or by different mechanisms to produce the same effect, or they may counteract each other at the same receptors or by completely different mechanisms. Further complication can arise from difficulty in quantifying the exact amount of drug effect. Do two drugs give twice the effect (usually termed *additive*) or more than twice (*potentiation* or *synergism*)? An **additive** effect describes the drugs giving an effect equal to the summation of their individual effects, or 1 + 1 = 2. **Synergism** and **potentiation** describe the same result: two drugs give an effect greater than the simple sum of their effects. However, synergism implies both drugs are active, or 1 + 1 = 3. Potentiation implies one of the drugs is inactive, or 1 + 0 = 3. **Antagonism** describes the situation of two drugs with opposing effects. For example, the effect of morphine can be reversed by use of its antagonist, nalorphine. Another example, of interest to respiratory care personnel, is the reversal of histamine by epinephrine.

Cumulation.   Cumulation occurs when a drug's rate of removal or inactivation is slower than the rate of administration (Fig 1–7). This can be dangerous depending on the drug's effect and is more likely when the drug has a long half-life in the body. The result of cumulation is toxicity, or a toxic as opposed to therapeutic level of the drug. For example, digitoxin is usually limited to 0.2 mg per day, and the electrocardiogram can be monitored for signs of toxicity (atrioventricular block).

Tolerance.   Tolerance is the phenomenon wherein increasing amounts of a drug are needed to produce the same effect. This is variable depending on the drug, but a well-known example is provided by the barbiturate group. Since barbiturates are metabolized in the liver by certain enzymes, a tolerance may develop due to *microsomal enzyme induction,* or the increase in enzyme levels that metabolize these agents. This is due to the increasing need for the enzymes with repeated doses of barbiturates in the body.

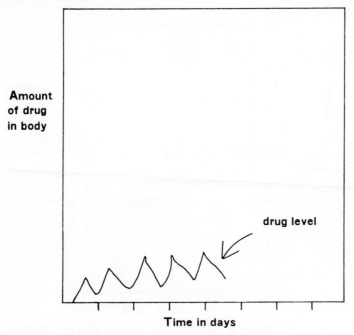

FIG 1–7. Cumulative amount of a drug given daily.

Tachyphylaxis.   Tachyphylaxis is the case of rapidly developing toler-ance, such as can occur with repeated doses of sympathomimetic com-pounds.

Therapeutic Index

By experimentation, one can determine the dosage of the drug that would be lethal to 50% of a test population of animals. This dose that is lethal to 50% of the population is termed the *lethal dose$_{50}$* (LD$_{50}$). One can also deter-mine the dose that is therapeutically effective for 50% of the test population, termed the *effective dose$_{50}$* (ED$_{50}$). The ratio of the LD$_{50}$ to the ED$_{50}$ is termed the *therapeutic index* (Fig 1–8).

$$\text{Therapeutic index} = LD_{50}/ED_{50}$$

In words this index indicates how close the effective dose is to the dose that is lethal for 50% of the test population. As the ED$_{50}$ approaches the LD$_{50}$, the danger of a drug increases significantly. If the LD$_{50}$ is 9 g and the ED$_{50}$ is 1 g, the therapeutic index is 9, but if the LD$_{50}$ dropped to 6 g with an ED$_{50}$ of 4 g, the therapeutic index would be 1.5. For example, penicillin has a therapeutic index greater than 100, which means the drug is relatively safe in terms of

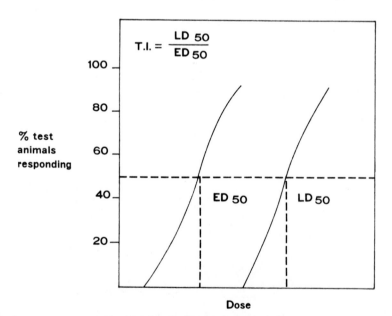

FIG 1–8. Therapeutic index *(T.I.)* indicating the effective dose and the lethal dose for 50% of the population.

toxic effects or overdosage. On the other hand, digitalis has a rather low index of 1.5 to 2.0, and the toxicity or lethal level of the dose is very close to the therapeutic dose. It is interesting to note that with the increase in drug usage, the therapeutic index seems to be decreasing on the average for all drugs.

THE PRESCRIPTION

The prescription is the written order for a drug, along with any specific instructions for compounding, dispensing, and taking the drug.

This order may be written by a physician, osteopath, dentist, veterinarian, and others, but not by chiropractors and opticians.

The detailed parts of a prescription are shown in Figure 1–9. It should be noted that both Latin and English, as well as metric and apothecary measures, have been used for drug orders. The directions (number 4 in the list that follows) to the pharmacist for mixing or compounding drugs have become less necessary with the advent of the large pharmaceutical firms and their prepared drug products. However, the importance of these directions is in no way diminished since misinterpretation is potentially lethal when dealing with drugs.

The most common abbreviations seen with prescriptions are listed in

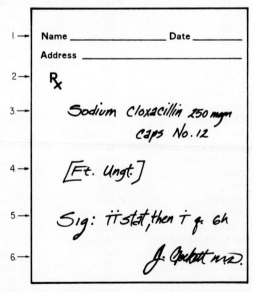

FIG 1–9. Prescription: an order for medication.

Table 1–2. Most abbreviations are derived from Latin, the mother tongue of medicine.

Ever since the Controlled Substances Act of 1971, physicians must include their registration numbers given by the Drug Enforcement Administration (and usually termed a *DEA Registration Number*) when prescribing

TABLE 1–2.

Abbreviations and Symbols Used in Prescriptions

Abbreviation	Meaning	Abbreviation	Meaning
a͞a	of each	p̄	after
a.c.	before a meal	part. aeq.	equal parts
ad lib.	as much as desired	p.c.	after meals
alt. hor.	every other hour	pil.	pill
aq. dest.	distilled water	placebo	I please
b.i.d.	twice daily	p.o.	by mouth
C, cong	gallon	p.r.n.	as needed
c̄	with	p.r.	rectally
caps.	capsule	pulv.	powder
cc	cubic centimeter	q.	every
dil.	dilute	q.h.	every hour
d.t.d.	give such doses	q.i.d.	four times daily
el.	elixir	q.o.d.	every other day
emuls.	emulsion	q.d.	every day
et	and	q2h	every 2 hours
ex aq.	in water	q3h	every 3 hours
ext.	extract	q4h	every 4 hours
fld.	fluid	q.s.	as much as required
ft.	make	qt	quart
gel.	a gel, jelly	px, Rx	take
g	gram	s̄	without
gr	grain	sig.	write
gtt.	a drop	sol.	solution
h.s.	at bedtime	solv.	dissolve
IM	intramuscular	s.o.s.	if needed (for one time)
IV	intravenous	spt.	spirit
L	liter	sp. frumenti	whiskey
lin.	a liniment	ss	half
liq.	liquid, solution	stat.	immediately
lot.	lotion	syr.	syrup
M	mix	tab.	tablet or tablets
mist., mixt.	Mixture	t.i.d.	three times daily
ml	milliliter	tr., tinct.	tincture
nebul.	a spray	ung.	ointment
non rep.	not to be repeated	ut dict.	as directed
n.p.o.	nothing by mouth	vin.	wine
o, ō	pint	(ʒ)	dram
O.D.	right eye	(M)	minim
ol.	oil	℥	ounce
O.S.	left eye	(℈)	scruple
O.U.	both eyes		

narcotics or controlled substances. Any licensed physician may apply for such a number.

The following parts of the prescription can be seen in Figure 1–9:

1. Patient's name and address; date.
2. Rx (meaning "recipe" or "take thou") directs the pharmacist to take the drugs listed and prepare the medication. This is called the *super-scription.*
3. The *inscription* lists the names and quantities of the drugs.
4. When applicable, the *subscription* directs the pharmacist in preparing the medication. In many cases, with precompounded drugs, counting out the correct number is the only requirement. In the example in Figure 1–9, the directions indicate that an ointment is to be made, which might be appropriate for certain medications.
5. Sig. (signa) means write. The pharmacist writes the *transcription* or signature on the label of the medication as instructions to the patient. *instructions to the pt. for taking the drug.*
6. Name of the prescriber.

RESPIRATORY CARE PHARMACOLOGY: AN OVERVIEW

One of the central themes of respiratory therapy has been care of the patient's airway, from acute emergency situations to chronic maintenance and rehabilitation. This theme has not only defined the field, including clinical responsibilities and equipment, but has proved definitive of that area known as *respiratory therapy pharmacology.* In particular, all drugs used in respiratory therapy can be considered as *bronchoactive,* with one purpose (i.e., *airway patency*) through three major modes of action:

1. Relaxation of bronchial smooth muscle.
2. Control/reduction of secretions.
3. Reduction/prevention of airway mucosal edema.

The relatively small group of bronchoactive drugs directly used by the therapist might be categorized as follows:

Bronchodilators
Epinephrine HCl 1:100
Racemic epinephrine (Micronefrin, Vaponefrin)
Isoproterenol 1:200 (Isuprel)
Isoetharine (Bronkosol)
Metaproterenol sulfate (Alupent, Metaprel)

Terbutaline sulfate (Bricanyl, Brethine)
Albuterol (Ventolin, Proventil)
Bitolterol mesylate (Tornalate)
Pirbuterol (Maxair)
Ipratropium bromide (Atrovent)
Mucolytics and Humidifying Agents
Acetylcysteine (Mucomyst)
Sodium bicarbonate
Normo-, hypo-, hypertonic saline
Distilled water
Surfactant Agents
Colfosceril palmitate (Exosurf)
Beractant (Survanta)
Corticosteroids
Dexamethasone sodium phosphate (Decadron Respihaler)
Beclomethasone dipropionate (Vanceril, Beclovent)
Triamcinolone acetonide (Azmacort)
Flunisolide (AeroBid)
Asthma Prophylactic
Cromolyn sodium (Intal, Aarane)
Nedocromil sodium (Tilade)
Antiinfective
Pentamidine isethionate (NebuPent)
Ribavirin (Virazole)

All the drugs mentioned above can be given either by the aerosol route or by direct tracheal instillation. In addition to these classes of drugs, the respiratory therapist is very closely involved with other classes including antibiotics, neuromuscular blocking agents, expectorants/antitussives, cardiovascular agents, and diuretics.

BIBLIOGRAPHY

Ariens EJ, Simonis AM: Drug action: target tissue, dose-response relationships, and receptors. In Teorell T, Dedrick RL, Condliffe PG, eds: Pharmacology and Pharmacokinetics, New York, 1974, Plenum Press.

Boyd EM: A review of studies on the pharmacology of the expectorants and inhalants, Int J Clin Pharmacol 3:55, 1970.

Covington TR: The ABCs of new drugs. Facts and Comparisons Newsletter 10(10):73, 1991.

Davies DS: Pharmacokinetics of inhaled substances, Postgrad Med J 51:69, 1975.

Flieger K: How experimental drugs are tested in humans, Pediatr Infect Dis J 8:160, 1989.

Gilman AG et al, eds: Goodman and Gilman's The pharmacological basis of therapeutics, ed 8, New York, 1990, Pergamon Press.

Gudmundsson JA, Nillins SJ, Berquist C: Intranasal peptide contraception by inhibition of ovulation with the gonadotropin-releasing hormone superagonist nafarelin: six months' clinical results, Fertil Steril 45:617, 1986.

Hassall TH, Fredd SB: A physician's guide to information available about new drug approvals, Am J Gastroenterol 84:1222, 1989.

Kaufmann DA, Swenson EW, Brickhouse GS: Effects of eucalyptol inhalation on pulmonary function, Respir Care 20:251, 1975.

La Du BN, Mandel HG, Way EL, eds: Fundamentals of drug metabolism and drug disposition, Baltimore, 1971, Williams & Wilkins.

Langley JN: On the physiology of the salivary secretion. Part II, J Physiol 1:339, 1988.

Lefkowitz RJ: β-adrenergic receptors: recognition and regulation, N Engl J Med 295:323, 1976.

Lehnert BE, Schachter EN: The pharmacology of respiratory care, St. Louis, 1980, CV Mosby.

Mathewson HS: Pharmacology for respiratory therapists, ed 2, St. Louis, 1981, CV Mosby.

Modell W, Schild HO, Wilson A: Applied pharmacology, ed 11, Philadelphia, 1976, WB Saunders.

Petrescu A et al: Dynamics of neutralizing secretory influenza antibodies after nasal administration of the NIVGRIP trivalent influenza vaccine, Virologie 36:187, 1985.

Pontiroli AE, Alberetto M, Pozza G: Metabolic effects of intranasally administered glucagon: comparison with intramuscular and intravenous injection. Acta Diabetol Lat 22:103, 1985.

Sahyoun N et al: Topographic separation of adenylate cyclase and hormone receptors in the plasma membrane of toad erythocyte ghosts, Proc Natl Acad Sci USA 74:2860, 1977.

Salzman R et al: Intranasal aerosolized insulin: mixed-meal studies and long-term use in type I diabetes, N Engl J Med 312:1078, 1985.

Shionoiri H, Kaneko Y: Intranasal administration of alpha-human natriuretic peptide produces a prolonged diuresis in healthy man, Life Sci 38:773, 1986.

Steer ML, Atlas D, Levitzki A: Inter-relations between β-adrenergic receptors, adenylate cyclase and calcium, N Engl J Med 292:409, 1975.

Ziment I. Respiratory pharmacology and therapeutics, Philadelphia, 1978, WB Saunders.

2

Administration of Aerosolized Agents

Chapter 2 presents technical aspects, including equipment, for the delivery of aerosolized drugs. The following topics are discussed:

- Physical principles of aerosol delivery of drugs
- Aerosol devices used for drug delivery
- Clinical application of aerosol delivery devices

Aerosol therapy may be defined as the delivery of aerosol particles to the pulmonary system for therapeutic purposes. One of the purposes of aerosol therapy is the deposition of bronchoactive agents such as bronchodilators, decongestants, and mucus-controlling, anti-inflammatory, or anti-infective agents in the lung.

The term *aerosol* has been ascribed to the German investigator Schmauss who around 1920 used this label generically for dusts, fogs, clouds, mists, fumes, and smoke in the air (Morrow, 1981).

The general advantages that support the use of aerosol therapy in respiratory care include the following:

1. Aerosol doses are smaller than those for systemic treatment.
2. Onset of drug action is rapid.
3. Drug delivery is targeted to the respiratory system.
4. Systemic side effects are fewer and less severe than with oral or parenteral therapy.
5. Inhaled-drug therapy is painless and relatively convenient.

Following are a number of potential complications in the apparently simple aerosol administration of drugs:

1. Difficulties in dosage estimation and dose reproducibility.
2. Difficulty in coordinating hand action and breathing with metered-dose inhalers (MDIs).
3. Lack of physician and therapist knowledge of administration protocols.
4. Lack of technical information on aerosol-producing devices.
5. Number of variables affecting aerosol delivery.

Both the 1974 and the 1979 conferences on the scientific bases of respiratory care recommended further studies on the deposition and distribution of and the clinical response to the aerosol delivery of agents, indicating the incomplete nature of knowledge in this area (Brain, 1980). The questions raised by these examinations of the scientific basis of aerosol therapy were further addressed by the Consensus Conference on Aerosol Delivery in January 1991. Proceedings of that conference are available in *Respiratory Care*, September 1991 (vol 36).

A rational approach to the aerosol delivery of drugs should be based on what is known of the variables affecting lung deposition in relation to the purpose of the agent. The emphasis in this chapter is placed on the physical principles of aerosol delivery and an understanding of aerosol delivery systems. Research findings on questions of the clinical application of aerosol therapy are summarized and include differences among delivery devices and methods of administration.

PHYSICAL PRINCIPLES OF AEROSOL DELIVERY OF DRUGS

The following definitions apply to inhaled therapeutic aerosols:

Aerosol: A suspension of liquid or solid particles in a carrier gas. For pulmonary diagnostic and therapeutic applications, the particle size range of interest is 1 to 10 μm. This range of sizes is small enough to exist as a suspension and enter the lung and large enough to deposit and contain the required amount of an agent (Morrow, 1974).

Stability: Tendency of aerosol particles to remain in suspension.

Penetration: Depth within the lung reached by particles.

Deposition: Process of particles depositing out of suspension to remain in the lung.

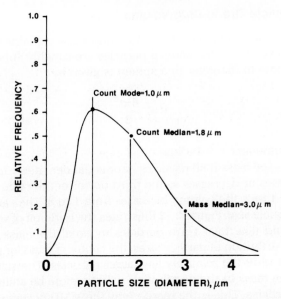

FIG 2–1. Hypothetical skewed frequency distribution of aerosol particle sizes illustrates the relative positions of the count mode, count median, and mass median. (From Rau JL Jr: Humidity and aerosol therapy. In Barnes TA, ed: Respiratory Care Practice, Chicago, 1988, Year Book Medical.)

Aerosol Size Distributions

The aerosol particles produced for inhalation into the lung include a range of sizes (polydisperse or heterodisperse) rather than a single size (monodisperse). As a result, a *distribution* of particle sizes is produced by nebulizing devices. To characterize a distribution of particle sizes, measures of central tendency and dispersion are needed. In fact, three measures of central tendency are often used with the typically skewed shape of particle size distributions seen with bronchoactive aerosols (Fig 2–1).

Count Mode: Most frequently occurring particle size in the distribution.

Count Median Diameter (CMD):   Particle size above and below which 50% of the particles are found (i.e., 50% of the particles in the distribution are larger than the count median diameter, and 50% are smaller).

Mass Median Diameter (MMD):   Particle size above and below which 50% of the mass of particles are found (i.e., the size particle that evenly divides the mass in the distribution).

Geometric Standard Deviation (GSD):   Measure of dispersion in the distribution; the ratio of particle size below which 84% of the particles occur to the particle size below which 50% occur, in a normal distribution.

Relation of Particle Size to Drug Volume

The relation of particle size to volume and mass explains why the MMD is larger, or above, the CMD. Aerosol particles are roughly spherical, and the relation of volume to diameter in a sphere is given by

$$V = \frac{4\pi r^3}{3}$$

where V = volume and r = radius.

The volume, or mass if all particles have equal densities (density = mass/volume), increases or decreases as the third power of the radius. If the radius increases from 1 to 2, the volume increases from 1 to 8. The same is true of a *decrease* in particle size. Figure 2–2 illustrates the trade-off of volume or mass for size. It would take 1000 1-μm particles to equal the mass of one 10-μm particle! In a distribution of particle sizes, the center of mass (or volume) therefore will be found in the relatively few larger particles. The size particle that evenly splits the *mass* in the distribution will therefore be shifted toward the larger-sized particles. This is the reason why the MMD occurs with the larger 3-μm size in the hypothetical distribution shown in Figure 2–1.

The point of application to aerosol delivery of drugs is this: It is the *volume* (mass) of the drug entering the lung on which the therapeutic effect is based. Therefore it is necessary to know where the volume or mass is centered in the range of particle sizes. This is given by the MMD. Notice also that the MMD will be larger than the CMD. Since small particle sizes are favored for lung penetration, as will be discussed, the CMD can make a nebulizer appear more efficient for pulmonary applications than the MMD would. Because of this, aerosol generators should be characterized by using the MMD for the

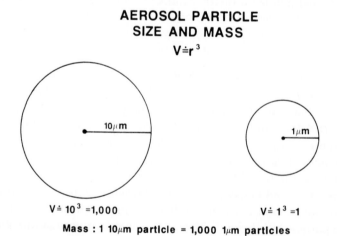

AEROSOL PARTICLE
SIZE AND MASS
$$V \doteq r^3$$

$V \doteq 10^3 = 1{,}000$ $V \doteq 1^3 = 1$

Mass : 1 10μm particle = 1,000 1μm particles

FIG 2–2.   Illustration of the relation of particle diameter size to mass.

center of distribution and either the standard deviation or GSD to indicate the range of variability of particle size.

Aerodynamic Mass Median Diameter

A term that may be used in place of the MMD is the *aerodynamic mass median diameter* (AMMD).

AMMD: Diameter of a sphere of unit density that settles at the same point, when projected horizontally, as the particle being tested.

The concept of AMMD is illustrated in Figure 2–3. The AMMD is actually an operational definition of particle size. It is difficult to measure the diameter of micrometer-sized objects, and this is a way of doing so by using known reference spheres. For practical purposes, the MMD and the AMMD can be interpreted as equivalent.

There are four major variables that can affect the use of aerosols for pulmonary deposition of drugs:

- Physical factors of aerosols
- Pattern of inhalation
- Delivery device used
- Status of the lung

Research has begun to provide more quantified information regarding each of these areas, and a number of references are provided at the end of this chapter on each factor affecting aerosol administration and deposition. Several general articles on the production and physical characteristics of aerosols used in respiratory care are provided.*

*Lourenco and Cotromanes (1982), Mercer (1973), Mitchell (1960), Morrow (1974, 1981), Newman (1985), and Newman and Clarke (1983b).

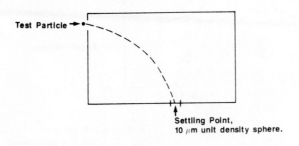

Test Particle ➡•

Settling Point,
10 μm unit density sphere.

AMMD =10 μm

FIG 2–3. Measurement of AMMD for a test particle settling at the same point as a reference 10-μm sphere.

Physical Factors of Aerosol Deposition

The goal of aerosol therapy intended to treat the lung is inhalation of a *stable* aerosol suspension, with *penetration* to the desired lung area, where the aerosol becomes unstable and *deposits* in the airway. A number of references offer more detailed information and extensive citations concerning the pulmonary deposition of inhaled aerosols: Lippman (1977), Newhouse and Ruffin (1978), Newman et al. (1981c), Swift (1980), and Task Group on Lung Dynamics (1966).

Particle Size

One of the major factors influencing aerosol deposition in the lung is particle size. The effect of particle size on deposition in the respiratory tract is illustrated in Figure 2–4.

The upper airway (nose, mouth) is efficient in filtering particulate matter so that generally there is 100% deposition in the nose and mouth of particles larger than 10 and 15 μm, respectively. Particle sizes in the 5 to 10 μm range tend to deposit out in the early airway generations, while 1- to 5-μm sizes are able to reach the lung periphery. The 1 to 5 μm range is often referred to as the *respirable range* for particle sizes, since such particles can reach the lung periphery.

It is not possible to specify exactly where a given sized particle will deposit in the lung. Other variables than size also affect deposition, so that the site of penetration is treated probabilistically and not deterministically. For example, tables often list the percentage of droplets of a given size that will

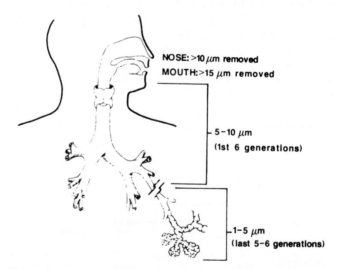

NOSE: >10 μm removed
MOUTH: >15 μm removed

5–10 μm
(1st 6 generations)

1–5 μm
(last 5–6 generations)

FIG 2–4. Effect of aerosol particle size on area of preferential deposition within the airway.

deposit in the lung at each bronchial level (Lippman, 1977). Figure 2–4 also illustrates an important therapeutic point concerning lung deposition: There is little or no deposition *between* the early and peripheral tracheobronchial branchings (Task Group on Lung Dynamics, 1966). As particle size decreases below 5 μm, deposition shifts from large airways to peripheral airways. It is not clear what therapeutic importance should be attached to this.

Autonomic receptors in airway smooth muscle differ in their location. Beta-adrenergic receptors have been identified throughout the airway but with greater density in bronchioles. In contrast, cholinergic receptors were numerous in proximal bronchial smooth muscle but rare in distal bronchioles (Barnes et al., 1983).

An interesting study by Clay et al. (1986) showed greater improvement in midmaximal expiratory flow rates from a beta-adrenergic bronchodilator by using an AMMD of 1.8 μm than with AMMDs of 4.6 or 10.3 μm. This was confirmed more recently by Johnson and associates (1989) who found a greater response to the beta-adrenergic bronchodilator albuterol with an MMD of 3.3 μm compared with 7.7 μm. Response to the anticholinergic agent ipratropium (see Chapter 6) was not significantly different for the two particle sizes, indicating that peripheral deposition with the smaller particle size did not enhance response.

Because anticholinergic (parasympatholytic) and beta-adrenergic (sympathomimetic) drugs comprise the two standard bronchodilator groups for aerosol use, the lack of midbronchial deposition may not pose a problem. Finally, because of the trade-off of size for volume, it is difficult to place large amounts of a drug in the lung periphery.

Mechanisms of Deposition

In the size range seen with current therapeutic aerosols, there are only two physical principles influencing deposition: inertial impaction and gravitational settling (sedimentation).

Inertial Impaction. Inertial impaction is the chief mechanism of deposition for larger particles (5 to 15 μm), which are filtered out in the upper airway and early bronchial generations below the larynx. In this area, particle velocity is highest, and overall cross-sectional area of the airway is smallest; both factors favor inertial impaction on the airway wall.

Gravitational Settling. Gravitational settling, or sedimentation, is more likely to occur with smaller particles down to the 1-μm size and is a function of decreased particle velocity and large cross-sectional area, which occurs in the lower tracheobronchial generations. Since the process of sedimentation is time dependent, the end-inspiratory breath hold should maximize deposition in the periphery. The rate of settling is proportional to the square of the particle size. For a 5-μm-diameter particle, the settling rate is reported to be 0.7 mm/sec (Newman, 1985).

Diffusion (brownian movement) affects particles of less than 1 μm, but this size particle is not currently useful for aerosol therapy.

Effect of Temperature and Humidity

Prediction of particle deposition with therapeutic aerosols is further complicated by the fact that the aerosol is generated at relatively dry ambient conditions and is then taken into the airway where temperature and humidity rapidly increase to saturation at 37° C. Several studies have shown that there is growth of particle size in high-humidity environments. For example, between ambient and BTPS (body temperature, pressure, saturated) conditions, cromolyn sodium powder particles increased from 2.31- to 3.02-μm AMMD (Hiller et al., 1980; Smith et al., 1980.)

Pattern of Inhalation

The pattern of inhalation includes lung volumes at the beginning and end of inspiration, inspiratory time and flow rates, mouth vs. nose breathing, and adjunct maneuvers such as an end-inspiratory pause. The pattern of inspiration can influence aerosol delivery of drugs to the lung. This has been shown by Dahlbäck and associates (1987) who found that a rapid, shallow breathing pattern with large particles (2 μm) increased aerosol deposition in central areas of the lung, while a slow, deep breathing pattern with smaller particles (0.5 μm) shifted aerosol deposition to the periphery. Because the optimal pattern of inhalation varies with the type of aerosol-generating device, the breathing pattern will be specified for each type of device considered.

AEROSOL DEVICES FOR DRUG DELIVERY

Several important questions arise concerning aerosol devices. How should they be quantitatively described for clinicians? Are there differences in clinical effect with different devices, including spacer and reservoir accessories? What is the correct or optimal use of different types of device?

Manufacturers do not uniformly characterize their aerosol generators, although helpful material is often provided. It would be extremely helpful for comparison purposes if the following specifications were provided when an aerosol-generating device is marketed:

- MMD or AMMD
- GSD
- Range of particle size (minimum, maximum)
- Either number or mass concentration per unit volume.

The MMD or AMMD is preferred to the CMD since the mass of drug produced is of therapeutic interest, and not the most frequent size, which is misleadingly lower, as previously illustrated. Either the standard deviation or the range will provide some idea of the particle size dispersion. Finally, the density of particles produced is useful and would have to be specified at given flow rates for devices using gas flow (e.g., ultrasonics, Babington, or gas-powered nebulizers). Table 2–1 gives a comprehensive listing of particle size

TABLE 2–1.

Comparison of Particle Size Distribution for Various Aerosol Generators

Aerosol Generator	Particle Size			
	CMD (μm)	MMD (μm)	GSD (μm)	Reference*
Babington and Ultrasonic				
Babington	—	1.2	—	1
DeVilbiss Pulmosonic	3.5	5.0	1.5	2
Fisons Fisoneb	—	2.5	2.0	3
Pneumatic Nebulizers				
Air Shields Jet	—	6.0	2.5	4
Raindrop	2.5	7.9	2.3	2
Acorn (Medic-Aid)	2.4	4.8	2.0	2
Mini-Neb (Inspiron)	—	5.5†	—	5
Micronebulizer (Bird)	—	7.0†	—	6
Acorn System 22	—	3.4	—	7
DeVilbiss 646 (6 L/min)	—	6.0	—	8
DeVilbiss 646 (12 L/min)	—	3.7	—	8
AeroTech II	—	1.0	1.9	3
RespirGard II	—	0.76	1.9	3
Ultravent	—	0.80	—	9
SPAG	—	6.8	—	10
Metered-Dose Inhalers				
Alupent (metaproterenol)	—	4.8	2.1	11
Metaprel (metaproterenol)	0.67	3.5	1.5	12
Proventil (albuterol)	—	2.4	1.7	11
Bronkometer (isoetharine)	—	5.5	2.3	11
Medihaler-Iso (isoproterenol)	—	3.9	2.1	11
Mistometer (isoproterenol)	—	4.2	2.5	11
Medihaler-Epi (epinephrine)	—	4.7	2.1	11
Beclovent (beclomethasone)	—	3.9	2.1	11
Vanceril (beclomethasone)	0.62	2.01	2.1	13
Azmacort (triamcinolone acetonide)	—	4.0	2.2	11
Dry-Powder Inhalers				
Aarane Spinhaler (cromolyn)	1.4	2.3	1.5	14
Cromolyn sodium (50 L/min)	—	5.6	2.2	15
Cromolyn sodium (80 L/min)	—	3.3	2.3	15

*Details of measurements can be found in the indicated references: 1, Swift (1980); 2, Hiller et al. (1981); 3, Smaldone et al. (1988); 4, Wolfsdorf et al. (1969); 5, Clay et al. (1983); 6, Newman et al. (1985); 7, Simonds et al. (1990); 8, Newman et al. (1987); 9, Flavin et al. (1986); 10, Cameron et al. (1990); 11, Sackner and Kim (1985); 12, Hiller et al. (1978); 13, Hiller et al. (1980); 14, Smith et al. (1980); 15, Kim et al. (1985).
†Measured at flow rate of 6 L/min.

specifications based on a variety of references. The sizes listed were measured in dry air. High-humidity environments will increase particle size, and this almost certainly occurs as particles enter the lung.

With all aerosol delivery devices, respiratory care personnel should carefully review instructional materials and package inserts to train patients in their correct use.

Nebulizers

The term *nebulizer* encompasses a variety of devices that operate on different physical principles to generate an aerosol from a drug solution. All of these aerosol generators contain a reservoir chamber to hold the drug solution, some form of baffling to produce a small and consistent particle size, and some mechanism by which the solution is shattered into a suspension of liquid particles in a carrier gas. The most common type of nebulizer used for aerosol delivery of drugs is the small-volume nebulizer.

Ultrasonic Nebulizer

The ultrasonic nebulizer is an electronic device that operates on the piezoelectric principle and is capable of high output. Particle sizes vary by brand. A generic illustration of an ultrasonic nebulizer is given in Figure 2–5. Although this device has not been used as routinely for aerosolization of drugs as others to be described on the following pages, it has recently been reintroduced as a portable, small unit that can operate on DC voltage. This unit has

UTRASONIC NEBULIZER

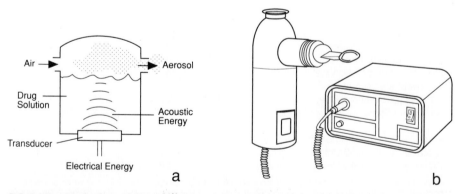

FIG 2–5.   Illustration of the principle of ultrasonic nebulization **(a),** with an example of a portable device used to aerosolize medications **(b).**

the advantages of small size, rapid nebulization with shorter treatment times, smaller amounts of medication solution without diluent for filling volume, and usability during car travel or camping.

Small-Particle Aerosol Generator

The small-particle aerosol generator (SPAG) is a large-reservoir nebulizer capable of holding 300 ml of solution for long periods of nebulization; it operates on a jet-shearing principle. The device was used during the clinical trials of the aerosolized antiviral drug ribavirin (Virazole) and is marketed by its manufacturer for delivery of that drug. The SPAG unit will be described more fully when ribavirin is discussed in Chapter 12.

Small-Volume Nebulizer

The small-volume nebulizer (SVN) is a small-reservoir, gas-powered (pneumatic) aerosol generator, also referred to as a hand-held nebulizer in the literature. A generic illustration is given in Figure 2–6. A jet-shearing principle is used for creation of an aerosol from the drug solution. A thumb control,

SMALL VOLUME NEBULIZER

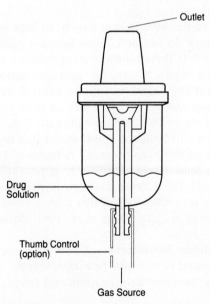

FIG 2–6. Generic illustration of a gas-powered SVN with a thumb control attachment to allow for inspiratory nebulization only when the control port is occluded.

pictured in Figure 2–6, allows routing of gas to the nebulizer during inspiration only, if this accessory is added.

Because the SVN is the most commonly used type of nebulizer for inhalation of aerosolized drugs, it will be reviewed in more detail.

Advantages.   The advantages of the SVN include the following:

1. Ability to aerosolize any drug solution or mixture.
2. Minimal coordination is required for inhalation.
3. Useful in very young patients or those in acute distress.
4. Effective with low-inspiratory flows or volumes.
5. Inspiratory pause (breath hold) is not required for efficacy.
6. Drug concentrations can be modified if desired.

Disadvantages.   The disadvantages of the SVN include the following:

1. Equipment required for use is expensive and cumbersome.
2. Treatment times are somewhat lengthy compared with other aerosol devices and other routes of administration.
3. Dose delivery is inefficient and wasteful.
4. Contamination is possible with inadequate cleaning.
5. Wet, cold spray occurs with mask delivery.

The inefficiency of the SVN is due largely to loss within the apparatus. Gas-powered nebulizers do not aerosolize below a minimal volume termed the *dead volume,* which is the amount of drug solution remaining in the reservoir when the device begins to "sputter" and aerosolization ceases. Kradjan and Lakshminarayan (1985) found that under clinical conditions of nebulization until sputter, approximately 35% to 60% of drug solution was delivered from the nebulizer. Even with vigorous agitation, this amount increased to only 53% to 72%. Shim and Williams (1984) found that only 40% to 52% of the total dose was delivered from gas-powered nebulizers. In a positive pressure circuit, this efficiency may decrease further to approximately 30% of the total dose (Rau and Harwood, 1992). Several reports have described significant variability in performance and efficiency of this type of nebulizer, including leakage of solution (Alvine et al., 1992; Hess et al., 1989; Hollie et al., 1991).

Use of Small-Volume Nebulizers.   There are several factors to be considered with gas-powered nebulizers: flow rate, volume, temperature, output rate, continuous vs. inspiratory nebulization, and length of treatment time.

Filling Volume and Treatment Time.   Figure 2–7 shows the relation of volume in a nebulizer to the time of nebulization. The measurements were

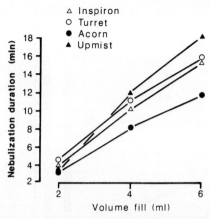

△ Inspiron
○ Turret
● Acorn
▲ Upmist

FIG 2–7. Effect of medication volume on time of nebulization for four gas-powered nebulizers using a flow rate of 8 L/min. (Based on Clay MM, et al: Assessment of jet nebulisers for lung aerosol therapy, Lancet 2:592, 1983.)

made with a power flow rate of 8 L/min. Below 2 ml, most pneumatic nebulizers do not perform well since the volume is close to the dead volume, that is, the residual amount that does not nebulize. At 6 ml, an excessively long time is required for treatment (over 10 minutes). Although 5 minutes seems to be a short time, even this can be inconveniently long as a way of taking medication 3 or 4 times a day. Some patients have difficulty in taking a pill 4 times a day, an approximately 2- to 3-second activity. Patient compliance is directly proportional to convenience. Given the volume requirements of nebulizers for efficient operation and the need for relatively brief treatments, a volume of 3 to 4 ml of solution is recommended. This is primarily the reason that diluent, which is really additional volume, is added to 0.5 ml of a bronchodilator solution. A 0.5-ml solution does not nebulize well, although the needed dose is present, and adding diluent does not alter the total dose contained. This point will be made again in Chapter 3.

Effect of Flow Rate. A second practical question concerns the flow rate at which to power pneumatic nebulizers. The flow rate will affect two variables: the length of treatment time and the size of the particles produced. Figure 2–8, *a*, gives the results of flow rates between 4 and 8 L/min on the time needed to nebulize 2 ml of solution. The results suggest that a minimum of 6 L/min is necessary to keep treatment times under 10 minutes. A flow rate of 8 L/min does not appreciably reduce nebulization time for 2 ml. However, in Figure 2–8, *b*, the effect of flow rate on particle size shows that a flow rate of 8 L/min *will* further decrease particle size below 5 μm. With the exception of the Inspiron Mini-neb, three of the four nebulizers deliver an average particle size below 5 μm at 6 L/min. Since it has been shown that a decrease in

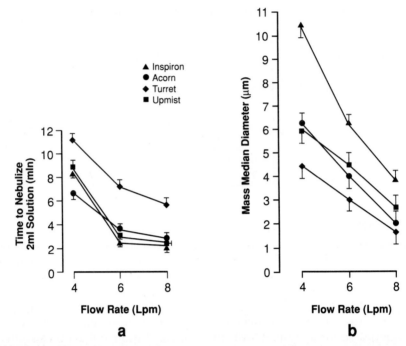

FIG 2–8. **a,** Effect of power gas flow rate on time of nebulization. (Based on Clay MM, et al.: Assessment of jet nebulisers for lung aerosol therapy. Lancet 2;592, 1983.) **b,** Effect of power gas flow rate on aerosol particle size from a gas-powered nebulizer. (Based on Clay MM, et al: Factors influencing the size distribution of aerosols from jet nebulisers, Thorax 38:755, 1983.)

size is costly with respect to *volume,* the 6-L/min flow rate would be preferred to obtain the maximal size (and therefore volume) to reach the lung periphery.

Recommended Use. On the basis of these results, as well as those of other studies referenced in the Bibliography, the following recommendations are suggested for optimal use of SVNs:

Filling Volume: 3 to 4 ml.

Flow Rate of Power Gas: 6 to 8 L/min.

Treatment Time: less than 10 minutes.

Inspiratory Nebulization Only: will increase delivery efficiency, although treatment time may lengthen.

Pattern of Inhalation: slow, deep breaths ideally with an occasional end-inspiratory pause if possible (tidal breathing with no breath hold is also effective).

Maintenance: rinse reservoir after each use to prevent medication accumulation.

These specifications are suitable for the bronchodilator solutions usually given with these devices. However, the volumes and flow rates suggested may need to be modified for some drug solutions such as pentamidine or antibiotics and will be described when these drugs are discussed.

Because SVNs are often used with infants or patients in acute respiratory distress, slow breathing and an inspiratory pause may not be feasible or obtainable. One of the main advantages of an SVN is that dose delivery occurs over 60 to 90 breaths, rather than in one or two inhalations. Thus, a poor breath will not destroy the efficacy of the treatment.

Metered-Dose Inhalers (MDI)

MDIs were first introduced for drug delivery around 1956. These devices are small, pressurized canisters for oral or nasal inhalation of aerosolized drugs and contain several hundred doses of an accurately metered drug. Dosage ranges of respiratory care drugs available in this type of device are from approximately 20 μg (ipratropium bromide) to 800 μg (cromolyn sodium).

Technical Description. There are five major components found in an MDI: drug, propellant/excipient mixture, canister, metering valve, and mouthpiece/actuator. An illustration of this device is given in Figure 2–9. The drug in an MDI is either a suspension of micronized powder in a liquefied propellant or a solution of the active ingredient in a solvent mixed with the propellant. Excipients are comparatively inert substances added most often to the formulation to keep a suitable consistency to the drug in suspension. These substances are surfactants, and those currently used include oleic acid, sorbitan trioleate, or lecithins. A detailed technical description of the complexities involved in producing an MDI is in Hallworth (1987).

When the canister is depressed into the actuator (Fig 2–9), the drug-propellant mixture in the metering valve is released under pressure. The liquid propellant rapidly expands and vaporizes or "flashes" as it ejects into ambient pressure. This expansion and vaporization shatters the liquid stream into an aerosol. The initial vaporization of propellant causes cooling of the liquid-gas aerosol suspension, which can be felt if discharged onto the skin. This can also cause users to stop inhaling as the cold aerosol hits the oropharynx.

The propellant used with MDIs as a power source to create an aerosol is a blend of liquefied gas chlorofluorocarbons ([CFCs] freon). This liquefied gas propellant is able to maintain a steady vapor pressure as the canister is exhausted, as long as ambient temperature does not fluctuate significantly. Di-

METERED DOSE INHALER

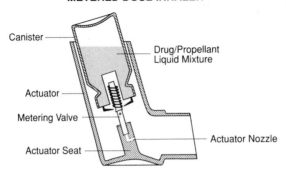

METERING VALVE FUNCTION

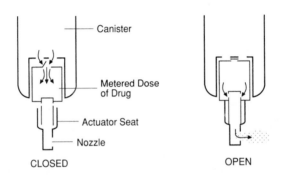

ADAPTERS

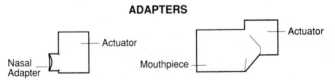

FIG 2–9.   The major components of an MDI, with an illustration of the function of the metering valve. Oral and nasal adapters are shown.

chlorodifluoromethane (propellant 12) is used as the basic driving force for atomizing the liquid solution or suspension, and trichlorofluoromethane (propellant 11) and/or dichlorotetrafluoromethane (propellant 114) are blended in to obtain the desired vapor pressure. The propellant is in a liquid state within the canister at the pressure maintained, which is around 400 kPa (Clarke and Newman, 1981).

The active drug, plus these other ingredients, can be found on the label of an MDI drug formulation. An example is provided by using the label for

Proventil brand of albuterol (Schering). The ingredients in the canister are the following:

Formulation: microcrystalline suspension of albuterol.
Propellants: trichloromonofluoromethane and dichlorodifluoromethane.
Surfactant (excipient): oleic acid.

The particle size of the aerosolized drug released is controlled by two factors: the vapor pressure of the propellant blend and the diameter of the actuator opening (Moren, 1981). Particle size will be reduced as vapor pressure increases and as diameter size of the nozzle opening decreases.

Although there is increasing concern over the destructive effect of CFCs on the ozone layer in the earth's atmosphere (Molina and Rowland, 1974), it is difficult and costly to find substitutions that work as well. CFCs have the features required for successful MDI function (i.e., low toxicity, good chemical stability, excellent vapor pressure characteristics, low cost, and acceptable taste). It is estimated that approximately 4500 tons (about 0.4% to 0.5% of annual production) of CFC gases are used worldwide in the MDIs (Balmes, 1991).

Advantages.   Listed below are the advantages of the MDI.

1. MDIs are portable and compact.
2. Drug delivery is efficient.
3. Treatment time is short.

Disadvantages.   The disadvantages of the MDI are as follows:

1. Complex hand-breathing coordination is required.
2. Drug concentrations are fixed.
3. There are possible reactions to the propellants in a small percentage of patients.
4. There is high oropharyngeal impaction and loss.
5. Foreign body aspiration of coins and debris from the mouthpiece can occur (Hannan, 1984; Schultz et al., 1991).
6. CFCs are released into the environment.

Procedure for Correct Use of an MDI.   The effectiveness of treatment with an aerosolized drug delivered by an MDI depends on correct use of the device. Unfortunately, there is evidence that 50% to 70% of patients do not use MDIs correctly, and physician knowledge of correct MDI use is often inadequate for patient education (Epstein et al., 1979; Kelling, 1983; Lee, 1983; Sackner and Kim, 1985). The work of Tobin et al. (1982) graphically illustrates that subjects often cannot coordinate actuation of an MDI with inhalation.

Rapid or nasal inhalation, lack of a breath hold, insufficiently deep inspiration, or activating the MDI at end inspiration or while exhaling are some of the problems seen. Patients may stop inhaling when the cold propellant spray hits the back of the throat, as previously noted, and patients may find it difficult to regulate their inspiratory flows to the 30 L/min or less needed for optimal bronchial deposition.

The following instructions for use of bronchodilator or corticosteroid aerosols with MDIs are written in terms that may be helpful for patient education. Package inserts on particular agents should always be checked and these protocols modified as needed.

To Inhale a Bronchodilator

1. Assemble the inhaler and remove the dust cap; push the canister nozzle into the jet hole of the mouthpiece. Before each use, shake the aerosol canister to thoroughly mix the suspended or dissolved ingredients. If the inhaler has not been used in over 24 hours, charge the inhaler for the first dose by holding the canister upside down and discharging it. Be sure it points away from everyone.
2. Open mouth wide and hold the MDI no more than 1 inch in front of your mouth. Keep tongue relaxed and down and teeth out of the way.
3. Breathe out normally.
4. Begin to take a slow, deep breath through your mouth and squeeze (activate) the MDI as you continue to breathe in.
5. Continue to breathe in until your lungs are full, then hold your breath for 10 seconds if possible.
6. Breathe out normally.
7. Wait 1 minute, then take the second puff from the MDI in the same manner. If a third puff is prescribed, wait 1 minute again before taking it.
8. Be sure to re-cap the mouthpiece to prevent foreign material from lodging in the actuator.

NOTE: If you have trouble aiming the MDI at your open mouth, you can place the mouthpiece directly in your mouth and rest it on the lower front teeth without sealing your lips around it. If you find it hard to coordinate breathing and activating the MDI, you may wish to ask your physician to prescribe a spacer device, such as the InspirEase (Key Pharmaceuticals), the Monaghan Aerochamber, or the Breathancer (Geigy).

To Inhale a Corticosteroid

Use the same procedure as for a bronchodilator, except

1. If you use both a bronchodilator and a corticosteroid, inhale the bronchodilator first and wait 1 to 2 minutes before inhaling the corticosteroid.

2. Always use an extension or spacer device when inhaling a corticosteroid. If you do not have such a device, try to hyperextend (straighten) your head and neck as much as possible when inhaling (in other words, look at the ceiling).
3. Rinse your mouth and throat with water when finished.

Care of Inhalers

1. Rinse mouthpiece daily in water to keep it clean.
2. Once a week disinfect the mouthpiece assembly by soaking it in a solution of one-half white vinegar and one-half water for 20 to 30 minutes, then rinse well with water and allow to dry thoroughly.
3. Float canister in a bowl of water to determine level of contents (about 200 puffs per canister):

Full: canister sinks or completely submerges, nozzle down.

Half Full: nozzle down in water, flat end above surface.

Empty: canister floats on side on surface of water.

These recommendations are based primarily on studies by Dolovich et al. (1981) and Newman et al. (1981b), as well as other studies that are referenced in the Bibliography (Blake et al., 1992a; Newman et al., 1981a, 1981c, 1982; Newman and Clarke, 1983a). These studies have shown that whole-lung deposition of aerosols with an MDI is inversely proportional to inspiratory flow rate. High inspiratory flow rates, above 30 L/min, increase inertial impaction in the oropharynx and decrease the amount of aerosol reaching the lung. A pause of 1 to 5 minutes between each puff of a bronchodilator from an MDI has been advocated in an attempt to improve distribution of the inhaled drug in the lung (Heimer et al., 1980). A study by Pedersen (1986b) showed no difference in forced expiratory volume in 1 second (FEV_1) with a 3- and 10-minute divided dose under nonacute, basic maintenance conditions. However, during attacks with acute wheezing, a pause between puffs resulted in substantially improved bronchodilatation, with greater effect using a 10-minute pause.

Extension or Auxiliary (Spacer) Devices.   A generic illustration of an extension device is given in Figure 2–10. Extension, reservoir, or more simply spacer devices were introduced primarily to simplify the complex coordination of aiming, actuation, and breathing with an MDI. Spacer devices actually offer three main advantages when used with an MDI:

1. Such devices allow space and time for more vaporization of the propellants and evaporation of initially large particles to smaller sizes. The initial particle size from an MDI can exceed 35 μm at the nozzle, which must be reduced to the 1 to 5 μm range for lung penetration (Clarke and Newman, 1981). This is seen conceptually in Figure 2–10.

MDI AUXILIARY DEVICES

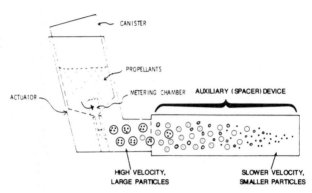

FIG 2–10. Effect of an extension device on aerosol particle size and velocity from an MDI.

2. Reservoirs reduce oropharyngeal impaction and loss of drug by extending the nozzle away from the mouth. Particles discharged from the actuator nozzle have velocities of 30 m/sec. By holding the actuator 4 cm in front of the mouth, or by using an extension device, this velocity is allowed to slow, and impaction in the back of the throat is reduced (Dolovich et al., 1981). This concept is also illustrated in Figure 2–10.

3. As holding chambers for the aerosol cloud, reservoir devices separate the actuation of the canister from the inhalation and simplify the coordination required for good use.

A disadvantage to reservoir devices is their size or in some cases the need for assembly, which elderly patients may find difficult.

There are a variety of reservoir devices now available, and the sizes range from 80 to over 750 ml. Figure 2–11 shows several units, illustrating the differences in size and design. The simplest units are little more than cylindrical extension tubes with a one-way valve at the mouthpiece. Units such as the InspirEase offer both a holding chamber and a flow-rate indicator to assist in maintaining a suitably low flow during inspiration. The loss of drug in reservoir devices can be as much as 60% to 65% of the total dose, but this is replacing the same amount previously lost in the oropharynx (Kim et al., 1987; Newman et al., 1986). Lung deposition can be improved, although it has not been shown to exceed 20% of the total dose and is probably in the 10% to 15% range. Variation limits for the 10% figure are clearly presented by Newman (1985) from studies of different devices.

Because of their ability to avoid misuse of MDI devices and improve drug

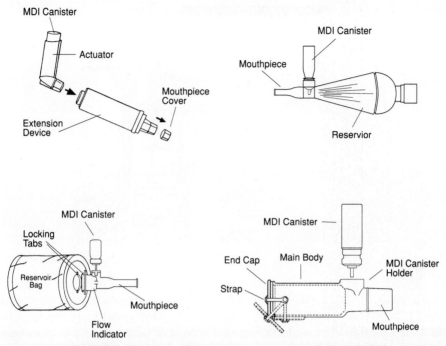

FIG 2–11. Representative MDI auxiliary reservoir devices. *Clockwise from upper left:* Monaghan Aerochamber, Aerosol Cloud Enhancer, InspirEase, and OptiHaler.

delivery, extension or reservoir devices are encouraged for all MDI prescriptions. With inhaled corticosteroids, reservoir devices are required to reduce oropharyngeal impaction and subsequent opportunistic throat infections such as candidiasis.

Several articles in the Bibliography provide excellent reviews of auxiliary spacer systems with detailed references (Konig, 1985; Newman et al., 1981d; Sackner and Kim, 1985).

Other MDI Auxiliary Devices. In addition to reservoir devices, which provide a holding chamber to decrease the need for close coordination between activating the MDI and inhaling, other devices have been developed to aid the user of MDIs. Two are illustrated in Figure 2–12.

The first of these, represented by the Vent Ease, is essentially a lever that fits over the entire canister-actuator assembly (Fig 2–12, *a*). By squeezing the handle, the canister is forced down into its actuator, and a metered dose of drug is released for inhalation. The advantage offered by this device is increased ease of physically actuating the pressurized canister, particularly for elderly patients with arthritis, reduced grip strength, or problems in gripping and squeezing the small canister.

MDI ACTUATING DEVICES

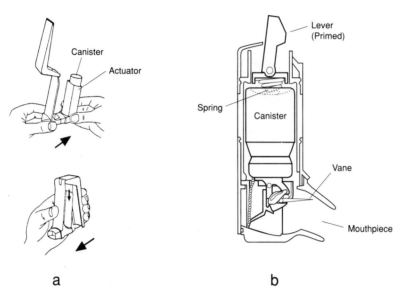

FIG 2–12. Devices intended to increase the ease of actuating an MDI. **a,** Lever type of device to squeeze the canister into the actuator. **b,** Breath-actuated inhaler.

The second type of device to simplify MDI use is a breath-actuated adapter (Fig 2–12, *b*). A conventional pressurized MDI canister is fitted within this actuator. The MDI canister is triggered by a spring, through a triggering mechanism activated when the patient inhales.

To use, the device is primed, or "cocked," by raising the lever on top of the adapter. This applies pressure to the canister. The canister cannot move downward because of a vane in the mouthpiece. As the patient inhales at flow rates of 22 to 26 L/min, the vane lifts, the canister is forced downward, and a metered dose is released. The device is reset by lowering the lever to its resting position, which allows the MDI valve to refill.

Devices such as the breath-actuated inhaler were described as early as 1971. An improved version, the Aerolin Autohaler produced by 3M Riker, is now available in the United Kingdom and contains salbutamol, which is known by the generic name of albuterol in the United States. The device is described by Newman and associates (1991) and by Baum and Bryant (1988). The corticosteroid beclomethasone is also available as Aerobec, in a breath-actuated inhaler, in the United Kingdom. Breath-actuated inhalers offer an alternative to spacer or reservoir devices for individuals who find it difficult to coordinate MDI actuation with inhalation. This device is now available in the United States for Maxair (Pirbuterol, 3M Pharmaceuticals).

Dry-Powder Inhalers

Dry-powder inhalers (DPIs) consist of a unit formulation of drug in a powder form and a small, MDI-sized apparatus for dispensing the powder during inspiration. These devices are breath actuated, with turbulent airflow from the inspiratory effort of the user providing the power to create an aerosol of microfine solid particles of drug as air is inhaled through a mouthpiece.

There are currently two drugs available as a dry-powder formulation in the United States: cromolyn sodium (Intal) and albuterol (Ventolin Rotacaps). Cromolyn sodium is dispensed in a device termed the *Spinhaler*, which has been available since 1971. The albuterol formulation is dispensed in a device termed the *Rotahaler*, which was introduced in the United States in 1989. Both of these devices use a single-dose, micronized-powder preparation of a drug in a gelatin capsule. Before inhalation, the capsule is inserted into the device and opened to release the powder (Fig 2–13). Powder flow properties depend on particle size distribution, and very small particles do not flow as well as larger sizes (Brown, 1987). For this reason, lactose and glucose powder are added to the finer drug particles as a coarse carrier substance. Particle sizes for the lactose carrier granules mainly range from 10 to 80 μm. The carrier substance improves the flow properties of the powder mixture and acts as a bulking agent to provide suitable volume to the unit dose. Lactose is the carrier substance added to current powder preparations of cromolyn and albuterol available in the United States.

DRY POWDER INHALERS

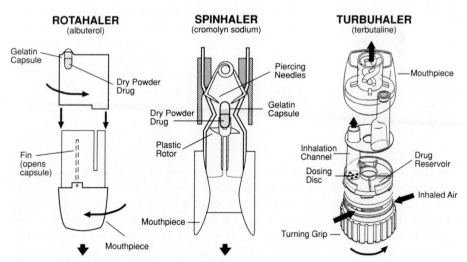

FIG 2–13. Three examples of delivery devices for inhalation of dry-powder aerosols: Rotahaler, Spinhaler, and Turbuhaler.

Advantages.   The advantages of a DPI are listed below:

1. Small, portable devices.
2. Short preparation and administration times.
3. Breath actuation removes the need for the hand-breathing coordination, inspiratory hold, or head-tilt needed with an MDI.
4. No CFC propellants (environmentally friendly).
5. No "cold freon effect" to cause bronchoconstriction or to inhibit full inspiration.
6. Count of remaining drug doses is simple.

Disadvantages.   Following are the disadvantages of the DPI:

1. Limited range of available drugs to date.
2. Possible reaction to the lactose or glucose carrier substance.
3. High inspiratory flow rates of 60 L/min or greater are needed with the two devices and formulations available.
4. Current devices must be loaded before use.

DPIs combine the advantages of both SVNs and MDIs, namely, ease of use with small, portable, efficient drug delivery, and eliminate the disadvantages. Pedersen (1986a) has shown that head tilting during inspiration and a breath hold do not add to the efficacy of use with the Rotahaler.

Limiting Factors.   The two major limiting factors for DPI formulations are the lack of available drugs in this form and the need for high inspiratory flow rates. With inspiratory flows below 50 L/min, there is significant reduction in clinical response with both the Rotahaler and the Spinhaler (Pedersen, 1986a; Richards et al., 1988). This affects use of a DPI by young children, especially below 5 years of age, and by any patient with an acute wheezing episode associated with airflow reduction. A third limitation is the need for loading each individual dose prior to use, which may be more difficult with anxiety during an asthma episode.

New DPI Formulations.   None of the limitations noted is inherent to the DPI device itself. Terbutaline is now available in a 200-dose powder inhaler known as the Turbohaler in the United Kingdom and the Turbuhaler in Europe (Persson et al., 1988). This device (see Fig 2–13) is effective at flow rates of approximately 30 L/min, which can be achieved by many children between 3 and 6 years of age (Pedersen et al., 1990). The Turbohaler was reported to be approximately 30% effective even with inspiratory flows as low as 13 L/min in the study by Pedersen et al., (1990). In addition, the powder preparation preloaded in the device contains no carrier substance, is disposable after the

200th dose, and gives a "20 doses left" warning signal (Crompton, 1988). Another multidose powder inhaler is the eight-dose reloadable Diskhaler (designed by the manufacturer of the Rotahaler), which can contain either albuterol (salbutamol) or beclomethasone dipropionate (Newman, 1990).

Other drugs that are either available outside the United States or are being investigated for dry-powder delivery include fenoterol, ipratropium, oxitropium (OxiVent), and salmeterol (Serevent).

Clinical Efficacy.   DPIs have been shown to be equivalent in efficacy to the pressurized aerosols with MDIs (Chambers et al., 1980; Hetzel and Clark, 1977; Towns et al., 1983; Vilsvik et al., 1991). As new devices and more drug formulations become available in the United States, DPIs could become the formulation of choice for aerosol delivery of drugs, replacing the complex MDI and the time-consuming, bulky SVN systems.

To Use the Cromolyn Spinhaler

1. Check the mouthpiece for any foreign debris prior to use.
2. Hold the Spinhaler vertically, with the mouthpiece downward, and unscrew the upper portion from the mouthpiece.
3. Place a gelatin capsule, colored end down, into the cup of the propeller and screw the upper portion back onto the mouthpiece.
4. With the Spinhaler still vertical, place fingers on the sides of the gray sleeve and slide the sleeve down and then back up once. Do not repeat this.
5. Exhale fully away from the Spinhaler to keep the powder from becoming moist.
6. Tilt the head backward, place lips around the mouthpiece, and inhale as deeply and rapidly as possible.
7. Remove the Spinhaler from the mouth, hold your breath for a few seconds, then exhale normally.
8. If necessary, inhale several times to empty the capsule of powder.
9. Open the Spinhaler, discard the empty capsule, and store the device.

CARE: Once or twice weekly, disassemble the unit and wash it in warm water to remove accumulated drug particles. Be sure to dry the pieces thoroughly before reassembly. Never lubricate the propellor shaft. Handle drug capsules with dry hands.

To Use the Rotahaler

1. Check the device for foreign objects in the mouthpiece prior to use.
2. Turn the Rotahaler vertically, with the darker mouthpiece end down, and turn the upper portion in one direction and then the other, as far as it will go.

3. Insert the clear end of a Ventolin Rotacaps capsule in the raised octagonal hole at the end opposite the mouthpiece and push the capsule in until it is level with the top of the hole. (If a previously used capsule is in the hole, force the old capsule in with the new one.)
4. Hold the Rotahaler horizontally with the white dot up and turn the upper portion as far as it will go. This will open the capsule.
5. With the Rotahaler horizontal, breathe out fully, place the mouthpiece in your mouth with teeth apart, and breathe in through your mouth as quickly and deeply as you can.
6. Hold your breath for a few seconds, remove the Rotahaler from your mouth, then exhale normally.
7. After use, open the device and discard previously used capsule fragments.

CARE: Once or twice a week, wash the device with warm water and allow to dry thoroughly before reassembling.

CLINICAL APPLICATION OF AEROSOL DELIVERY DEVICES

Criteria for Choosing an Aerosol Delivery Device

The assumption of correct use with each type of delivery device cannot be made in every patient. However, the differences among the available devices can be used as the basis for choosing the type of device to match the patient's needs. The following criteria are qualitative but may assist practitioners in selecting aerosol devices for patient use.
1. Use a **nebulizer** if an individual
   a. is unable to follow instructions or is disoriented.
   b. has a poor inspiratory capacity.
   c. is incapable of a breath hold.
   d. is tachypneic (>25 breaths per minute) or has an unstable respiratory pattern.
   e. needs to aerosolize a drug not in MDI or DPI form.
2. Use an **MDI** if an individual
   a. is able to follow instructions.
   b. has an adequate inspiratory capacity.
   c. is capable of a breath hold.
   d. has a stable respiratory pattern.
   e. needs a drug available in MDI form.
3. Use **auxiliary (spacer) devices** for individuals
   a. inhaling aerosolized corticosteroids.
   b. with poor hand-breathing coordination in use of an MDI.

    c. simply to enhance MDI use and reduce oropharyngeal loss with all MDI aerosols.
4. Use **DPIs** for individuals
    a. if the drug is available in DPI form.
    b. with poor MDI coordination.
    c. sensitive to CFC propellants.
    d. capable of high inspiratory flow rates (>60 L/min).
    e. who need accurate dose count monitoring.

Nebulizers and MDIs are currently the most used devices for drug delivery in respiratory care, and all aerosolized drugs are available in one form or the other, or both. There is a trend to shift aerosol treatments from nebulizer delivery to MDI delivery, especially for hospitalized patients, to reduce costs (Bowton et al., 1992; Jasper et al., 1987). Table 2–2 summarizes a conversion protocol based on a model published by Tenholder and associates (1992) that offers more quantitative criteria for use of an MDI than those given previously, and that practitioners in other institutions may find helpful. Patients must be capable of meeting the criteria listed to substitute MDI aerosol delivery for an SVN.

TABLE 2–2.

Criteria for Changing from Nebulizer to MDI

Vital Capacity: ≥900 ml
Breath Hold at Vital Capacity: ≥5 seconds
Respiratory Rate: <25 breaths per minute
Orientation: What is your name? What year is it?
Coordination: full use of arm and hand needed for actuating MDI; demonstrate adequate hand actuation of MDI coordinated with early inspiratory phase.

Efficiency and Loss Patterns of Aerosol Delivery Devices

Many studies have examined the question of differences among MDIs, MDIs with auxiliary devices, and gas-powered SVNs.* Studies comparing the efficacy of MDI use with that of DPIs were previously noted. The consensus is that all of these devices, including an MDI alone or with an auxiliary spacer attachment, can be equally effective assuming proper training and correct use.

The overall efficiency in dose delivery to the lung does not differ greatly among the MDI, MDI with spacer, DPI, and SVN, although there are differences. All devices deliver approximately 10% of the total drug dose to the lung. However, the pattern of loss to the mouth and stomach, to the apparatus, and through exhalation does differ among the devices.

Figure 2–14 illustrates both the percentage of dose deposited in the lung

---

*Christensson et al. (1981), Dolovich et al. (1983), Kemp et al. (1986), Pedersen (1983), Stauder and Hidinger (1983), Toogood et al. (1982).

Pattern of Aerosol Deposition
Aerosol Delivery Device Types

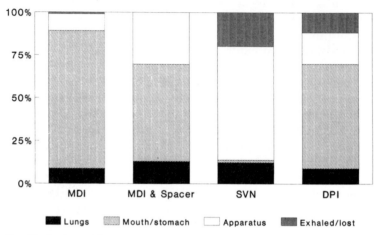

FIG 2–14. Illustration of the patterns of aerosol loss for four drug delivery systems.

and the pattern of loss, based on separate studies of four delivery systems: MDI, Newman et al. (1981c); MDI and spacer, Newman et al. (1981d); SVN, Lewis and Fleming (1985); DPI, Zainudin et al. (1990). The four systems of aerosol delivery each gave the following lung deposition:

MDI: 8.8%
MDI and Spacer: 13.0%
SVN: 12.4%
DPI: 9.1%

The average amount of lung deposition for each device varies in different studies. One cannot conclude that an SVN will always deliver a higher percentage of dose to the lungs than will an MDI. Spiro and associates (1984) showed that an MDI delivered an average of 11.1% to the lungs, while the study by Zainudin and others (1990) found that an SVN delivered 9.9% of the total dose, in contrast to the percentages given above. Individual subjects also vary in their efficiency of use. Newman and others (1986) reported that the usual technique of patients in their study delivered 6.5% of a dose from an MDI to the lungs; improved technique, without addition of a spacer, increased this to 11.2%. One patient with good MDI technique was able to achieve a 12.1% lung deposition without a spacer. Another patient with very poor technique had a 6.2% deposition even with use of an InspirEase spacer device. Differences in administration technique and efficiency of particular brands, especially among nebulizers, can alter the aerosol dose reaching the lung.

The MDI and the SVN show the greatest contrast in the loss pattern of aerosol drug. Most of the loss with an MDI occurs in the mouth and stomach (approximately 80%), whereas the SVN loses only 1.5% to the mouth and stomach. Most of the loss with an SVN is in the delivery apparatus (66%), with most of that remaining in the nebulizer, while an MDI loses approximately 10% in the actuator.

Adding a spacer device to an MDI lowers the amount lost in the oropharynx and stomach to around 57% and increases the amount left in the reservoir to 30% (Newman et al., 1981d). In a different study by Newman et al. (1986) to evaluate the InspirEase, these amounts shifted to a 9.5% loss in the oropharynx, with 59% lost in the spacer reservoir. The type and size of spacer can influence the pattern of loss, based on these results.

The DPI is similar to the MDI in its pattern of aerosol loss. In the study by Zainudin and others (1990), 61% of the aerosolized drug was lost in the mouth or stomach, approximately 18% in the apparatus, with almost 12% apparently lost to the air during opening of the drug gelatin capsule.

Equivalent Doses Among Device Types

If an MDI, SVN, and DPI all deliver approximately the same amount of drug to the lungs, a question arises concerning the difference in dose between devices. For example, the dose of albuterol (a beta-adrenergic bronchodilator) by MDI vs. nebulizer is as follows:

MDI: Two puffs or 0.18 mg
SVN: 0.5 ml or 2.5 mg

If 10% of the dose reaches the lungs, then very different doses are being delivered. A number of studies have examined this question of equipotent doses between delivery devices.

Equipotent Dose: Dose by each delivery method that produces an equivalent degree of effect (for bronchodilators, this would be bronchodilatation).

The standard difference in dose between the MDI and the SVN delivery methods for albuterol is in the ratio of 1:14. However, at least two studies suggest MDI:SVN dose ratios of 1:3 and 1:4 to achieve equal bronchodilatation (Tarala et al., 1980) or equivalent amounts of drug delivery to the lung (Blake et al., 1992b). These equipotent dose ratios of 1:3 and 1:4 are achieved by increasing the number of puffs from the MDI to 7 and 10, respectively, in the two studies.

One of the clearest statements on the question of delivery efficiency among types of aerosol devices resulted from a study by Zainudin and others (1990). The study examined drug delivery by MDI, DPI, and SVN, and the results are summarized graphically in Figure 2–15. These results are particularly helpful

Lung Deposition & Response
3 Bronchodilator Delivery Methods

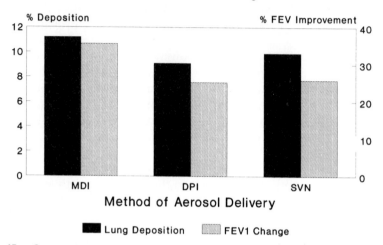

FIG 2–15. Comparison of lung deposition as percentage of total dose and clinical response to aerosol delivery of the same dose of albuterol (400 μg) from three types of aerosol devices. (Based on Zainudin BMZ, Biddiscombe M, Tolfree SEJ, Short M, Spiro SG: Comparison of bronchodilator responses and deposition patterns of salbutamol inhaled from a pressurised metered dose inhaler, as a dry powder, and as a nebulised solution, *Thorax* 45:469, 1990.)

because the investigators used the *same* dose of 400 μg of albuterol (salbutamol) delivered by each type of device. The percentage of lung deposition is shown in Figure 2–15, with MDI delivery of 11.2%, DPI delivery at 9.1%, and SVN delivery at 9.9%. The dose delivered to the lung from the MDI was substantially higher than that from the DPI but not from the SVN. However, clearly the amounts are close to the usual figure of 10% given for lung deposition of an inhaled aerosolized drug. The results show that the same approximate amount of drug is delivered to the lung with the same loading dose, regardless of the type of device used.

The clinical response measured by the improvement in FEV_1 is also similar, although the change with the MDI (35.6%) is statistically significantly greater than that seen with the DPI (25.2%) or the SVN (25.8%).

These results support the view that when the amount of aerosolized drug delivered to the lung is similar with the three types of devices, the clinical response is similar. The greater response with the MDI correlates with the greater amount of drug delivered by the MDI in the study. The amount of bronchodilatation obtained is a reflection of the dose of drug given and not the method of delivery (Mestitiz et al., 1989). The reason that two puffs from a standard-dose MDI is not always effective is due to the probability that this dose is suboptimal especially when airflow obstruction is present (Newhouse and Dolovich, 1987). There are subjects who are able to maintain their bronchodilatation with a small, two-puff MDI dose, as shown in a study by Jenkins and others (1987), where 10 of 19 patients were maximally bronchodilated with two puffs. This contrasted with six puffs needed for two other patients in the study.

Patient-Device Interface

Most methods of aerosol delivery of drugs use oral inhalation, that is, the subject inhales the aerosol through the open mouth. However, other types of interface occur in clinical practice and raise questions concerning efficacy and drug delivery. These are administration by intermittent positive pressure breathing (IPPB), aerosol administration with a face mask, and administration of aerosolized drugs through endotracheal tubes (ETTs).

Intermittent Positive Pressure Breathing. IPPB is a lung inflation technique that has been used to deliver aerosolized drugs from an SVN. As illustrated in Figure 2–16, the SVN receives its power gas from the IPPB device to nebulize a drug solution. The nebulizer is incorporated in the inspira-

AEROSOL DELIVERY BY IPPB

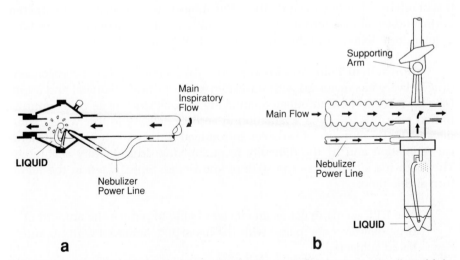

FIG 2–16. Use of gas-powered nebulizers with an IPPB breathing circuit. **a,** Mainstream nebulizer. **b,** Side-stream nebulizer.

tory limb of the IPPB breathing circuit, often forming part of an assembly with the exhalation valve. The aerosol is then delivered with the positive pressure breath through a mouthpiece (not pictured).

Although a popular form of aerosol therapy in past years, the consensus of research on this method of delivery has been that IPPB delivery of aerosolized medication is no more clinically effective than simple, spontaneous, unassisted inhalation from SVNs (Chester et al., 1972; Dolovich et al., 1977; Loren et al., 1977). As a result, the use of IPPB for delivery of aerosolized drugs is not supported for general clinical or at-home use.

Face Mask Administration.   Use of a face mask with an aerosol generator usually occurs with infant and pediatric applications or with debilitated, unresponsive patients. Clinical efficacy has been demonstrated with a face mask in a pediatric application by Conner and associates (1989) and by Kraemer and coworkers (1991). Both of these studies examined bronchodilator administration with an MDI-spacer assembly attached to a face mask. However, Salmon and others (1990) investigated lung delivery with a face mask in both adults and children, and they found that much less than the usual 10% dose of drug reaches the lungs. The following amounts of drug delivery to the lung were estimated from urinary measurements of cromolyn sodium:

SVN and Mask (child):   0.76%
MDI/Spacer and Mask (child):   0.3%
SVN and Mask (adult):   1.5%

It is of interest that in this study the adult subjects were instructed to breathe normal tidal volumes through their noses rather than their mouths. The 1.5% of total dose delivered to the lung represents this method of inhalation.

Endotracheal Tube Administration.   An increasing use of aerosolized-drug delivery has occurred with intubated subjects, both neonatal and adult. Data have begun to accumulate quantifying the efficiency of aerosol administration with this interface. Evaluation of aerosol delivery in this way is complicated by the number of variables introduced if the patient is on mechanical ventilation and by the difficulty in quantifying drug delivery accurately. The following summarizes the state of knowledge represented in the literature at this time:

1. The ETT seems to act as an efficient baffle to reduce the amount of drug delivered compared with the usual 10% achieved with nonintubated subjects.
2. The effect of ventilatory variables remains unclear, although in a study by Benson et al. (1991) these variables did not exert a major influence on delivery.

3. Both MDIs and SVNs have been used, and both can produce clinical effects (Gay et al., 1991; Fernandez et al., 1990).
4. Use of an extension tube or other reservoir, or placement of the aerosol generator upstream from the ETT adapter, improves aerosol delivery (Fuller et al., 1990; Hughes and Saez, 1987; Rau et al., 1992).

Results of a number of studies quantifying lung deposition with both adults and neonates, and in vivo as well as in vitro models, are given in Table 2–3. The studies indicate that less aerosol is delivered with smaller-sized ETTs, and this would be consistent with increased inertial baffling of particles. Larger delivery efficiencies seem to occur with bench studies than with human or in vivo methods. This may be due to an overestimation by some of the methods used to quantify aerosol delivery, particularly when weighing of filters is used. In addition, the amount of control over extraneous variables, such as coordination with respiratory patterns, is far greater in the laboratory than with an actual patient, and this type of control tends to maximize delivery.

Status of the Lung

The presence or absence of pulmonary disease adds another variable to deposition of aerosols in the lung. Pulmonary disease probably affects the *pat-*

TABLE 2–3.

Summary of Studies Measuring the Amount of Aerosol Dose Delivered Through an Endotracheal Tube

Study*	Device	ETT Size (mm)	% Delivered
Crogan (In vitro)	MDI	6.0	3.0
	MDI	7.5	4.7
	MDI	9.0	6.5
Fraser (In vitro)	SVN	8.0	1.62
Fuller (In vivo)	MDI	—	5.65
	SVN	—	1.22
MacIntyre (In vivo)	SVN	≥7.0	2.9
Ahrens (In vitro)	SVN	3.0	8.5
Banks (In vivo)	SVN	—	0.28
Benson (In vitro)	SVN	2.5	2.11
	SVN	3.0	2.0
	SVN	3.5	2.14
Cameron (In vitro)	SVN	3.5	0.22–1.52
	SPAG	3.5	0.15
	USN†	3.5	0.60
Flavin (In vivo)	SVN	3.0	0.19–1.96
Rau (In vitro)	SVN	3.0	0.97–1.78

*The first author of the study is listed, with complete citation in the Bibliography.
†USN, ultrasonic nebulizer.

tern of deposition seen with therapeutic aerosols, rather than the overall amounts, although studies differ on the question. Newhouse and Ruffin (1978) examined a healthy subject, an asymptomatic smoker, and a patient with severe emphysema (chronic obstructive pulmonary disease) who was using radioactive-tagged particles with an AMMD of 3 μm. The following results were obtained:

Healthy Subject: uniform, diffuse peripheral deposition of aerosol.

Smoker: poor aerosol penetration presumably due to small airway narrowing, although pulmonary function was normal.

Patient With Emphysema: very poor distribution of particles to the periphery.

A central, patchy, hilar pattern of deposition has been confirmed in other studies when obstructive disease is present (Goldberg and Lourenco, 1973; Itoh et al., 1981; Swift, 1980).

The results of a study by Spiro and coworkers (1984) differed with the preceding findings. They delivered radiolabeled ipratropium bromide to both healthy subjects and those with chronic bronchitis by using a reconstituted MDI. The results showed no difference in either total lung delivery (11.2% for healthy subjects and 11.7% for bronchitic patients) or deposition pattern between central and peripheral lung zones.

Application of Variables to Aerosol Therapy

On the basis of evidence currently available concerning each of the major variables affecting lung deposition of aerosols, some general patterns of treatment can be suggested. The purpose of the aerosol should be considered in relation to the variables affecting lung deposition, and those variables (particle size, pattern of inhalation, device) should be tailored to achieve the desired purpose, taking into account the status of the patient. Table 2–4 presents a configuration of the key variables intended to optimize aerosol treatment for the nasopharynx, the upper and central airway, and the lower airway.

Several comments should be made concerning the suggested tailoring of variables in Table 2–4. Gas-powered nebulizers will generally produce an MMD of less than 5 μm, which is not ideal for treating the upper or central airway. In such a case, it is important that the patient inhale rapidly to promote more inertial impaction in the upper airway. Alternatively, the atomizer would be preferred for strictly upper airway (above the larynx) application. Lowering flow rates on pneumatic nebulizers will increase particle size, but treatment time becomes unacceptably long.

Large amounts of mixed particle sizes (1 to 30 μm) can be obtained with large-reservoir jet nebulizers for treatment of the entire lung. In the past, this has been done with water aerosols to hydrate secretions. This use of a bland

TABLE 2–4.

Configuration of Variables Affecting Pulmonary Deposition of Aerosols for Treating Various Portions of the Airway

Variable	Nasopharynx	Upper/Central Airway	Peripheral Airway
Problem	Intubation; bronchoscopy; rhinitis; nasal congestion	Postextubation edema; bronchoscopy; croup; epiglottitis; sputum induction	Asthma; acute or chronic bronchitis; respiratory infections
Agent	Topical anesthetic; decongestant; corticosteroid	Decongestant; topical anesthetic; distilled water; saline	Bronchodilator; corticosteroid; antibiotic; mucus-controlling
Particle size	10–15 μm	5–10 μm	1–5 μm
Pattern of inhalation	Nasal breathing; high flow rates (>30 L/min); end-inspiratory pause	Mouth breathing; normal-to-high flow rate (30–60 L/min); end-inspiratory pause	Mouth breathing; slow flow rate (<30 L/min); vital or inspiratory capacity; 10-second inspiratory pause
Aerosol generator	Atomizer; nasal inhaler	Atomizer; pneumatic hand-held nebulizer; Babington; ultrasonic	MDI, with extension if needed; pneumatic hand-held nebulizer; DPI (flow rate as needed)

aerosol is probably ineffective, can create runny secretions, and should be advised against in favor of systemic hydration. This question is discussed more completely in Chapter 8.

The use of ultrasonic and Babington nebulizers can cause relatively large amounts of small particles to reach the lung periphery. However, this is not usually necessary with therapeutic aerosols currently used. Furthermore, the dense, fine particles produced by these devices have long been known to cause significant airway constriction. References supporting this point can be found in the Bibliography (Flick et al., 1977; Malik and Jenkins, 1972; Pflug et al., 1970).

BIBLIOGRAPHY

Ahrens RC et al: The delivery of therapeutic aerosols through endotracheal tubes, Pediatr Pulmonol 2:19, 1986.

Alvine GF et al: Disposable jet nebulizers: how reliable are they? Chest 101:316, 1992.

Asmundsson T: Efficiency of nebulizers for depositing saline in human lung. Am Rev Respir Dis 108:506, 1973.

Balmes JR: The environmental impact of chlorofluorocarbon use in metered dose inhalers, Chest 100:1101, 1991.

Banks JL et al: Pulmonary aerosol deposition in the mechanically ventilated newborn piglet, Pediatr Res 27:295A, 1990 (abstract).

Barnes PJ, Basbaum CB, Nadel JA: Autoradiographic localization of autonomic receptors in airway smooth muscle, Am Rev Respir Dis 127:758, 1983.

Baum EA, Bryant AM: The development and laboratory testing of a novel breath-actuated pressurized inhaler, J Aerosol Med 1:219, 1988.

Benson JM et al: The impact of changing ventilator parameters on availability of nebulized drugs in an in vitro neonatal lung system, Drug Intell Clin Pharmacol 25:272, 1991.

Blake KV, Harman E, Hendeles L: Evaluation of a generic albuterol metered-dose inhaler: importance of priming the MDI, Ann Allergy 68:169, 1992a.

Blake KV et al: Relative amount of albuterol delivered to lung receptors from a metered-dose inhaler and nebulizer solution, Chest 101:309, 1992b.

Bowton DL, Goldsmith WM, Haponik EF: Substitution of metered-dose inhalers for hand-held nebulizers: success and cost savings in a large, acute-care hospital, Chest 101:305, 1992.

Brain J: Aerosol and humidity therapy, Am Rev Respir Dis 122:17, 1980.

Brown K. The formulation and evaluation of powders for inhalation. In Ganderton D, Jones T, eds: Drug delivery to the respiratory tract, Chichester, England, 1987, Ellis Horwood.

Cameron D, Clay M, Silverman M: Evaluation of nebulizers for use in neonatal ventilator circuits, Crit Care Med 18:866, 1990.

Chambers S, Dunbar J, Taylor B: Inhaled powder compared with aerosol administration of fenoterol in asthmatic children, Arch Dis Child 55:73, 1980.

Chester EH et al: Bronchodilator therapy: comparison of acute response to three methods of administration, Chest 62:394, 1972.

Christensson P, Arborelius M, Lilja B: Salbutamol inhalation in chronic asthma bronchiale: dose aerosol vs jet nebulizer, Chest 79:416, 1981.

Clarke SW, Newman SP: Differences between pressurized aerosol and stable dust particles, Chest 80(suppl):907, 1981.

Clay MM et al: Factors influencing the size distribution of aerosols from jet nebulisers, Thorax 38:755, 1983.

Clay MM, Pavia D, Clarke SW: Effect of aerosol particle size on bronchodilation with nebulised terbutaline in asthmatic subjects, Thorax 41:364, 1986.

Conference on the Scientific Basis of Respiratory Therapy: Final report: aerosol therapy, Am Rev Respir Dis 110:7, 1974.

Conner WT et al: Reliable salbutamol administration in 6- to 36-month-old children by means of a metered dose inhaler and aerochamber with mask, Ped Pulmonol 6:263, 1989.

Crogan SJ, Bishop MJ: Delivery efficiency of metered dose aerosols given via endotracheal tubes, Anesthesiol 70:1008, 1989.

Crompton GK: New inhalation devices, Eur Respir J 1:679, 1988 (editorial).

Dahlbäck M et al: Deposition of tracer aerosols in the rabbit respiratory tract, J Aerosol Sci 18:733, 1987.

Dolovich MB et al: Pulmonary aerosol deposition in chronic bronchitis: intermittent positive pressure breathing versus quiet breathing, Am Rev Respir Dis 115:397, 1977.

Dolovich M et al: Optimal delivery of aerosols from metered dose inhalers, Chest 80(suppl):911, 1981.

Dolovich M et al: Clinical evaluation of a simple demand inhalation MDI aerosol delivery device, Chest 84:36, 1983.

Epstein SW et al: Survey of the clinical use of pressurized aerosol inhalers, Can Med Assoc J 120:813, 1979.

Fernandez A et al: Bronchodilators in patients with chronic obstructive pulmonary disease on mechanical ventilation: utilization of metered-dose inhalers, Am Rev Respir Dis 141:164, 1990.

Ferron GA, Kerrebijn KF, Weber J: Properties of aerosols produced with three nebulizers, Am Rev Respir Dis 114:899, 1976.

Flavin M et al: Aerosol delivery to the rabbit lung with an infant ventilator, Pediatr Pulmonol 2:35, 1986.

Flick MR, Moody LE, Block AJ: Effect on ultrasonic nebulization on arterial oxygen saturation in chronic obstructive pulmonary disease, Chest 71:366, 1977.

Fraser I et al: Therapeutic aerosol delivery in ventilator systems. Am Rev Respir Dis 123:107, 1981 (abstract).

Fuller HD et al: Pressurized aerosol versus jet aerosol delivery to mechanically ventilated patients, Am Rev Respir Dis 141:440, 1990.

Gay PC et al: Metered dose inhalers for bronchodilator delivery in intubated, mechanically ventilated patients, Chest 99:66, 1991.

Goldberg IS, Lourenco RV: Deposition of aerosols in pulmonary disease, Arch Intern Med 131:88, 1973.

Hallworth GW: The formulation and evaluation of pressurised metered-dose inhalers. In Ganderton D, Jones T, eds: Drug delivery to the respiratory tract, Chichester, England, 1987, Ellis Horwood.

Hannan SE et al: Foreign body aspiration associated with the use of an aerosol inhaler, Am Rev Respir Dis 129:1025, 1984.

Heimer D, Shim C, Williams MH Jr: The effect of sequential inhalation of metaproterenol aerosol in asthma, J Allergy Clin Immunol 66:75, 1980.

Hess D, Horney D, Snyder T: Medication-delivery performance of eight small-volume, hand-held nebulizers: effects of diluent volume, gas flowrate, and nebulizer model. Respir Care 34:717, 1989.

Hetzel MR, Clark TJH: Comparison of salbutamol Rotahaler with conventional pressurized aerosol, Clin Allergy 7:563, 1977.

Hiller C et al: Aerodynamic size distribution of metered-dose bronchodilator aerosols, Am Rev Respir Dis 118:311, 1978.

Hiller FC et al: Physical properties, hygroscopicity and estimated pulmonary retention of various therapeutic aerosols, Chest 77(suppl):318, 1980.

Hiller FC et al: Physical properties of therapeutic aerosols. Chest 80(suppl):901, 1981.

Hollie MC et al: Extreme variability in aerosol output of the DeVilbiss 646 jet nebulizer. Chest 100:1339, 1991.

Hughes JM, Saez J: Effects of nebulizer mode and position in a mechanical ventilator circuit on dose efficiency, Respir Care 32:1131, 1987.

Itoh H et al: Clinical observations of aerosol deposition in patients with airways obstruction, Chest 80(suppl):837, 1980.

Jasper AC et al: Cost-benefit comparison of aerosol bronchodilator delivery methods in hospitalized patients, Chest 91:614, 1987.

Jenkins SC et al: Comparison of domiciliary nebulized salbutamol and salbutamol from a metered-dose inhaler in stable chronic airflow limitation, Chest 91:805, 1987.

Johnson MA et al: Delivery of albuterol and ipratropium bromide from two nebulizer systems in chronic stable asthma: efficacy and pulmonary deposition, Chest 96:1, 1989.

Kelling JS et al: Physician knowledge in the use of canister nebulizers, Chest 83:612, 1983.

Kemp JP et al: Comparison of bronchodilator responses with bitolterol mesylate solution with the use of two different nebulizer systems in asthma. J Allergy Clin Immunol 77:509, 1986.

Kim CS, Eldridge MA, Sackner MA: Oropharyngeal deposition and delivery aspects of metered-dose inhaler aerosols, Am Rev Respir Dis 135:157, 1987.

Kim CS, Trujillo D, Sackner MA: Size aspects of metered-dose inhaler aerosols, Am Rev Respir Dis 132:137, 1985.

Konig P: Spacer devices used with metered-dose inhalers: breakthrough or gimmick? Chest 88:276, 1985.

Kradjan WA, Lakshminarayan S: Efficiency of air compressor-driven nebulizers, Chest 87:512, 1985.

Kraemer R et al: Short-term effect of albuterol, delivered via a new auxiliary device, in wheezy infants, Am Rev Respir Dis 144:347, 1991.

Lee HS: Proper aerosol inhalation technique for delivery of asthma medications, Clin Pediatr 22:440, 1983.

Lewis RA, Fleming JS: Fractional deposition from a jet nebulizer: how it differs from a metered dose inhaler, Br J Dis Chest 79:361, 1985.

Lippman M: Regional deposition of particles in the human respiratory tract. In Lee DHK, Falk HL, Murphy SD, eds: Handbook of physiology, section 9, Bethesda, Md, 1977, American Physiological Society.

Loren M et al: Comparison between simple nebulization and intermittent positive-pressure in asthmatic children with severe bronchospasm, Chest 72:145, 1977.

Lourenco RV, Cotromanes E: Clinical aerosols. I. Characterization of aerosols and their diagnostic uses, Arch Intern Med 142:2163, 1982.

MacIntyre NR et al: Aerosol delivery in intubated, mechanically ventilated patients, Crit Care Med 13:81, 1985.

Malik SK, Jenkins DE: Alterations in airway dynamics following inhalation of ultrasonic mist, Chest 62:660, 1972.

Mercer TT: Production and characterization of aerosols, Arch Intern Med 131:39, 1973.

Mestitz H, Copland JM, McDonald CF: Comparison of outpatient nebulized vs metered dose inhaler terbutaline in chronic airflow obstruction, Chest 96:1237, 1989.

Mitchell RI: Retention of aerosol particles in the respiratory tract. A review, Am Rev Respir Dis 82:627, 1960.

Molina MJ, Rowland FS: Stratospheric risk for chlorofluoromethanes: chlorine atom-catalyzed destruction of ozone, Nature 249:810, 1974.

Moren F: Pressurized aerosols for oral inhalation, Int J Pharmacol 8:1, 1981.

Morrow PE: Aerosol characterization and deposition, Am Rev Respir Dis 110(suppl):88, 1974.

Morrow PE: An evaluation of the physical properties of monodisperse and heterodisperse aerosols used in the assessment of bronchial function, Chest 80(suppl):809, 1981.

Newhouse M, Dolovich M: Aerosol therapy: nebulizer vs metered dose inhaler, Chest 91:799, 1987, (editorial).

Newhouse MT, Ruffin RE: Deposition and fate of aerosolized drugs, Chest 73(suppl):936, 1978.

Newman SP: Aerosol deposition considerations in inhalation therapy, Chest 88(suppl):152S, 1985.

Newman SP: Aerosol inhalers, Br Med J 300:1286, 1990.

Newman SP, Clarke SW: Inhalation technique with aerosol bronchodilators: does it matter? Pract Cardiol 9:157, 1983a.

Newman SP, Clarke SW: Therapeutic aerosols 1—physical and practical considerations, Thorax 38:881, 1983b, (editorial).

Newman SP, Pavia D, Clarke SW: How should a pressurized beta-adrenergic bronchodilator be inhaled? Eur J Respir Dis 62:3, 1981a.

Newman SP, Pavia D, Clarke SW: Improving the bronchial deposition of pressurized aerosols, Chest 80(suppl):909, 1981b.

Newman SP et al: Deposition of pressurized aerosols in the human respiratory tract, Thorax 36:52, 1981c.

Newman SP et al: Deposition of pressurized suspension aerosols inhaled through extension devices, Am Rev Respir Dis 124:317, 1981d.

Newman SP et al: Effects of various inhalation modes on the deposition of radioactive pressurized aerosols, Eur J Respir Dis 119(suppl):57, 1982.

Newman SP et al: Effect of InspirEase on the deposition of metered-dose aerosols in the human respiratory tract, Chest 89:531, 1986.

Newman SP, Pellow PGD, Clarke SW: In vitro comparison of DeVilbiss jet and ultrasonic nebulizers, Chest 92:991, 1987.

Newman SP et al: Improvement of drug delivery with a breath actuated pressurised aerosol for patients with poor inhaler technique, Thorax 46:712, 1991.

Pedersen S, Hansen OR, Fuglsang G: Influence of inspiratory flow rate upon the effect of a Turbuhaler. Arch Dis Child 65:308, 1990.

Pedersen S: Aerosol treatment of bronchoconstriction in children with or without a tube spacer, N Engl J Med 308:1328, 1983.

Pedersen S: How to use a rotahaler. Arch Dis Child 61:11, 1986a.

Pedersen S: The importance of a pause between the inhalation of two puffs of terbutaline from a pressurized aerosol with a tube spacer, J Allergy Clin Immunol 77:505, 1986b.

Persson G, Gruvstad E, Stahl E: A new multiple dose powder inhaler, (Turbuhaler), compared with a pressurized inhaler in a study of terbutaline in asthmatics, Eur Respir J 1:681, 1988.

Pflug AE, Cheney FW Jr, Butler J: The effects of an ultrasonic aerosol on pulmonary mechanics and arterial blood gases in patients with chronic bronchitis, Am Rev Respir Dis 101:710, 1970.

Popa VT: How to inhale a whiff of pressurized bronchodilator, Chest 76:496, 1979, (editorial).

Rau JL Jr, Harwood RJ: Comparison of nebulizer delivery methods through a neonatal endotracheal tube: a bench study, Respir Care 37:1233, 1992.

Rau JL, Harwood RJ, Groff JL: Evaluation of a reservoir device for metered-dose bronchodilator delivery to intubated adults: an in vitro study, Chest 102:924, 1992.

Richards R et al: Inhalation rate of sodium cromoglycate determines plasma pharmacokinetics and protection against AMP-induced bronchoconstriction in asthma. Eur Respir J 1:896, 1988.

Sackner MA, Kim CS: Auxiliary MDI aerosol delivery systems. Chest 88(suppl):161S, 1985.

Salmon B, Wilson NM, Silverman M: How much aerosol reaches the lungs of wheezing infants and toddlers? Arch Dis Child 65:401, 1990.

Schultz CH, Hargarten SW, Babbitt J: Inhalation of a coin and a capsule from a metered-dose inhaler, N Engl J Med 325:432, 1991, (letter).

Shim CS, Williams MH Jr: Effect of bronchodilator therapy administered by canister versus jet nebulizer, J Allergy Clin Immunol 73:387, 1984.

Simonds AK et al: Alveolar targeting of aerosol pentamidine, Am Rev Respir Dis 141:827, 1990.

Smaldone GC, Perry RT, Deutsch DG: Characteristics of nebulizers used in the treatment of AIDS-related *Pneumocytis carinii* pneumonia. J Aerosol Med 1:113, 1988.

Smith G et al: Aerodynamic size distribution of cromolyn sodium at ambient and airway humidity. Am Rev Respir Dis 121:513, 1980.

Spiro SG et al: Direct labelling of ipratropium bromide aerosol and its deposition pattern in normal subjects and patients with chronic bronchitis. Thorax 39:432, 1984.

Stauder J, Hidinger KG: Terbutaline aerosol from a metered dose inhaler with a 750-ml spacer or as a nebulized solution: comparison of two delivery systems for bronchodilator aerosol. Respiration 44:237, 1983.

Swift DL: Generation and respiratory deposition of therapeutic aerosols. Am Rev Respir Dis 122(part 2):71, 1980.

Tarala RA, Madsen BW, Paterson JW: Comparative efficacy of salbutamol by pressurized aerosol and wet nebulizer in acute asthma, Br J Clin Pharmacol 10:393, 1980.

Task Group on Lung Dynamics: Deposition and retention models for internal dosimetry of the human respiratory tract. In Health physics, vol 12, Elmsford, NY, 1966, Pergamon Press.

Tenholder MF, Bryson MJ, Whitlock WL: A model for conversion from small volume nebulizer to metered dose inhaler aerosol therapy, Chest 101:634, 1992.

Tobin MJ et al: Response to bronchodilator drug administration by a new reservoir aerosol delivery system and a review of other auxiliary delivery systems, Am Rev Respir Dis 126:670, 1982.

Toogood JH et al: Clinical use of spacer systems for corticosteroid inhalation therapy: a preliminary analysis, Eur J Respir Dis 122(suppl):100, 1982.

Towns SJ et al: Bronchodilator effects of salbutamol powder administered via Rotahaler and of terbutaline aerosol administered via Misthaler, Med J Aust 1:633, 1983.

Vilsvik J et al: Comparison between Bricanyl Turbuhaler and Ventolin metered dose inhaler in the treatment of exercise-induced asthma in adults, Ann Allergy 67:315, 1991.

Wolfsdorf J, Swift DL, Avery ME: Mist therapy reconsidered: an evaluation of the respiratory deposition of labelled water aerosols produced by jet and ultrasonic nebulizers, Pediatrics 43:799, 1969.

Zainudin BMZ et al: Comparison of bronchodilator responses and deposition patterns of salbutamol inhaled from a pressurised metered dose inhaler, as a dry powder, and as a nebulised solution, Thorax 45:469, 1990.

3

Calculating Drug Dosages

Chapter 3 presents calculations used for drug dosages, with an emphasis on dealing with percentage-strength solutions. The following topics are discussed:

- Systems of measure
- Calculating dosages from prepared-strength liquids, tablets, and capsules
- Calculating dosages from percentage-strength solutions

Practice problems and answers are included.

One of the necessary skills in administering drugs is the calculation of correct dosages and amounts. Although three different systems of measure have been used in drug calculations, metric units of measure are currently employed with formulations in the United States. Therefore, all of the examples in this chapter will be based on the metric system. For completeness as a reference, the older apothecary system, the avoirdupois system, and a set of equivalents between these systems and the metric system are given in Appendix A.

SYSTEMS OF MEASURE

Metric System

The metric system is based on the decimal system, using multiples or fractions of ten. Table 3-1 provides metric units of measure for length, volume, and mass or weight.

TABLE 3–1.

Metric System of Length, Volume, and Mass (Weight)

Word	Abbreviation
Length	
10 millimeters = 1 centimeter	10 mm = 1 cm
10 centimeters = 1 decimeter	10 cm = dm
10 decimeters = 1 meter	10 dm = 1 m
10 meters = 1 dekameter	10 m = 1 Dm
10 dekameters = 1 hectometer	10 Dm = 1 Hm
10 hectometers = 1 kilometer	10 Hm = 1 km
Volume	
10 milliliters = 1 centiliter	10 ml = 1 cl
10 centiliters = 1 deciliter	10 cl = 1 dl
10 deciliters = 1 liter	10 dl = 1 L
10 liters = 1 dekaliter	10 L = 1 Dl
10 dekaliters = 1 hectoliter	10 Dl = 1 Hl
10 hectoliters = 1 kiloliter	10 Hl = 1 kl
Mass	
1000 micrograms (gammos) = 1 milligram	1000 μg = 1 mg
10 milligrams = 1 centigram	10 mg = 1 cg
10 centigrams = 1 decigram	10 cg = 1 dg
10 decigrams = 1 gram	10 dg = 1 g
10 grams = 1 dekagram	10 g = 1 Dg
10 dekagrams = 1 hectogram	10 Dg = 1 Hg
10 hectograms = 1 kilogram	10 Hg = 1 kg

The primary units in the metric system are the following:

Length: meter (m)
Volume: liter (L)
Mass: gram (g)

Fractional parts, or multiples of these primary units, are expressed by adding Latin prefixes for sizes smaller than the primary unit and Greek prefixes for sizes larger than the primary unit.

Decreasing Prefixes (Latin)

micro = 1/1,000,000

milli = 1/1,000

centi = 1/100

deci = 1/10

Increasing Prefixes (Greek)

deka = 10

hecto = 100

kilo = 1,000

In calculating drug dosages, the metric units for volume and mass (weight) are needed. The most commonly encountered unit of volume in respiratory care is the milliliter (ml) or 0.001 L. Common units of weight are the kilogram (kg), the gram (g), the milligram (mg), and with recent aerosolized drugs, the microgram (μg). Conversions within the metric system should be familiar, such as converting 1 mg to 0.001 g, 500 ml to 0.5 L, or 0.4 mg to 400 μg. Facility with such conversions, with decimal fractions, and with the other basic rules of arithmetic are necessary before attempting calculation of drug dosages. Appendix B provides an arithmetic self-test and practice problems with answers as a review.

The *gram* is defined as the weight of 1 ml of distilled water at 4° C in vacuo. Under these conditions, 1 g of water and 1 ml of water are equal. This should not be used to convert from weight to volume, however, as a gram of liquid is not always equal to a milliliter of liquid depending on the temperature, pressure, and nature of the substance.

Système International d'Unites

The International System of Units, or Système International d'Unites (SI), was adopted in 1960 and is the modern metric system. The SI system is well presented by Chatburn (1988) with conversion factors between older metric units for volume and the English system of measurement units. The SI system is based on the meter-kilogram-second system, with volume as a derived unit of length. The primary units of interest in pharmacology calculations are as follows:

Mass: kilogram (kg)
Volume: cubic meter (m^3)
Equivalence: $10^{-3}m^3 = 1$ L

Although the base unit of measure in the SI system for volume is the cubic meter (m^3), the liter (L), as well as its fractions or multiples, is currently accepted and is still common in measures of liquid volume in respiratory care.

Drops as Units of Volume

Orders in respiratory care may often involve drops, such as four drops of racemic epinephrine with 2.5 cc (or ml) of distilled water. The following equivalence is used:

$$16 \text{ drops (gtt)} = 1 \text{ ml}$$

In this example then, four drops (4 gtt) would equal 0.25 ml [1 ml/(16 gtt × 4 gtt) = 4/16 ml]. Therefore 0.25 ml is drawn up into a small accurate syringe, such as a tuberculin syringe, to obtain the four drops.

It should be noted that drops are not standardized and can vary in size due to the physical properties of the particular fluid (specific gravity, viscosity) and the orifice of the dropper. Since drops can vary in amount delivered, physicians should be diplomatically cautioned to prescribe in metric units (cubic centimeters or milliliters) unless a dropper calibrated specifically for the particular medication is supplied by the manufacturer.

Household Units of Measure

Household units of measure are useful when instructing patients to take medications at home and are based on common kitchen measures, such as the teaspoon, tablespoon, and cup. Metric equivalents to these household measures are given in Appendix A. Although the teaspoon is equivalent to 5 ml, not every teaspoon used for eating will actually equal 5 ml. However, measuring spoons and cups will more accurately give the volumes indicated, such as 5 ml per teaspoon or 240 ml per cup.

CALCULATING DOSAGES FROM PREPARED-STRENGTH LIQUIDS, TABLETS, AND CAPSULES

Once the therapist is able to freely convert within the metric system, it is possible to begin calculating drug dosages. In general, such calculations will be of two types:

1. Those involving fluids, tablets, or capsules of a given strength (e.g., 5 mg/ml).
2. Those involving solutions of a percentage strength.

Because there are definite conventions regarding solutions, and because solutions for aerosol delivery are the primary dosage form for respiratory care, they are treated separately and in detail.

When using a prepared-strength liquid, tablet, or capsule, you are always trying to determine how much liquid or how many tablets or capsules are needed to give the amount, or dose, of the drug ordered. For example, if one tablet of a drug contains 5 mg and you want to give 2.5 mg, you immediately realize that one-half tablet must be given.

Calculating With Proportions

The simplest, and therefore probably the most accurate, error-free method of calculation when using a vial of a prepared-strength drug (or a tablet or capsule) involves two steps at most:

1. Convert to consistent units of measure.
2. Set up a straightforward proportion:

$$\frac{\text{original dose}}{\textit{per} \text{ amount}} = \frac{\text{desired dose}}{\textit{per} \text{ amount}}$$

or, original dose:*per* amount : : desired dose:*per* amount.

In step one, this conversion may be from grams to milligrams within the metric system, or even from apothecary to metric, if an apothecary dosage strength has been ordered. In step two, either format for the proportion is correct. In the second form, the extremes and means are each multiplied together (see Appendix B, Ratios and Proportions). If one arrangement is more intuitively clear, that should be preferred by the user.

Consider an example of oxytetracycline tablets, each 250-mg strength. If you need 0.5 g of the drug, either convert 250 mg to 0.25 g or 0.5 g to 500 mg. Once the units are consistent, set up the proportion to find the unknown (i.e., how many tablets are needed to deliver the desired dose to the patient). By using the previous formula, we set up the following:

$$\text{original drug dose} = 250 \text{ mg}$$

$$\textit{per} \text{ amount} = \text{per tablet (tab.)}$$

$$\text{desired drug dose} = 0.5 \text{ g} = 500 \text{ mg}$$

$$\textit{per} \text{ amount} = \text{unknown } (x)$$

$$\frac{250 \text{ mg}}{1 \text{ tab.}} = \frac{500 \text{ mg}}{x \text{ tab.}}$$

$$250 \times x = 500 \times 1$$

$$x = \frac{500}{250} = 2 \text{ tabl.}$$

While this calculation is trivially clear and can be performed mentally, others may require calculation for the sake of accuracy.

EXAMPLE: You have 120 mg of phenobarbital in 30 ml of phenobarbital elixir. How many milliliters of elixir will you use to give a 15-mg dose?

$$\frac{120 \text{ mg (original dose)}}{30 \text{ ml } (per \text{ amount})} = \frac{15 \text{ mg (desired dose)}}{x \ (per \text{ amount})}$$

$$120 \times x = 15 \times 30$$

$$x = \frac{450}{120} = 3.75 \text{ ml}$$

Simplification is possible, such as reducing 120 mg/30 ml to 4 mg/1 ml. Then knowing that there are 4 mg in every 1 ml, simply divide 4 mg/1 ml into 15 mg to determine how many milliliters are needed. Often, reducing a fluid to its dosage strength per milliliter allows quick mental computation of the dose. Caution and care should be observed in the initial reduction, however. An error at that point causes a subsequent dosage error. **Do not hesitate to write out a calculation.** In a busy clinical setting, a patient's well-being should take precedence over a therapist's mathematical pride!

Drug Amounts in Units

Note that some drugs are manufactured in units (U) rather than in grams or milligrams. Examples are penicillin, insulin, and heparin. Solving dosage problems for these drugs is exactly the same as for the other units of measure previously mentioned.

EXAMPLE: A brand of sodium heparin is available in 1000 U/ml. How many milliliters do you need for 500 U of the drug?

By using the second form of the proportion (extremes and means), we set up the following:

$$\text{Original dose}:per \text{ amount} :: \text{Desired dose}: per \text{ amount}$$

$$1000 \text{ U}:1 \text{ ml} :: 500 \text{ U}:x \text{ ml}$$

By multiplying the extremes and the means, we obtain the following:

$$1000 \times x = 500$$

$$x = 0.5 \text{ ml}$$

The amount required for 500 U, given the prepared-strength liquid, is 0.5 ml.
There is no universal equivalence between units as a measure of amount

and the metric weight system. Units are used with biological standardization and are defined for each drug by a standard preparation of that drug, when the drug is measured in units. For example, there is a standard preparation of digitalis that consists of dried, powdered digitalis leaves, and 100 mg of this preparation equals one USP *(United States Pharmacopeia)* unit of activity. In this way, when drugs are extracted from animals, plants, or minerals, there is a standard, reference preparation. Note that 100 mg is not 1 U for every drug with units: insulin has a standard preparation of 0.04 mg = 1 U. When a drug is isolated as a pure chemical form, either extracted as the active substance in a natural source or synthesized in the laboratory, biological standardization based on a standard preparation from the natural source is no longer necessary. The specific chemical amount is given in metric weight or volume measure.

Calculations With a Dosage Schedule

There are times when the dose of a drug must be obtained from a *schedule*, which may be based on the size of a person. For example, a suggested schedule for atropine sulfate by aerosol is 0.05 mg/kg body weight. This means that first the *dose* must be calculated after the body weight is obtained, then the amount of the drug preparation needed for treatment can be calculated. EXAMPLE: Using a dosage schedule of 0.05 mg/kg for atropine by aerosol and a prepared-strength vial with 0.4 mg/ml, how much of the drug preparation will be needed for a 60-kg woman?

1. Calculate the dose needed.

$$\text{Dose} = 0.05 \text{ mg/kg} \times 60 \text{ kg} = 3.0 \text{ mg}$$

2. Calculate the amount of the preparation.

$$\frac{0.4 \text{ mg}}{1 \text{ ml}} = \frac{3.0 \text{ mg}}{x \text{ ml}}$$

$$0.4 \times x = 3.0$$

$$x = 7.5 \text{ ml}$$

Sample Calculations With Prepared-Strength Drugs

EXAMPLE 1. An injectable solution of glycopyrrolate with a prepared-strength of 0.2 mg/ml is used for nebulization. How many milliliters are needed for a 1.5-mg dose?

a. Solution.

Original dose per amount: 0.2 mg/ml
Desired dose: 1.5 mg
Amount needed: x ml

b. Substituting.

$$\frac{0.2 \text{ mg}}{1 \text{ ml}} = \frac{1.5 \text{ mg}}{x \text{ ml}}$$

c. Solving for x.

$$0.2 \text{ mg} \times x = 1.5 \text{ mg} \times 1 \text{ ml}$$

$$x = 1.5 \text{ ml}/0.2$$

$$x = 7.5 \text{ ml}$$

ANSWER. An amount of 7.5 ml will contain the desired dose of 1.5 mg, using the prepared-strength given.

EXAMPLE 2. You have a corticosteroid in a vial, with a prepared-strength of 4 mg/ml. How much of the liquid do you need for a 1-mg dose?

a. Solution.

Original dose per amount: 4 mg/ml
Desired dose: 1 mg
Amount needed: x ml

b. Substituting.

$$\frac{4 \text{ mg}}{1 \text{ ml}} = \frac{1 \text{ mg}}{x \text{ ml}}$$

c. Solving for x:

$$4 \text{ mg} \times x = 1 \text{ mg} \times 1 \text{ ml}$$

$$x = 1 \text{ ml}/4$$

$$x = \text{¼ ml, or } 0.25 \text{ ml}$$

ANSWER. Give 0.25 ml for the desired dose of 1 mg.

EXAMPLE 3. A dosage schedule of a surfactant calls for 5 ml/kg body weight. If a premature infant weighs 1200 g, how many milliliters are needed?

a. Convert body weight to kilograms.

$$1 \text{ kg}/1000 \text{ g} \times 1200 \text{ g} = 1.2 \text{ kg}$$

b. Multiply the weight in kilograms by the schedule of 5 ml/kg.

$$1.2 \text{ kg} \times 5 \text{ ml/kg} = 6 \text{ ml}$$

ANSWER: Based on the dosage schedule and weight, 6 ml should be given.

EXAMPLE 4. The prepared-strength of a drug is 100 mg/4 ml. The dosage schedule is 100 mg/kg birth weight. A premature newborn weighs 1100 g. Based on the weight, what dose is needed? Second, how many milliliters of the drug should be given to achieve this dose?

a. Solution: dose needed.

(1) Convert birth weight to kilograms.

$$1 \text{ kg/1000 g} \times 1100 \text{ g} = 1.1 \text{ kg}$$

(2) Multiply the birth weight by the dosage schedule.

$$100 \text{ mg/kg} \times 1.1 \text{ kg} = 110 \text{ mg}$$

The dosage needed is 110 mg of drug.

b. Solution: amount needed for dose.

(1) Solve for amount using a proportion.
  Original dose per amount: 100 mg/4 ml
  Desired dose: 110 mg
  Amount needed: x ml

c. Substituting.

$$\frac{100 \text{ mg}}{4 \text{ ml}} = \frac{110 \text{ mg}}{x \text{ ml}}$$

$$100 \text{ mg} \times x = 110 \text{ mg} \times 4 \text{ ml}$$

$$x = (110 \text{ mg} \times 4 \text{ ml})/100 \text{ mg}$$

$$x = 4.4 \text{ ml}$$

ANSWER: Based on the dosage schedule, weight of the newborn, and the prepared-strength, 4.4 ml will give the needed dose of 110 mg.

Practice Problems and Answers: Prepared-Strength Dosage Calculations

Answers to the practice problems follow. The solution to each problem is set up and the answer given. Details of the algebraic solution are not given; the preceding examples should be used as a guide, along with the exercises in Appendix B if necessary.

Problems

1. A bottle is labeled Demerol (meperidine) 50 mg/cc. How many cubic centimeters are needed to give a 125-mg dose?
2. Promazine HC1 comes as 500 mg/10 ml. How many milliliters are needed to give a 150-mg dose?
3. Hyaluronidase comes as 150 U/cc. How many cubic centimeters are needed for a 30-U dose?
4. Morphine sulfate 4 mg is ordered. You have a vial with 10 mg/ml. How much do you need?
5. You have a morphine sulfate vial with 15 mg/cc. How many cubic centimeters for a 10-mg dose?
6. Diphenhydramine (Benadryl) elixir contains 12.5 mg of diphenhydramine HCl in each 5 ml of elixir. How many milligrams are there in one-half teaspoonful dose (1 teaspoon = 5 ml)?
7. A pediatric dose of oxytetracycline 100 mg is ordered. The dosage form is an oral suspension containing 125 mg/5 cc. How much of the suspension contains a 100 mg dose?
8. How much heparin is in 0.2 ml if you have 1000 U/ml?
9. If you have a vial of dexamethasone with 4 mg/ml, how much do you need for a 1-mg dose?
10. If Cogentin is available as 0.5 mg/tab., how many tablets do you need for a 1-mg dose?
11. If Tempra is available as 120 mg/5 ml, how much dose is there in ½ teaspoon?
12. If Dalmane is available as 15-mg capsules, what dosage is given with two capsules?
13. Terbutaline sulfate is available as 1 mg/ml in an ampule. How many milliliters are needed for a 0.25-mg dose?
14. A patient is told to take 4 mg of albuterol 4 times daily. The medication comes in 2-mg tablets. How many tablets are needed for one 4-mg dose?
15. Metaproterenol is available as a syrup with 10 mg/5 ml. How many teaspoons should be taken for a 20-mg dose?
16. If you have 3 mg/ml of d-tubocurarine, how many milliliters are needed for a dose of 9 mg?
17. If a dosage schedule requires 0.25 mg/kg body weight, what dose is needed for an 88-kg person?
18. Using 0.05 mg/kg body weight for atropine by aerosol, what dose is needed for a 75-kg man?
19. How much drug is needed for a 65-kg adult, using 0.5 mg/kg?
20. Pediatric dosage of an antibiotic is 0.5 g/20 lb body weight not to exceed 75 mg/kg per 24 hours.

a. What is the dose for a 40-lb child?

b. If this dose is given twice in 1 day, is the maximum dose exceeded?

Answers

1. 50 mg/1 cc = 125 mg/x cc; x = 2.5 cc
2. 500 mg/10 ml = 150 mg/x ml; x = 3 ml
3. 150 U/cc = 30 U/x cc; x = 0.2 cc
4. 10 mg/ml = 4 mg/x ml; x = 0.4 ml
5. 15 mg/cc = 10 mg/x cc; x = 0.67 cc
6. ½ teaspoon = 2.5 ml
   12.5 mg/5 ml = x mg/2.5 ml; x = 6.25 mg
7. 125 mg/5 cc = 100 mg/x cc; x = 4 cc
8. 1000 U/ml = x U/0.2 ml; x = 200 U
9. 4 mg/ml = 1 mg/x ml; x = 0.25 ml
10. 0.5 mg/1 tab. = 1 mg/x tab; x = 2 tablets
11. ½ teaspoon = 2.5 ml
    120 mg/5 ml = x mg/2.5 ml; x = 60 mg
12. 15 mg/caps. = x mg/2 caps.; x = 30 mg
13. 1 mg/ml = 0.25 mg/x ml; x = 0.25 ml
14. 2 mg/tab. = 4 mg/x tab.; x = 2 tablets
15. 1 teaspoon = 5 ml
    10 mg/5 ml = 20 mg/x ml; x = 10 ml
    10 ml × 1 tsp/5 ml = 2 teaspoons
16. 3 mg/ml = 9 mg/x ml; x = 3 ml
17. 0.25 mg/kg × 88 kg = 22 mg
18. 0.05 mg/kg × 75 kg = 3.75 mg
19. 0.5 mg/kg × 65 kg = 32.5 mg
20. a. 0.5 g/20 lb × 40 lb = 1.0 g
    b. 2 doses = 2 × 1.0 g = 2.0 g = 2000 mg
       40 lb × 1 kg/2.2 lb = 18 kg
       2000 mg/18 kg = 111.1 mg/kg
       Yes. Two doses give 2000 mg/40 lb, which is 2000 mg/18 kg, or 111.1 mg/kg a day.

CALCULATING DOSAGES FROM PERCENTAGE-STRENGTH SOLUTIONS

Since the respiratory therapist deals almost exclusively with the inhalation route, aerosols, solutions, and percentage strengths are fundamental to the calculation of a drug dose.

A solution contains a *solute* that is dissolved in a *solvent*, giving a homogeneous mixture.

The *strength* of a solution is expressed in percentage of solute to total solvent and solute. *Percentage* means parts of the active ingredient (solute) in a preparation contained in 100 parts of the total preparation (solute *and* solvent).

Types of Percentage Preparations

Weight to Weight. Percent in weight (W/W) expresses the number of grams of a drug or active ingredient in 100 g of a mixture (W/W: grams per 100 g of mixture).

Weight to Volume. Percent may be expressed for the number of grams of a drug or active ingredient in 100 ml of a mixture (W/V: grams per 100 ml of mixture).

Volume to Volume. Percent volume in volume expresses the number of milliliters of drug or active ingredient in 100 ml of a mixture (V/V: milliliters per 100 ml of mixture).

NOTE: Calculating percentage strengths of solutions *either* by weight of a drug in grams, *or* by volume of a drug in milliliters, and taking percentages of grams to milliliters, is based on or allowed because 1 g H_2O = 1 ml H_2O, 4° C in vacuo.

Solutions by Ratio

Frequently when diluting a medication for use in an aerosol or IPPB treatment, a solute-to-solvent ratio is given (e.g., isoproterenol 1:200 or Bronkosol 1:8).

Ratio by Grams:Milliliters. In the isoproterenol 1:200 example, what is indicated is 1 g/200 ml of solution = 0.5% strength. Other examples include epinephrine 1:100 = 1% strength and epinephrine 1:1000 = 0.1% strength. Generally, grams per milliliters, or grams:milliliters, are the intended units.

Ratio by Simple Parts. In the Bronkosol 1:8 example, actual parts medication to parts solvent are indicated: 1:8 = one part to eight parts, which is the same as 0.25 cc to 2 cc. However, part-to-part ratios do not indicate actual amounts or specific units, although usually milliliters:milliliters are meant. It is assumed you know that 0.25 cc or 0.5 cc of Bronkosol is given and not a 1-cc amount as far as the absolute amount is concerned. An order such as Bronkosol 1:8 is not precise without further specifications of the amount of drug to be given.

Note on Mixing Solutions

One determines the amount of active ingredient needed for the percent-age strength desired, then adds enough solvent to "top off" to the total solu-tion amount needed. When ordering a solution, this is indicated by *q.s.*, or "quantity sufficient" for the total needed.

For example, to obtain 30 cc of 3% procaine HCl, we calculate 0.9 cc of the active ingredient and water q.s. for 30 cc of solution.

One does not merely give the difference between solute and total solu-tion (30 cc − 0.9 cc = 29.1 cc) because certain solutes can change volume (e.g., alcohol "shrinks" in water).

Solving Percentage-Strength Solution Problems

For solutions when the active ingredient itself is **undiluted** (pure 100% strength), the following formula is easily used:

$$\text{Percentage strength (in decimals)} = \frac{\text{Solute (in grams or cubic centimeters)}}{\text{Total amount (solute and solvent)}} \quad (1)$$

Alternatively, a ratio format can be used:

$$\frac{\text{Amount of solute}}{\text{Total amount}} = \frac{\text{Amount of solute}}{100 \text{ parts (grams or milliliters)}} \quad (2)$$

When the active ingredient, or solute, is already **diluted** (less than pure), the following formula may be used to calculate the amount of solute needed:

$$\text{Percentage strength (in decimals)} = \frac{\text{Dilute solute} \times \text{Percentage strength of solute}}{\text{Total amount (solution)}} \quad (3)$$

In brief, the solute (active ingredient) multiplied by the percentage strength gives the amount of pure active ingredient in the dilute solution. Equation 3 adds only one modification to the formula given in Equation 1, that is, to multiply the dilute solute by its actual percentage strength, with the result indicating the amount of active ingredient at a 100% (pure) strength. For example, 10 ml of 10% solute means you have 1 ml of pure solute. Put another way, you would need 10 ml of dilute solute to have 1 ml of pure sol-ute (active ingredient). When used in Equation 3, the unknown is usually how much of the dilute solute, or active ingredient, is needed in the total solution to give the desired strength. This is illustrated in the following examples:

EXAMPLE 1. Undiluted Active Ingredient: How many milligrams of active ingre-dient are there in 2 cc of 1:200 isoproterenol?

a. Using Equation 1.
   Percentage strength = 1:200 = 0.5% = 0.005
   Total amount of solution = 2 cc
   Active ingredient = x
b. Substitutions.

$$0.005 = x \text{ g/2 cc}$$

$$x \text{ g} = 0.005 \times 2$$

$$x = 0.01 \text{ g}$$

c. Converting.

$$0.01 \text{ g} = 10 \text{ mg.}$$

ANSWER: In 2 cc of 1:200 solution there is 10 mg of active ingredient.

EXAMPLE 2. Diluted Active Ingredient: How much of 20% of Mucomyst (brand of acetylcysteine) is needed to prepare 5 cc of 10% Mucomyst?
   a. Using Equation 3 (here the acetylcysteine is only 20% strength, not pure).
      Desired percentage strength = 10% = 0.10
      Total solution amount = 5 cc
      Active ingredient percentage strength = 20%
      = 0.20
      Amount of active ingredient needed = x
   b. Substituting.

$$0.10 = x \times (0.20)/5 \text{ cc}$$

$$x = 5 \times (0.10)/0.20$$

$$x = 2.5 \text{ cc}$$

ANSWER: You need 2.5 cc of 20% Mucomyst mixed with enough normal saline to give a total of 5 cc of solution. This 5 cc will be a 10% strength solution.

NOTE. While diluting a 20% solution to a 10% solution is obviously a half-and-half procedure and need not require use of a formula, less intuitive dilutions will need to be calculated. The reader might try diluting 20% Mucomyst to obtain 5 cc of a 5% strength solution, using the preceding approach.

Percent Strengths in Milligrams per Milliliter

The basic definition of percent strength in solutions involves grams or milliliters. However, the amount of active ingredient in most aerosolized respiratory drugs is in milligrams. It may be a useful clinical reference, and one that is easily remembered, to define percent strengths in terms of milligrams per single milliliter, using a 1% strength reference point.

Recall that 1% strength is 1 g/100 ml. Using the formula for percent strength (Equation 1), you have the following:

$$0.01 = \frac{1\,g}{100\,ml}$$

For 1ml of a 1% strength, the above formula would give the following:

$$0.01 = \frac{x\,g}{1\,ml}$$

$$x = 0.01\ grams$$

$$0.01\,g \times 1000\,mg/g = 10\,mg$$

Since 0.01 g equals 10 mg, you then have 10 mg/1 ml in a 1% solution.

In general, the percentage formula will give any percentage strength in grams per single milliliter, and then grams can be converted to milligrams. For several common percentage strengths, the following milligrams per milliliter amounts would be obtained:

Percentage strength	mg/ml
20%	200 mg/ml
10%	100 mg/ml
5%	50 mg/ml
1%	10 mg/ml
0.5%	5 mg/ml
0.1%	1 mg/ml
0.05%	0.5 mg/ml

The 1% strength is an easily learned reference point. Note the relationships of 1% to 10%: If there are 10 mg/ml in a 1% solution, there would be 10 times that amount in a 10% solution, or 100 mg/ml. Likewise, a 0.5% solution has one-half as much active ingredient as 1%: one half of 10 mg/ml would be 5 mg/ml. This amount of 5 mg/ml could have been used to solve Example 1, the undiluted active ingredient percentage problem. In that example, it was found that a 1:200 solution (a 0.5% strength) has 10 mg/2 ml (or, cc) which is the same as 5 mg/1 ml.

The formula should be known and represents a more general statement of percentage strengths for solving any problem. However, knowledge of milligrams per milliliters for a 1% solution can be very helpful in many problems, to know how many milligrams of the active ingredient are being given. For example, metaproterenol is available as a 5% solution, an ampule of terbutaline (1 mg/cc) is a 0.1% strength, and 0.05% strength isoproterenol is compounded with 10% acetylcysteine.

Diluents and Drug Dosage Strengths

A common misconception persists that the amount of diluent added to a liquid drug to be aerosolized "weakens" the dosage strength. This is not necessarily the case. One-half cubic centimeter of a 1% drug solution has the same amount (5 mg) of active ingredient, whether it is diluted with 2 cc of normal saline or 10 cc. The amount of diluent simply affects the time required to nebulize a given solution. Practicality dictates that 2.5 cc of solution nebulizes in a reasonable time limit of 10 minutes or so, whereas 10 cc may take much longer. Theoretically, given a suitable nebulizing device, there is no reason that the original 0.5 cc of 1% drug could not be nebulized undiluted. This is essentially what is accomplished with two puffs from a metered-dose inhaler. It is the amount of the active ingredient, determined by the percentage strength and quantity in cubic centimeters of the drug that gives a dosage strength. For this reason it makes little sense to ask students to calculate the resulting percentage strength when 0.5 cc of 1% drug is diluted with 2 cc of isotonic saline. Although technically the percentage strength of the resulting solution is weaker, the dosage strength remains unchanged at 5 mg. It is the dosage strength in milligrams that should be of concern to the clinician. The percentage strength of the drug as supplied is of interest only because it allows one to calculate the dosage strength in milligrams per cubic centimeter.

Definitions and Terms

Solution: A solution is a physically homogeneous mixture of two or more substances (liquid).

Isotonic solutions: Solutions with equal osmotic pressures.

Buffer solution: Aqueous solution able to resist changes of pH with addition of acid/base.

Strength of Solutions

Normal: one gram-equivalent weight (GEW) of solute per liter of solution.

Molar: one mole of solute per liter of solution.

Molal: one mole of solute per 1000 g of solvent.

Osmole: molarity times number of particles per molecule.

Osmolar: one osmole per liter of solution.

Osmolal: one osmole per kilogram of solvent.

Following is an example of the strength of normal vs. physiological (isotonic) saline solution:

1 Normal Solution, NaCl

$$1 \text{ GEW, NaCl} = 58.5 \text{ g}$$
$$.. \ 1 \text{ N solution} = 58.5 \text{ g/L or}$$
$$= 5.85 \text{ g/100 ml}$$
$$= 5.85\% \text{ solution}$$

Therefore, a 1 normal solution of NaCl is a 5.85% strength solution. Physiological saline = 0.9% NaCl (isotonic to body fluid) = 0.9 g/100 ml. One ml has .009 grams of NaCl, which is a 0.9% strength. The 0.9% saline solution is isotonic to body fluid, and is usually termed "normal saline." This is not the same strength as a one normal solution of NaCl.

Sample Calculations With Percentage-Strength Solutions

EXAMPLE 1. How many milligrams of active ingredient are in 3 cc of a 2% solution of procaine HCl?
a. Use Equation 1.

$$\frac{\text{Percentage strength}}{\text{(in decimals)}} = \frac{\text{Solute}}{\text{Total amount}}$$

b. Substituting.

$$0.02 = \frac{x \text{ g}}{3 \text{ cc}}$$
$$x \text{ g} = 0.02 \times 3 \text{ cc}$$
$$x = 0.06 \text{ g}$$

c. Converting.

$$0.06 \text{ g} \times 1000 \text{ mg/g} = 60 \text{ mg}$$

ANSWER: 60 mg

EXAMPLE 2: A resident wants to dilute 20% acetylcysteine to a strength of 6% for a research study. How many milliliters of 20% drug solution are needed to have 10 ml of 6% strength?
a. Use Equation 3.

$$\frac{\text{Percentage strength}}{\text{(in decimals)}} = \frac{\text{Dilute solute} \times \text{Percentage strength}}{\text{Total solution}}$$

Desired percentage strength = 6% = 0.06

Dilute solute = unknown = x ml

Percentage strength = 20% = 0.20

Total solution = 10 ml

b. Substituting.

$$0.06 = \frac{x\ ml \times 0.20}{10\ ml}$$

$$0.06 \times 10\ ml = x\ ml \times 0.20$$

$$x = 0.06 \times 10/0.20$$

$$x = 3\ ml$$

ANSWER: Draw up 3 ml of the 20% strength and add saline, quantity sufficient, for a total of 10 ml. Check your calculation for correctness: 3 ml of 20% strength solution has 600 mg of active ingredient (20% = 200 mg/ml); 600 mg is 0.6 grams, and 0.6 g/10 ml (or 6 g/100 ml) is in fact a 6% strength. So you obtained the needed amount of drug with 3 ml of the 20% solution.

EXAMPLE 3: The usual dose of albuterol sulfate is 0.5 ml of a 0.5% strength solution. How many milligrams is this?

    a. Use Equation 1.

        Percentage in decimals = 0.5% = 0.005
        Active ingredient = unknown = x g
        Total solution = 0.5 ml

    b. Substituting.

$$0.005 = \frac{x\ g}{0.5\ ml}$$

$$x\ g = 0.005 \times 0.5 = 0.0025\ g$$

    c. Converting.

$$0.0025\ g = 2.5\ mg$$

ANSWER: 2.5 mg of active ingredient.

EXAMPLE 4. Albuterol sulfate is also available as a unit dose, with 3 ml, and a percentage strength of 0.083%. If the entire amount of 3 ml is given, is this the same as the usual dose of 2.5 mg?

a. Use Equation 1.
   Percentage in decimals = 0.083% = 0.00083
   Active ingredient = unknown = x g
   Total solution = 3 ml

b. Substituting.

$$0.00083 = \frac{x\ g}{3\ ml}$$

$$x\ g = 3 \times 0.00083 = 0.00249\ g$$

c. Converting.

$$0.00249\ g = 2.49\ mg$$

ANSWER. 2.49 mg is approximately 2.5 mg, the usual dose.

EXAMPLE 5. Terbutaline sulfate is available as 1 mg in 1 ml of solution. What percentage strength is this?

a. Convert 1 mg to 0.001 g.

$$1\ mg \times 1\ g/1000\ mg = 0.001\ g$$

b. Substitute.

$$x = \frac{0.001\ g}{1\ ml}$$

$$x = 0.001 = 0.1\%$$

ANSWER. The strength is 0.1%

Summary of Method for Solving Percentage Problems

Undiluted Drug Solute:

$$\%\ (decimals) = \frac{Solute\ (g,\ ml)}{Total\ solution\ (g,\ ml)}$$

Diluted Drug Solute:

$$\%\ (decimals) = \frac{Solute\ (g,\ ml) \times \%\ strength\ (decimals)}{Total\ solution\ (g,\ ml)}$$

1. Convert to metric units and decimal expressions.
2. Substitute knowns in the appropriate percentage equation.
3. Express answer in units or system requested.

Remember the definition of percentage strength: Percentage equals parts (g, ml) per 100 parts. *You must use grams or milliliters in the percentage equation.*

Practice Problems and Answers: Percentage-Strength Solutions

Problems

1. How many grams of calamine are needed to prepare 120 g of an ointment containing 8% calamine?
2. One milliliter of active enzyme is found in 147 ml of solution. What is the percentage strength of active enzyme in the solution?
3. If Valium contained 2% active ingredient, how many grams of the active ingredient would be needed to make 20 g of Valium?
4. If you have Isuprel 1:100, how many milliliters of Isuprel would be needed to contain 30 mg of active ingredient?
5. A dose of 0.4 ml of epinephrine HCl 1:100 is ordered. This dose contains how many milligrams of epinephrine HCl? (the active ingredient?)
6. If you administer 3 ml of a 0.1% strength solution, how many milligrams of active ingredient have you given?
7. The maximum dose of Isuprel that may be given by aerosol for a particular patient is 3 mg. The drug is available as a 1:200 solution. What is the maximal amount of solution (in milliliters) of isoproterenol that may be used?
8. How many milliliters of 1:100 epinephrine are needed for a 5-mg dose?
9. How many milligrams are there in a 1-cc dose of 2% Xylocaine?
10. How many milligrams of sodium chloride are needed for 10 ml of a 0.9% solution?
11. If you have 5 mg/ml of Xylocaine, what percentage strength is this?
12. A 0.5% strength solution contains how many milligrams in 1 ml?
13. Cromolyn sodium contains 20 mg in 2 ml of water. What is the percentage strength?
14. How much active ingredient of acetylcysteine (Mucomyst) have you given with 4 cc of a 20% solution?
15. How many milliliters of 20% acetylcysteine are needed to form 4 ml of an 8% solution?

16. The recommended dose of metaproterenol 5% is 0.3 cc. How many milligrams of solute are there in this amount?
17. Mucomyst brand of acetylcysteine is marketed as 10% acetylcysteine with 0.05% isoproterenol. How many milligrams of each ingredient are there in a 4-cc dose of solution?
18. Which contains more drug: 0.5 cc of a 1% drug solution with 2 ml of saline, or 0.5 cc of a 1% drug solution with 5 ml of saline?
19. How many milligrams per milliliter are in a 20% solution?
20. On an emergency cart, you have sodium bicarbonate solution ($NaHCO_3$), 44.6 mEq/50 ml. A physician orders an aerosol of 5 cc and 3.25% strength. How many milliliters of the bicarbonate solution do you need?
    1 mEq = 1/1000 GEW; GEW = gram formula wt/valence
    Atomic weights: Na, 23; H, 1; C, 12; 0, 16

Answers

1. $0.08 = x\ g/120\ g;\ x = 9.6\ g$
2. $x = 1\ ml/147\ ml;\ x = .0068 = 0.68\%$
3. $0.02 = x\ g/20\ g;\ x = 0.4\ g$
4. $0.01 = 0.03\ g/x\ ml;\ x = 3ml$
5. $0.01 = x\ g/0.4\ ml;\ x = 0.004\ g = 4\ mg$
6. $0.001 = x\ g/3\ ml;\ x = 0.003\ g = 3\ mg$
7. $1:200 = 0.5\% = 0.005;\ 3\ mg = 0.003\ g$
   $0.005 = 0.003\ g/x\ ml;\ x = 0.6\ ml$
8. $1:100 = 1\% = 0.01;\ 5\ mg = 0.005\ g$
   $0.01 = 0.005\ g/x\ ml;\ x = 0.5\ ml$
9. $0.02 = x\ g/1\ cc;\ x = 0.02\ g = 20\ mg$
10. $0.009 = x\ g/10\ ml;\ x = 0.09\ g = 90\ mg$
11. $x = 0.005\ g/ml;\ x = 0.005 = 0.5\%$
12. $0.005 = x\ g/ml;\ x = 0.005\ g = 5\ mg$
13. $x = 0.02\ g/2\ ml;\ x = 0.01 = 1\%$
14. $0.2 = x\ g/4\ cc;\ x = 0.8\ g = 800\ mg$
15. $0.08 = 0.2\ (x)\ ml/4\ ml;$
    $0.2\ (x) = 0.32$
        $x = 1.6\ ml$, and saline q.s. for 4 ml
16. $0.05 = x\ g/0.3\ cc;\ x = 0.015\ g = 15\ mg$
17. Acetylcysteine: $0.10 = x\ g/4\ cc;\ x = 0.4\ g = 400\ mg$
    isoproterenol: $0.0005 = x\ g/4\ cc;\ x = 0.002\ g = 2\ mg$
18. They each contain the same amount of drug: 5 mg $(0.01 = x\ g/0.5cc;\ x = 0.005\ g = 5\ mg)$. The different amounts of diluent (2 ml, 5 ml) will change the resulting percentage strength and the total amount of new solution but not the amount of drug.

19. $0.20 = x$ g/ml; $x = 0.2$ g $= 200$ mg
20. Step 1: Percentage strength of 44.6 mEq/50 cc:

$$NaHCO_3 - GEW = 84 \text{ g/l} = 84 \text{ g}$$

$$1 \text{ mEq} = 0.084 \text{ g}$$

$$44.6 \text{ mEq} \times 0.084 \text{ g/mEq} = 3.75 \text{ g}$$

$$\text{Percentage strength} = 3.75 \text{ g/50 cc} = 0.0075 = 7.5\%$$

Step 2: Calculate how much of a 7.5% solution is needed to form 5 cc of

3.25% strength using the formula for dilute solution:

$$0.0325 = 0.075 \text{ (x)/5 cc}$$

$$x = 5(0.0325)/0.075 = 2.17 \text{ ml}$$

ANSWER: Take 2.17 ml of the bicarbonate solution and add saline q.s. for a total of 5 cc. Resulting strength will be 3.25%.

BIBLIOGRAPHY

Carr JJ, McElroy NL, Carr BL: How to solve dosage problems in one easy lesson, Am J Nurs 76:1934, 1976.

Chatburn RL: Measurement, physical quantities, and le Systeme International d'Unites (SI units). Respir Care 33:861, 1988.

Fitch GE, Larson MA, Mooney MP: Basic arithmetic review and drug therapy, ed 4, New York, 1977, Macmillan Publishing Co.

McDermid GL: Calculating the amount of solute in a solution, Respir Care 21:861, 1976.

Medici GA: Drug dosage calculations: a guide for current clinical practice, Englewood Cliffs, NJ, 1980, Prentice-Hall.

Plein JD, Plein EM: Fundamentals of medication, ed 2, Hamilton, Ill, 1974, The Hamilton Press.

Richardson LI, Richardson JK: The mathematics of drugs and solutions with clinical applications, New York, 1976, McGraw-Hill.

Saxton DF, Walter JF: Programmed instruction in arithmetic, dosages and solutions, ed 3, St. Louis, 1974, CV Mosby.

4

Central and Peripheral
Nervous Systems

Chapter 4 presents the nervous system as a background to understanding drugs that exert their effects through actions in this system. Emphasis is placed on the autonomic nervous system. The following topics are discussed:

- Organization of the nervous system
- Autonomic nervous system
- Parasympathetic branch
- Sympathetic branch
- Autonomic control in lungs

ORGANIZATION OF THE NERVOUS SYSTEM

The best approach to understanding principles of drug action is through a clear, well-organized grasp of the central and peripheral nervous systems, since numerous drugs in respiratory care exert their effects by altering this system.

The basic organization of the nervous system can be outlined as follows:

1. Central Nervous System
   a. Brain
   b. Spinal cord
2. Peripheral Nervous System
   a. Sensory (afferent)
   b. Motor (efferent)
   c. Autonomic nervous system
      (1) Parasympathetic branch
      (2) Sympathetic branch

Figure 4–1 indicates a functional, but not anatomically accurate, diagram of the central and peripheral nervous system.

Impulses to the brain (afferent) from sensory receptors, and from the brain (efferent) to skeletal muscle, are conveyed by a sequence of electrical and chemical means, which will be examined in detail for each junction of the system. Very generally, the **sensory** input from heat, light, pressure, and pain

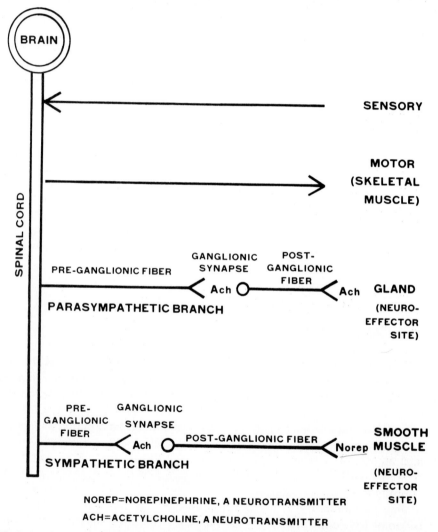

FIG 4–1. Functional diagram of the central and peripheral nervous systems, indicating the somatic branches (sensory, motor) and the autonomic branches (sympathetic, parasympathetic) with their synapses and neurotransmitters. (From Rau JL: Autonomic airway pharmacology, *Respir Care* 22:263, 1977.)

receptors and the skeletal muscle **motor** functions are largely under conscious, **voluntary** control. The sensory and motor branches are also known in combination as the somatic system.

Neither the motor nor the sensory branches have synapses outside of the spinal cord before reaching the muscle or sensory receptor site. This is in contrast to the synapses occurring in the sympathetic and parasympathetic divisions of the autonomic system. The additional synapses of the autonomic system offer potential sites for drug effect besides the terminal, neuroeffector sites.

It should be noted that the neurotransmitter at the motor (skeletal muscle) sites is acetylcholine, which is the same for the parasympathetic branch and all ganglionic synapses. The motor, or efferent division, is of great importance when considering neuromuscular agents.

AUTONOMIC NERVOUS SYSTEM

The autonomic nervous system is the **involuntary,** unconscious control mechanism of the body, sometimes said to control vegetative functions. It is divided into the parasympathetic and sympathetic branches, which maintain a balance of opposing effects on the body's smooth muscle (such as the myocardium, gastrointestinal [GI] tract, sphincters) and glands (lacrimal, salivary, mucosal).

General Description of Parasympathetic and Sympathetic Branches

Efferent and Afferent Fibers

The autonomic system is generally considered an **efferent** system; that is, impulses in the sympathetic and parasympathetic branches travel *from* the brain and spinal cord out *to* the various neuroeffector sites, such as the heart, GI tract, or lungs. However, there are **afferent** nerves, which run alongside the sympathetic and parasympathetic efferent fibers, that carry impulses *to* the cord *from* to the periphery. The afferent fibers convey impulses due to visceral stimuli and can form a reflex arc of stimulus input/autonomic output analogous to the well-known somatic reflex arcs, such as the knee-jerk reflex. The mechanism of a vagal reflex arc mediating bronchoconstriction will be further discussed in Chapter 6, in conjunction with drugs used to block the parasympathetic impulses (parasympatholytics). Figure 4–2 illustrates the portions of the spinal cord where the parasympathetic and sympathetic nerve fibers originate. The parasympathetic branch arises from the craniosacral portion, while the sympathetic branch leaves from the thoracolumbar portion of the cord.

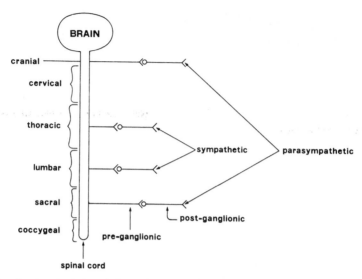

FIG 4–2. Anatomical description of parasympathetic and sympathetic branches. This can be contrasted with the functionally organized diagram in Figure 4–1.

Midbrain Control Centers

Much of the control of the autonomic nervous system lies in midbrain and medullary centers. These include the respiratory center, the vasomotor center controlling blood pressure, the cough center, and the chemoreceptor trigger zone responsible for vomiting. Well-known clinical effects of ventilatory depression or nausea and vomiting are mediated by drug action on such centers.

Contrasts Between Parasympathetic and Sympathetic Effects

Although both the parasympathetic and sympathetic branches of the autonomic system will each be presented in some detail, a general overview shows contrasts between the two branches. The parasympathetic control is essential to life and is considered a more discrete, finely regulated system than the sympathetic. Parasympathetic effects control day-to-day body functions of digestion, bladder and rectum discharge, and basal secretion of bronchial mucus. Overstimulation of the parasympathetic branch would prevent violent action for the body and would result in what is termed the *SLUD* syndrome: salivation, lacrimation, urination, and defecation. These reactions are definitely counterproductive to fleeing or fighting!

By contrast, the sympathetic branch reacts as a general alarm system and does not exercise discrete controls. This is sometimes characterized as a "fight-or-flight" system: Heart rate and blood pressure increase, blood flow shifts from the periphery to muscles and the heart, blood sugar rises, and bronchi dilate. The organism prepares for maximum physical exertion. The sympathetic branch is not essential to life; sympathectomized animal models can survive but of course are not prepared to cope with violent stress.

Autonomic Neurotransmitters

Another general feature of the autonomic nervous system, both sympathetic and parasympathetic branches, is the mechanism of neurotransmitter control of nerve impulses. This is the *chemical* transmission of the electrical impulse at the ganglionic synapses and at the end of the nerve fiber called the *neuroeffector site*. Identification of the chemical transmitters dates back to Loewi's experiments in 1921 and is fundamental to understanding autonomic drugs and their classifications.

The usual neurotransmitters at the ganglionic synapses and terminal sites in the autonomic branches are indicated in Figure 4–1, where *Ach* is acetylcholine and *Norep* is norepinephrine.

Although it is an oversimplification, an easy way to initially learn the various neurotransmitters is to remember that acetylcholine is the neurotransmitter *everywhere* (skeletal, all ganglionic synapses, and parasympathetic terminal nerve sites) *except* at sympathetic terminal nerve sites. Then the exceptions provided by cholinergic sympathetic fibers can be remembered as exceptions to that general rule.

Terminology of Drugs Affecting the Autonomic Nervous System

The terms used to classify drugs that act on the autonomic nervous system are based on the type of nerve fiber (parasympathetic or sympathetic) or, alternatively, the type of neurotransmitter. Cholinergic refers to acetylcholine, and adrenergic is derived from adrenalin, another term for epinephrine, which can stimulate sympathetic neuroeffector sites.

With agonists and antagonists, there are four classes of drug affecting the autonomic system end sites.

Parasympathomimetic (cholinergic): Agent causing stimulation of the parasympathetic nervous system.

Parasympatholytic (anticholinergic): Agent blocking or inhibiting effects of the parasympathetic nervous system.

Sympathomimetic (adrenergic): Agent causing stimulation of the sympathetic nervous system. Such agents are alpha stimulants (phenylephrine), beta stimulants (isoproterenol), β_2 stimulants (isoetharine), or alpha and beta stimulants (epinephrine).

Sympatholytic (antiadrenergic): Agent blocking or inhibiting the effect of the sympathetic nervous system.

Muscarinic and Nicotinic Effects

Alkaloid muscarine, from the mushroom plant *Amanita muscaria,* stimulates acetylcholine receptor sites, but only at parasympathetic neuroeffector sites: exocrine glands (lacrimal, salivary, bronchial mucous glands), cardiac muscle, smooth muscle (GI tract). Therefore, stimulation of parasympathetic sites by any drug similar to acetylcholine in effect is termed a *muscarinic effect.* Receptors at these sites are considered *muscarinic* receptors. A muscarinic effect well known to respiratory care clinicians is the increase in airway secretions following administration of acetylcholine-like drugs such as neostigmine. There is also a fall in blood pressure caused by slowing of the heart and vasodilatation.

The other acetylcholine receptor sites at the ganglionic synapses and at the skeletal muscles are termed *nicotinic* receptors and cause nicotinic effects. This is based on the action of nicotine with acetylcholine receptors at ganglia (both sympathetic and parasympathetic) and skeletal muscle sites. Stimulation of these sites results in increased activity followed by a depolarization blockade (inactivation). Practical effects of stimulating these nicotinic receptors include a rise in blood pressure due to stimulation of sympathetic ganglia, causing vasoconstriction when the postganglionic fibers discharge (an alpha effect), and stimulation of the adrenal medulla, which has acetylcholine receptors. This last site releases circulating epinephrine.

Summary

Muscarinic Effect.   The muscarinic effect results from stimulation of parasympathetic neuroeffector sites. EFFECTS: mucous and salivary gland discharge, decreased heart rate, vasodilatation, and lowered blood pressure.

Nicotinic Effect.   The nicotinic effect results from stimulation of ganglionic (sympathetic and parasympathetic) sites and skeletal muscle receptors. EFFECTS: increased blood pressure with vasoconstriction and increased heart rate.

PARASYMPATHETIC BRANCH

The parasympathetic branch arises from the craniosacral portions of the spinal cord and consists of two neurons—a preganglionic fiber leading from the cord to the ganglionic synapse outside the cord, and a postganglionic fiber from the ganglionic synapse to the gland or smooth muscle being innervated (Fig 4–2).

The parasympathetic branch has good specificity with the postganglionic fiber arising very near the effector site (gland, smooth muscle). This is a discrete system whose effects are listed below.

Site	Effect
Heart	Slows rate of sinoatrial node via vagus (tenth cranial) nerve
Bronchial muscle	Constricts
Bronchial mucous glands	Stimulates to secrete
Lacrimal, salivary, sweat glands	Increased secretion
Peripheral (dermal), pulmonary circulation	Vasodilatation
Urinary bladder	Detrusor contracts; trigone and sphincter relax
Intestines	Increased motility; relaxed sphincters

Parasympathetic Neurotransmitter

Nervous impulses are conducted by electrical and chemical means. Chemical transmission of the impulse occurs at synapses and can be understood by considering the mode of action of the neurotransmitter acetylcholine at the parasympathetic effector site. This action is illustrated in Figure 4–3. The term *neurohormone* has also been used in place of *neurotransmitter*.

Vesicles containing acetylcholine *(Ach)* are present in the end of the nerve fiber. The electrical nerve impulse releases acetylcholine, formerly synthesized and stored, which attaches to receptors on the postsynaptic membrane. In somatic motor nerve endings, membrane permeability to Na^+ and K^+ is altered, depolarizing or "firing" the cell. Acetylcholine is then inactivated through hydrolysis by cholinesterase enzymes, to terminate stimulation of the neuroeffector site. In effect the nerve impulse is "shut off."

A similar event occurs in both the parasympathetic and sympathetic ganglionic synapses and at the end of the parasympathetic postganglionic fibers.

Drugs can use this neurotransmitter mechanism to stimulate parasympathetic nerve endings (parasympathomimetics) or to block the transmission of such impulses (parasympatholytics). Both categories of drugs affecting the parasympathetic branch are commonly seen clinically and can be exemplified with specific drugs. The effects of the parasympathetic system, listed previously, on the heart, bronchial smooth muscle, and exocrine glands should be mentally reviewed prior to considering parasympathetic agonists or antagonists (blockers):

Heart: slows rate.

Bronchial Smooth Muscle: constriction.

Exocrine Glands: increased secretion.

Parasympathomimetic Agents

Parasympathomimetic agents mimic the action caused by acetylcholine at its receptor sites. Such agents can cause stimulation at the terminal nerve site (neuroeffector junction) by two distinct mechanisms, leading to their classification as direct or indirect acting.

Direct Acting

Drugs in this group are structurally similar to acetylcholine. In reference to Figure 4–3, the direct acting parasympathomimetics would occupy the receptor sites and cause depolarization. Examples of this group include methacholine, carbachol, bethanechol, and pilocarpine. Methacoline has been used in bronchial challenge tests by inhalation to assess the degree of airway reactivity in asthmatics and others. The parasympathetic effect being used is bronchoconstriction, and the question of interest is the difference in severity of bronchoconstriction among different types of individuals. Carbachol and bethanechol (Urecholine) have been used to relieve postoperative urinary retention. Pilocarpine has been used to cause miosis in ophthalmology.

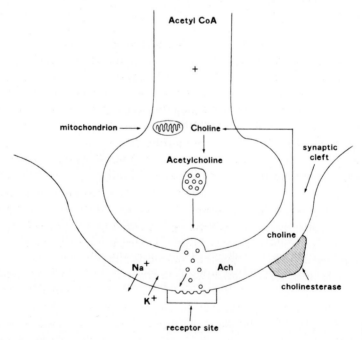

FIG 4–3. Storage, release, and inactivation of the parasympathetic neurotransmitter acetylcholine.

Indirect Acting

Some parasympathomimetics inhibit the cholinesterase enzyme seen in Figure 4–3. Since cholinesterase usually inactivates the acetylcholine neurotransmitter, inhibiting this enzyme results in accumulation of endogenous acetylcholine, which is continuously released at parasympathetic nerve endings. This makes more acetylcholine available to attach to receptor sites and produces parasympathetic effects. If acetylcholine receptors have been blocked by a parasympatholytic drug, this increase in neurotransmitter can reverse the block by competing with the parasympatholytic for the receptors. Nerve transmission can then resume.

Drugs that inhibit cholinesterase thus cause parasympathetic effects but do not themselves directly stimulate the receptor site. Cholinesterase inhibitors are therefore termed *indirect-acting parasympathomimetics.* Such drugs are also called *anticholinesterase* agents and can be classified into two types: reversible and irreversible inhibitors.

Reversible Inhibitors. Reversible inhibitor agents combine reversibly with the cholinesterase enzyme, and their duration of effect is limited to hours. Examples of drugs in this group are physostigmine (Eserine), neostigmine (Prostigmin), edrophonium (Tensilon), pyridostigmine (Mestinon), ambenonium (Mytelase), and demecarium (Humorosol). Neostigmine is used to reverse neuromuscular blockade caused by curare-type drugs, which block acetylcholine receptors, and in treating myasthenia gravis, a disease of impaired nerve transmission at the neuromuscular junction. Edrophonium is used in the Tensilon test for the diagnosis of myasthenia gravis.

Irreversible Inhibitors. Irreversible inhibitors include organophosphates such as parathion, malathion, diisopropylfluorophosphates (Floropryl), and echothiophate (Phospholine). The last two agents are used in ophthalmology for miotic effect on the pupil (pupillary constriction). The irreversible bond eliminates the need for continued eye drops. The iris of the eye has a radial muscle, innervated by the sympathetic system, that causes pupillary dilatation when stimulated. The iris also has a circular smooth muscle, innervated by parasympathetic fibers, that causes pupillary constriction when stimulated. Parasympathomimetics (e.g., pilocarpine) or parasympatholytics (e.g., atropine, homatropine, or hyoscine) are often used for their constricting and dilating effects on the iris. The eye itself, with its radial and circular muscles of the iris and its ciliary muscle, together with its sympathetic and parasympathetic innervation, has often been used as a model organ when explaining autonomic effects. To be useful as a model, the anatomy of the eye must be understood, and this can distract from the understanding of the autonomic nervous function. However, such an approach is incorporated in texts such as Modell et al. (1976) and can be helpful.

The organophosphates are used as insecticides, and occasionally patients are seen with toxic exposure and absorption. The effects of these agents can be lethal, and because of this, they have also been used as nerve gas. Since they affect acetylcholine, they have an effect on neuromuscular function and muscarinic receptors: There is initial stimulation, then blockade if a high enough dosage is absorbed. The military practice of carrying 1 cc of atropine in a Syrette was to counteract these indirect-acting, irreversible parasympathomimetic nerve gas agents.

The general symptoms of toxicity with organophosphates, whether used as insecticide or in warfare, include nausea, vomiting, diarrhea, GI cramping, salivation and drooling, miotic pupils, bronchoconstriction, increased blood pressure (due to ganglionic stimulation of sympathetic nerves) and decreased heart rate, sweating, skeletal muscle fasciculation (crawling appearance under the skin), central nervous system effects (hallucination, disorientation), and finally death due to paralysis of the respiratory muscles.

The bonding of irreversible inhibitors with the cholinesterase is slow, taking up to 24 hours. However, once formed, the duration is limited only by the body's ability to produce new cholinesterase, which takes 1 to 2 weeks. Therefore treatment of organophosphate toxicity can use a drug such as pralidoxime (Protopam), a cholinesterase reactivator, in the first 24 hours. After this time the bond of cholinesterase and cholinesterase inhibitors cannot be reversed, but atropine (a parasympatholytic) can be used to block the overly available acetylcholine neurotransmitter at the receptor sites. Supportive ventilation and airway maintenance would be required for the duration of the effects.

Most of the toxic effects are typical parasympathetic effects, except for the neuromuscular symptoms and the increase in blood pressure. This increase is explained by excess acetylcholine stimulating the sympathetic ganglia. Because indirect-acting agents simply inhibit cholinesterase, they do not directly stimulate acetylcholine receptors, as the direct-acting agents do. Consequently, there is no direct stimulation of acetylcholine receptors found on blood vessels, and therefore no drop in blood pressure such as is usually seen with direct-acting parasympathomimetics. Instead, the activity of acetylcholine at the sympathetic ganglia leads to the sympathetic effect of increased blood pressure.

Parasympatholytic Agents

Parasympatholytic agents, typified by atropine, block acetylcholine receptors and are therefore antagonists. They act primarily at the parasympathetic neuroeffector junction and not at neuromuscular receptors. Technically, the term *anticholinergic* is broader than *parasympatholytic* because it refers to all receptors stimulated by the neurotransmitter acetylcholine. Drug classes considered anticholinergic would also include neuromuscular blockers and ganglionic blockers, because of the neurotransmitter being blocked. The parasympatholytics could be termed, and are by some, *antimuscarinic* because of the limitation to parasympathetic terminal fiber sites.

Parasympatholytic drugs can be grouped into three classes: the belladonna alkaloids (atropine, scopolamine), synthetic compounds (methantheline [Banthine], propantheline [Pro-Banthine]), and semisynthetics (homatropine and methscopolamine, which are modifications of atropine). The duration of action of the semisynthetics is much shorter than that of atropine, which can cause pupillary dilation for 7 to 14 days.

Atropine as a Prototype Parasympatholytic

Atropine is usually considered the prototype parasympatholytic, and there is renewed interest in use of aerosolized analogues to atropine in respiratory care. This is discussed more fully in Chapter 6. Atropine is a *competitive antagonist* to acetylcholine at muscarinic receptor sites (glands, GI tract, heart, eyes) and can form a reversible bond with these cholinergic receptors. In the respiratory system, atropine decreases secretion by mucous glands and relaxes bronchial smooth muscle by blocking parasympathetically maintained basal tone. Atropine blocks vagal innervation of the heart to produce increased heart rate. There is no effect on blood vessels since these do not have parasympathetic innervation, only the acetylcholine receptors. Vascular resistance would not increase with atropine. Of course, if a parasympathomimetic *were* given, then atropine would block the effect on blood vessel receptor sites. There is pupillary dilatation (mydriasis) due to blockade of the circular iris muscle, and the lens is flattened (cycloplegia) by blockade of the ciliary muscle.

Atropine has significant central nervous system effects, with stimulation in low doses and depression of the CNS in high doses. Delirium and hallucinations can be seen with therapeutic dosage ranges. Scopolamine produces depression in all doses and is combined with a narcotic such as Demerol to produce "twilight sleep." In the GI tract, atropine decreases acid secretion, tone, and mobility.

Parasympatholytic Effects

If the basic effects of the parasympathetic system are known, the effects of an antagonist such as atropine can be deduced. For example, if the parasympathetic system (vagus nerve) slows the heart rate, a parasympatholytic should increase heart rate by blocking that innervation.

The primary uses of parasympatholytics are based on these effects:

- Bronchodilatation
- Preoperative drying of secretions
- Antidiarrhea
- To prevent bed-wetting in children (increase urinary retention)
- To treat peptic ulcer
- To treat organophosphate poisoning (previously mentioned)
- To treat mushroom *(A. muscaria)* ingestion
- To treat bradycardia

The use of atropine to block muscarinic effects when reversing curare with an indirect-acting parasympathomimetic provides a useful application and integration of the concepts presented. Curare acts to block acetylcholine receptors at the neuromuscular junction, causing paralysis, but has no effect at the parasympathetic neuroeffector junction. A cholinesterase inhibitor such as neostigmine is a parasympathomimetic but also acts at the neuromuscular site to inhibit cholinesterase, facilitating neuromuscular nerve transmission by allowing acetylcholine to displace the blocking curare. However, neostigmine would also have muscarinic effects, particularly increased airway secretions. Therefore atropine is given *before* reversing the curare with neostigmine. The atropine only blocks neostigmine at the muscarinic sites but not at the neuromuscular sites. The selectivity of atropine for muscarinic (parasympathetic) sites and curare for neuromuscular sites, and the general effect of the anticholinesterase neostigmine all interact to create the desired result.

SYMPATHETIC BRANCH

The sympathetic branch arises from the thoracolumbar portion of the spinal cord and has a short preganglionic fiber and a long postganglionic fiber, with acetylcholine as the ganglionic neurotransmitter and norepinephrine as the neurotransmitter at the neuroeffector site. The effects of this system are listed below.

Site	Effect
Heart	Increased rate, conduction, force; β_1
Bronchial muscle	Dilates, relaxes; β_2
Coronary and skeletal blood vessels	Relax; β
Pulmonary and cerebral blood vessels	Contract/relax; α and β
Peripheral (dermal) blood vessels	Constrict; α
Sweat glands	Increased secretion; cholinergic effect

NOTE: When alpha and beta receptors are equally distributed, as is the case with pulmonary and cerebral blood vessels in the preceding table, the physiological effect depends on which receptor type is more stimulated by a given drug. For example, norepinephrine will tend to cause vasoconstriction, because of greater alpha stimulation; isoproterenol will cause vasodilatation, with little alpha effect (constriction); epinephrine may cause no net effect since equal alpha and beta stimulation will cancel each other.

Sympathetic Neurotransmitter

The sympathetic system is the site of much pharmacological manipulation in respiratory care and offers a certain amount of complexity. The synapse at the effector site seems to be functionally similar to that of the parasympathetic. However, instead of inactivation by enzymes, reuptake of the transmitter is most important for termination of the impulse, with catechol-O-methyltransferase (COMT) and monoamine oxidase (MAO) serving to metabolize any remaining norepinephrine.

In somewhat more detail, the sequence of production, storage, release, and inactivation of norepinephrine at the sympathetic effector site can be visualized in Figure 4–4.

Phenylalanine is converted to tyrosine by a hydroxylase enzyme, which in turn converts tyrosine to dopa; dopa is changed to dopamine by dopa decarboxylase; dopamine then converts to norepinephrine, by action of dopamine β-monooxygenase. Norepinephrine is a precursor to epinephrine. This sequence may end with dopamine, norepinephrine, or epinephrine at actual sites.

Terminating Neurotransmitter Action

At sympathetic neuroeffector junctions, the action of norepinephrine is terminated primarily by a reuptake mechanism in which the neurotransmitter is reabsorbed through the neuronal membrane by an actively mediated process. This mechanism of reuptake at the sympathetic sites can be contrasted with the mechanism of enzyme activity at parasympathetic sites.

In addition to the neuronal reuptake process, which is fairly specific to the levorotatory isomer of norepinephrine, there are several other mechanisms in the body for inactivating chemicals similar to norepinephrine. Such chemicals are termed *catecholamines*, and their general structure will be outlined in Chapter 5 when considering sympathomimetic bronchodilators. These mechanisms of inactivation include a second uptake process and enzyme activity.

Uptake-1 and Uptake-2.   In 1965, Iversen published results of research and made a distinction between two types of uptake processes. The neuronal

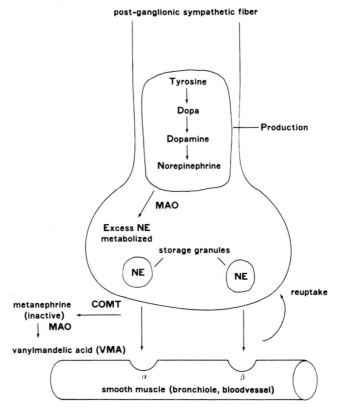

FIG 4—4. Storage, release, and inactivation of the sympathetic neurotransmitter norepinephrine.

reuptake process just described was called *uptake-1.* A second type of uptake process was discovered and called *uptake-2.* The uptake-2 process is a mediated uptake of exogenous amines (chemicals such as norepinephrine) in *nonneuronal* tissues (e.g., cardiac muscle cells). Iversen distinguished a number of details of the uptake-2 process:

1. It is a mediated transport system.
2. It is a low-affinity but high-capacity system.
3. It is not as stereochemically specific as uptake-1.
4. It is specific to catecholamines.
5. The order of affinity for uptake of specific agents, in *decreasing* order, is isoproterenol > epinephrine > norepinephrine.
6. Finally, and of extreme therapeutic importance, certain corticosteroids can inhibit the uptake-2 process, thereby potentiating catecholamines.

The last effect of uptake-2 inhibition by corticosteroids is discussed more fully in Chapter 10, when dealing with such drugs. The uptake-2 process is active throughout the range of external (exogenous) catecholamine concentrations, occurring at low perfusion concentrations and apparently not at critical concentrations as previously theorized. It is thought that the uptake-2 mechanism removes circulating catecholamines into the nonneuronal storage sites, where the enzymes COMT and MAO can metabolize them. At low perfusion concentrations, there would be no accumulation of catecholamines in the storage sites since enzyme degradation is constantly breaking them down into other forms.

Enzyme Inactivation.   There are two enzymes available that can inactivate catecholamines. These are COMT and MAO. The action of both enzymes on epinephrine is illustrated in Figure 4–5 and is of importance because COMT is responsible for ending the action of catecholamine bronchodilators.

Catechol-O-Methyltransferase.   The name of the enzyme, COMT, describes its action: A methyl group is transferred to the oxygen at the carbon-3 site of the catechol nucleus. To avoid being vulnerable to COMT, catechol-

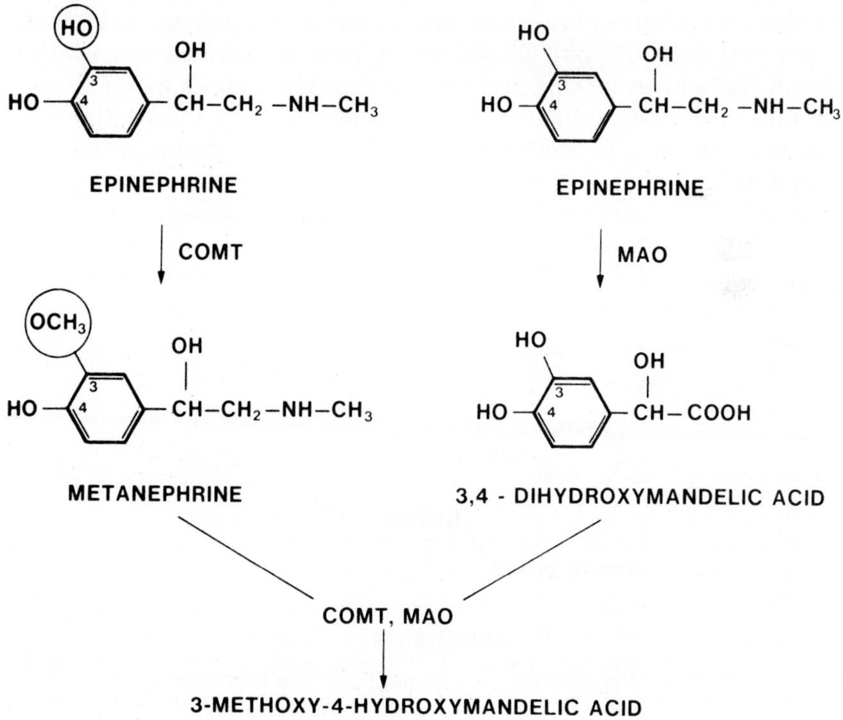

FIG 4–5. Chemical action of COMT and MAO on the catecholamine epinephrine.

amine bronchodilators would have to be modified. This is of clinical interest since COMT is very rapid in inactivating drugs such as epinephrine or isoproterenol. For instance, it is estimated that isoproterenol by aerosol, using 1:200 strength solution in therapeutic dosages, peaks in 20 minutes, and total duration is, on the average, 1½ hours. These kinetics are not useful for long-term maintenance therapy.

Monoamine Oxidase.   A second enzyme, MAO, is also capable of degrading catecholamines, as seen in Figure 4–5. When there is a single amine group (NH) on a terminal carbon atom in the side chain, MAO can deaminate, or remove, the amine group, leaving an acid. MAO is found in the GI tract, together with additional sulfatase enzymes, which makes oral use of catecholamines such as epinephrine or isoproterenol very ineffective. Catecholamines are primarily metabolized by COMT, but also by MAO, and these enzymes ultimately convert the catecholamines to a product, 3-methoxy-4-hydroxymandelic acid, which is excreted in urine.

Part of the action of ephedrine, a bronchodilator, is due to the way in which MAO metabolizes monoamines, such as the catecholamines. The chemical structure of ephedrine is seen in Figure 4–6 and should be compared with that of epinephrine seen in Figure 4–5. Two differences in its structure give noticeably different clinical effects. First, ephedrine is not a catecholamine: It has a benzene ring and not the catechol with its two hydroxyl attachments. Therefore ephedrine is not metabolized by COMT; there is no hydroxyl on the ring to methylate. Second, the amine group, or NH, is not attached to the *terminal* carbon in the side chain but instead to the second carbon. Ephedrine combines with MAO but is not metabolized, and acts as a competitive inhibitor of MAO. By tying up MAO, more endogenous epinephrine and norepinephrine are available to stimulate sympathetic receptor sites. Ephedrine can also *directly* stimulate adrenergic receptors, so there is both a direct and indirect action.

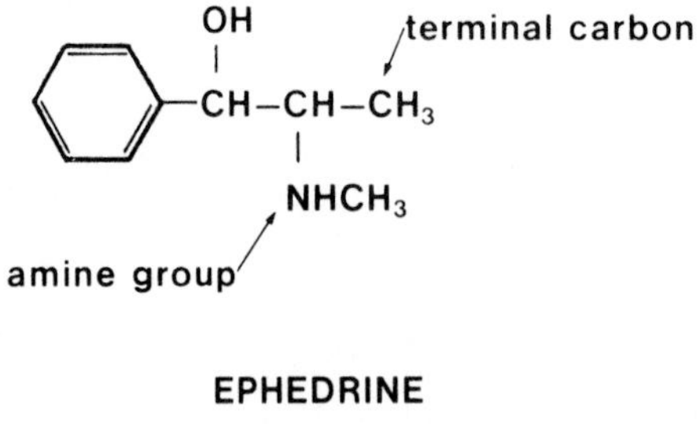

EPHEDRINE

FIG 4–6.   Structure of ephedrine, a noncatecholamine bronchodilator.

Summary of Neurotransmitter Inactivation

1. Uptake mechanisms.
   a. Uptake-1: Reuptake into the nerve ending; usual method of inactivating endogenous neurotransmitter norepinephrine.
   b. Uptake-2: Extraneuronal uptake for storage and breakdown of exogenous circulating catecholamines, such as epinephrine.
2. Enzyme degradation.
   a. COMT: inactivates catecholamines by methylating the carbon-3 oxygen.
   b. MAO: deaminates catecholamines, removing the amine group (NH) on the terminal carbon atom.

Sympathetic (Adrenergic) Receptor Types

Adrenergic receptors (receptors responding to norepinephrine) have been differentiated according to a spectrum of effects elicited by different drugs.

Alpha and Beta Receptors

In 1948, Ahlquist distinguished *alpha* and *beta* sympathetic receptors on the basis of their differing responses to phenylephrine, norepinephrine, epinephrine, and isoproterenol.

Alpha Receptors. Alpha receptors generally *excite*, with the exception of the intestine and central nervous system receptors where inhibition or relaxation occurs.

Beta Receptors. Beta receptors generally inhibit or *relax*, with the exception of the heart where stimulation occurs.

Certain sites were considered as alpha, for example peripheral blood vessels, while others were designated as beta, such as bronchial smooth muscle. Drug activity of sympathetic stimulants (sympathomimetics) ranges along the spectrum seen in Figure 4–7.

As illustrated in Figure 4–7, phenylephrine is one of the purest alpha stimulants, and isoproterenol is an almost pure beta stimulant. It is stressed that "pure" reactions do not occur with any drug; that is, even phenylephrine may affect other sites. Epinephrine stimulates both alpha and beta sites equally, but norepinephrine has more of an alpha than beta effect.

β_1 and β_2 Receptors

In 1967, Lands et al. further differentiated beta receptors into β_1 and β_2. β_1 receptors are found in cardiac muscle, and β_2 are all other beta receptors, including bronchial, vascular, and skeletal muscle.

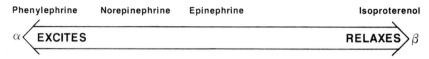

FIG 4–7. Spectrum of activity of common sympathomimetics, ranging from alpha to beta stimulants.

β₁ Receptors. β_1 receptors increase the rate and force of cardiac contraction.

β₂ Receptors. β_2 receptors relax bronchial smooth muscle and vascular beds of skeletal muscle.

β_1 receptors constitute the exception to the general rule that beta receptors cause relaxation.

α_1 and α_2 Receptors

Alpha receptors have also been differentiated into α_1 and α_2 receptor types. This classification has been on a *morphological* basis (location of the receptors) and a *pharmacological* basis (response differences to various drugs). The pharmacological differentiation of α_1 and α_2 receptors is similar to the distinction of alpha and beta receptors and is illustrated in Figure 4–8. This differentiation is based on a response continuum ranging from excitation (α_1) to inhibition (α_2) as different drugs are administered. For example, phenylephrine causes vasoconstriction, as previously mentioned, whereas clonidine (Catapres) causes a lowering of blood pressure and sympathetic activity. *Both* agents are considered alpha-receptor agonists. Other agents such as prazosin (Minipress) or labetalol (Normodyne) cause a lowering of blood pressure, but yohimbine causes a rise in blood pressure. Yet these agents are *all* considered alpha-receptor antagonists. Since different alpha agonists can cause opposite effects, and different alpha blockers do the same, alpha receptors were subdivided into the two types given.

The location or morphological differentiation of α_1 and α_2 receptors is more complex. In **peripheral** nerves, α_1 receptors are located on postsynaptic sites such as vascular smooth muscle, and α_2 receptors are presynaptic.

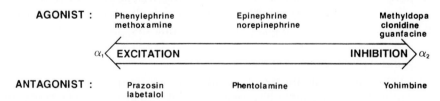

FIG 4–8. Spectrum of activity for common alpha-receptor agonists and antagonists, ranging from α_1 to α_2 effects.

This is illustrated in Figure 4–9. Stimulation of these peripheral α_1 receptors causes excitation and vasoconstriction; activation of peripheral (presynaptic) α_2 receptors causes inhibition of further neurotransmitter release. Peripheral α_2 receptors thereby perform a negative feedback control mechanism, which has been demonstrated with sympathetic (adrenergic) neurons (Langer, 1980). This autoregulation of norepinephrine is also illustrated in Figure 4–9. Norepinephrine released from the nerve ending can activate both α_1 (postsynaptic) and α_2 (presynaptic) receptors. The postsynaptic stimulation causes the cell response such as vasoconstriction, but the presynaptic stimulation leads to inhibition of further neurotransmitter release. In other words, release of norepinephrine from the nerve leads to inhibition of further norepinephrine release.

In the **central** nervous system, α_2 receptors are generally considered to be on postsynaptic sites; this is the reverse of their location peripherally where they are presynaptic. These central postsynaptic α_2 receptors are the site of action for antihypertensive agents such as clonidine (Catapres) or methyldopa (Aldomet). These are further discussed and illustrated in Chapter 17.

In summary, α_1 and β_1 receptors *excite,* and α_2 and β_2 receptors *inhibit.*

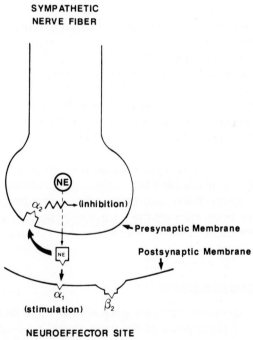

SYMPATHETIC
NERVE FIBER

NE

α_2 (inhibition)

Presynaptic Membrane

Postsynaptic Membrane

NE

α_1
(stimulation) β_2

NEUROEFFECTOR SITE
(e.g. blood vessel)

FIG 4–9. Presynaptic autoregulation of neurotransmitter release at adrenergic nerve terminal by α_2 receptors.

This consistency of subscripts for excitation (1) vs. inhibition (2) aids in remembering their effects.

Dopaminergic Receptors

There are other receptors in the central nervous system (brain) that respond to dopamine, a chemical precursor of norepinephrine, and are therefore termed *dopaminergic*. Since dopamine is chemically similar to epinephrine, which is also known as adrenalin (hence the term *adrenergic*) and which stimulates alpha and beta receptors, dopaminergic receptors are classified as a type of adrenergic receptor.

Summary of Autonomic Receptor Types

1. Cholinergic (respond to acetylcholine).
    a. Muscarinic: parasympathetic neuroeffector sites (exocrine glands, smooth muscle, cardiac muscle).
    b. Nicotinic: autonomic ganglia and skeletal muscle (neuromuscular) junctions.
2. Adrenergic (respond to dopamine, norepinephrine, or epinephrine [adrenalin]).
    a. α_1: postsynaptic peripheral neuroeffector sites (e.g., vascular smooth muscle).
    b. α_2: presynaptic peripheral nerve terminal; postsynaptic sites in central nervous system.
    c. β_1: cardiac smooth muscle.
    d. β_2: smooth muscle other than the heart (bronchioles, blood vessels), skeletal muscle.
    e. Dopaminergic: brain, renal vascular smooth muscle.

It should be recalled that receptors are characterized by the type of neurotransmitter they respond to, rather than the presence of parasympathetic or sympathetic fibers. Receptors may be present without any autonomic fibers, as exemplified by β_2 receptors in human bronchial smooth muscle, where no sympathetic fibers have been discovered. Adrenergic receptors responding to the sympathetic neurotransmitter norepinephrine are more widely found in the body than are the sympathetic fibers themselves. For this reason, the term *adrenergic* is more comprehensive than the term *sympathetic* when applied to receptors.

Cholinergic Sympathetic Nerves

The terms *parasympathomimetic, sympatholytic,* and so forth are derived from the anatomical description of the nerve fibers involved. For example, a parasympathomimetic drug stimulates sites innervated by parasympathetic nerve fibers. The terms *cholinergic* and *adrenergic* are derived from the neurotransmitter involved, with cholinergic or anticholinergic drugs acting where acetylcholine is the neurotransmitter, and adrenergic or antiadrenergic drugs acting where norepinephrine is the neurotransmitter. The two sets of terms are roughly synonymous, but not completely. Their differences bring out some detail of autonomic innervation.

Generally, adrenergic drugs stimulate sympathetic neuroeffector sites, and thus "sympathomimetic" is usually synonymous with "adrenergic." This is because norepinephrine is the usual neurotransmitter at the ends of the sympathetic branch. However, certain sympathetic neuroeffector sites, namely, the sweat glands, have *acetylcholine* as the neurotransmitter. In addition, sympathetic preganglionic fibers directly innervate the adrenal medulla, with acetylcholine as the neurotransmitter. Sympathetic control of the adrenal medulla does not involve a postganglionic fiber or a norepinephrine neurotransmitter.

Sympathetic fibers that have acetylcholine at the neuroeffector sites are *cholinergic sympathetic* fibers. This would be an apparent contradictory combination of terms if not for the exceptions to the rule of norepinephrine as the sympathetic neurotransmitter. Sweating can be caused by giving a cholinergic drug although this effect is under sympathetic control, along with the release of epinephrine from the adrenal medulla into the bloodstream. "Breaking out in a sweat," along with sweaty palms, and increased heart rate due to circulating epinephrine are common effects of stress or fright mediated by sympathetic discharge.

Beta Receptor Pathway

The beta receptor is probably a surface protein complex on the cell. Detailed research on the nature of the beta receptor and its interaction with the enzyme adenyl cyclase is referenced (Fraser and Venter, 1990). When a beta-sympathomimetic drug attaches to this surface receptor, the enzyme adenyl cyclase found in the cell membrane is activated. Adenyl cyclase, once activated, then catalyzes the conversion of intracellular adenosine triphosphate (ATP) to cyclic adenosine $3',5'$-monophosphate (cyclic AMP). It is the level of intracellular cyclic AMP that is responsible for relaxation of smooth muscle, whether in the bronchioles or in the blood vessels. A second important effect of cyclic AMP is the inhibition of mast cell degranulation, which releases histamine and other chemicals causing bronchoconstriction and mucosal edema. The schema of this pathway is given in Figure 4–10. A detailed consideration of cyclic AMP and its chemical mechanism with cardiac and bronchial smooth muscle cells is given by Darin (1981). Cyclic AMP is metabolized by another enzyme, phosphodiesterase, to an inactive form.

When beta receptors become unresponsive to stimulation, beta-blockade is said to exist. As a physiological occurrence, the cause or causes of this are not known. However, the same blockade can be induced pharmacologically

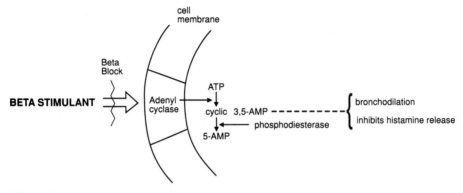

FIG 4–10. Beta receptor pathway. Beta stimulants combine with the beta receptor to activate the enzyme adenyl cyclase in the cell membrane, which catalyzes the conversion of ATP to cyclic AMP.

with a beta-blocking drug such as propranolol (Inderal). A comprehensive summary of autonomic effects in the cardiopulmonary system is given in Table 4–1.

AUTONOMIC CONTROL IN THE LUNG

The human pulmonary system is under control of the nervous system by means of nerve fibers innervating the lung and by the presence of receptors with or without accompanying nerve fibers. A diagrammatic representation of autonomic control in the lung is seen in Figure 4–11.

TABLE 4–1.
Autonomic Effects in the Cardiopulmonary System

	Effect	
System	Parasympathetic	Sympathetic
Lungs		
Bronchial smooth muscle	Constricts	Relaxes, dilates; β_2
Circulation	Vasodilatation	$\alpha = \beta$
Bronchial mucous glands	Vagus, increased secretion	—
Heart		
Atrium, sinoatrial and atrioventricular nodes	Decreased force, rate, conduction	Increased force, rate, conduction; β_1
Ventricle	—	Increased rate, force; β_1
Systemic Circulation		
Peripheral (dermal)	Vasodilatation	Constricts; α
Skeletal muscle	—	Dilates; β
Coronary	—	Dilates; β
Cerebral	—	Constrict/dilate; $\alpha = \beta$

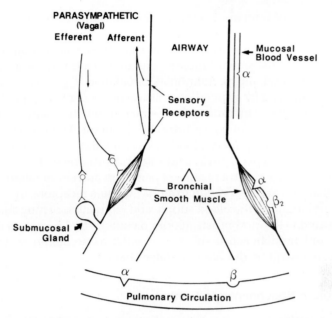

FIG 4–11. Diagrammatic representation of autonomic control mechanisms in the human lung.

Cholinergic Control

Parasympathetic innervation of the lung is from the tenth cranial (vagus) nerve, which enters the lung at the hilum and branches along with the bronchi and blood vessels. Parasympathetic innervation affects larger airways, such as the trachea and bronchi, as well as mucous glands. Stimulation of the parasympathetic nerve supply to the lung or, alternatively, administration of an agent similar to the neurotransmitter acetylcholine would cause bronchial smooth muscle constriction and mucous gland secretion. This is the mechanism for bronchial challenge tests using methacholine, a parasympathomimetic (Parker et al., 1965). There are also sensory nerve endings in smooth muscle at bronchial bifurcations that supply portions of the airway epithelium. These sensory nerves are thought to be afferent vagus nerves that can be triggered by irritants to the airway; other sensory nerves may play a role in the Hering-Breuer reflex. The concept of a vagal reflex arc (afferent-efferent) causing bronchoconstriction is presented in Chapter 6 when discussing parasympatholytic (anticholinergic) bronchodilators.

Adrenergic Control

Sympathetic (adrenergic) nerve fibers are present in the tracheobronchial smooth muscle of many animal species, but most studies indicate they are not found in that of humans. No morphological evidence has been offered to contradict this. There is pharmacological evidence, based on response to various sympathomimetics and sympatholytics, for the presence of alpha and beta receptors on bronchial smooth muscle, mucosal blood vessels, and on blood vessels in the gas-exchanging pulmonary circulation (Fig 4–11). These receptors can be stimulated by sympathetic release of circulating epinephrine from the adrenal medulla or by exogenous sympathomimetic agents, such as epinephrine, isoproterenol, phenylephrine, or albuterol. There is evidence that alpha receptors on pulmonary blood vessels mediate a vasoconstricting response to hypoxia, hypercapneic acidosis, and histamine. This would allow the lung to selectively control regions of perfusion and shunt blood away from poorly ventilated areas. In addition to alpha and beta receptors, there are other receptor types found in the blood supply and circulation of lung tissue. These include histamine (H_1) and prostaglandin receptors, and receptors for various vasoactive and bronchoactive substances such as serotonin or bradykinin. Such substances will be discussed in later chapters.

Nonadrenergic-Noncholinergic Control

There is evidence of a third type of nervous control in the lung that is neither cholinergic nor adrenergic. Normally, parasympathetic (cholinergic) activity will constrict bronchial smooth muscle, and sympathetic (adrenergic) activity will dilate or relax the same smooth muscle. There is an additional inhibitory neural pathway in human airways that can relax airway smooth muscle. Stimulation of these nerves results in inhibition of smooth muscle, that is, bronchodilatation. Therefore, the term *nonadrenergic inhibitory* has been used to describe this third neural control. The term *purinergic* has also been used, since a purine has been proposed as a possible neurotransmitter in this system.

Evidence for the third system is based on the following type of experimentation. When parasympathetic (cholinergic) receptors are blocked with an antagonist such as atropine, and sympathetic (adrenergic) receptors are also blocked with a beta blocker such as propranolol, electric field stimulation of the lung will produce relaxation of bronchial smooth muscle. This is illustrated in Figure 4–12. In the presence of beta-blockade, this would be the sole inhibiting system to prevent bronchoconstriction. The defective function of this third system could contribute to abnormal airway sensitivity in asthma (Barnes, 1987).

The exact neurotransmitter and function of this system are under investigation. Possible neurotransmitters that have been proposed include vasoactive intestinal peptide and peptide histidine isoleucine, in addition to a purine. The nonadrenergic inhibitory nervous system found in the GI tract is

NONADRENERGIC INHIBITORY NERVES

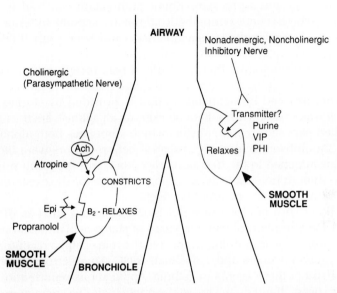

FIG 4–12. Illustration of a third type of nervous control and possible neurotransmitters in human airways that can inhibit or relax smooth muscle. *Ach,* acetylcholine; *Epi,* epinephrine; *VIP,* vasoactive intestinal peptide; *PHI,* peptide histidine isoleucine.

primarily responsible for the relaxation of peristalsis and the internal anal sphincter. In the GI tract, this system develops in conjunction with the parasympathetic branch. Embryologically, the GI and respiratory tracts share a common origin, and the separation of the trachea and gut occurs around the fourth or fifth week of gestation. This adds plausibility to the presence of a nonadrenergic inhibitory system in the lungs similar to that in the GI tract. The clinical relevance of such a system for pharmacology awaits development of drugs capable of modifying its usual function.

Although a gross description of the nerve supply to the human lung was given 300 years ago by Thomas Bartholinus and Thomas Willis, at least one respected researcher commented that our understanding of nerves in the lung is little better today (Richardson, 1979). Most of the data in physiology texts is based on animal studies, and very little human material is available. A number of references in the Bibliography discuss or report the results of research on the nerve supply and presence of receptors in the lung (Adolphson et al., 1971; Richardson, 1979; Richardson and Beland, 1976; Simonsson et al., 1972).

Autonomic Effects in the Airway

The clinical effect of stimulating each type of autonomic receptor in the lung is well known and is illustrated in Figure 4–13. Parasympathetic (cholinergic) stimulation and alpha-sympathetic stimulation can lead to bronchial constriction, whereas beta-sympathetic stimulation results in bronchial relaxation. The evidence for the parasympathetic and beta-sympathetic effect is well known.

It has also been shown that blockade of beta receptors can cause bronchoconstriction in subjects such as asthmatic patients. Evidence for alpha-sympathetic–induced bronchoconstriction is provided by studies in which lung tissue was treated with a beta blocker, or antagonist, such as propranolol, and then exposed to epinephrine, which stimulates both alpha and beta receptors (Adolphson et al., 1971). Because beta receptors were blocked, the epinephrine attached to the free alpha receptors, and the result was contraction of the smooth muscle, thus providing evidence for the existence of alpha receptors and showing a contractile effect.

The clinical use of alpha-receptor blocking agents such as dibenamine, thymoxamine, and phentolamine in cases of status asthamticus has been reported for over 35 years, lending support to the role of alpha receptors in bronchial contraction (Falliers and Tinkelman, 1986). There are no clear-cut indications for use of these agents in asthma. Applications reported in the literature have been limited to investigational trials or refractory cases of bronchoconstriction (Gaddie et al., 1972; Gross, et al., 1974; Simonsson et al., 1972; Walden et al., 1984). However, note that there is disagreement on the

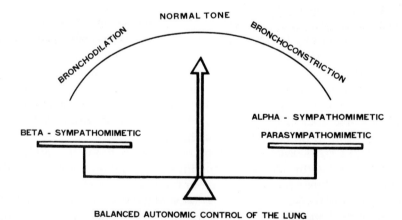

FIG 4–13.   Illustration of the interplay of alpha, beta, and parasympathetic innervation in the bronchial tree. (From Rau JL: Autonomic airway pharmacology, *Respir Care* 22:263, 1977.)

presence, number, and effect of alpha receptors in human airways (see for example Rosenthal et al., 1976).

In a more recent study of 15 patients with asthma, 3 patients responded to phentolamine (an alpha-blocking drug) with definite bronchodilatation; whereas 2 patients experienced severe bronchoconstriction (Shiner and Molho, 1983). Such apparently conflicting evidence points to a need for more carefully controlled investigation of the nature and exact function of alpha receptors in both diseased and normal airways.

In the normal lung, it is probable that a basal parasympathetic activity causes a certain amount of *tone* (a bronchiole that is neither flaccid and maximally dilated, nor tightly contracted). In subjects with hyperreactive airways, that is, airways that constrict from various stimuli, the constriction could be caused by any of three possible mechanisms:

Parasympathetic (cholinergic) stimulation
Alpha-sympathetic stimulation
Beta-receptor blockade

Intracellular Control: Cyclic AMP and GMP

At the cellular level, it is thought that the effects of each type of stimulation or blockade are mediated through a balance of cyclic AMP and an analogous substance, cyclic GMP (guanosine monophosphate). Figure 4–14 illustrates the pathways of these two opposing nucleotides. The cyclic AMP path has already been discussed with beta-receptor stimulation (Fig 4–10).

The importance of the autonomic system for pulmonary pathologic conditions and drug treatment is evident when the biological activity of these nucleotides is considered:

1. Cyclic AMP.
   a. Relaxes smooth muscle to cause bronchodilatation.
   b. Inhibits mast cell degranulation, which can release histamine to cause bronchoconstriction, secretions, and mucosal edema.
2. Cyclic GMP.
   a. Contracts smooth muscle to cause bronchoconstriction.
   b. May enhance mast cell release of histamine and other bronchoconstricting mediators.

Autonomic effects mediated by the intracellular nucleotides can then be summarized as follows:

Parasympathetic Stimulation: results in an increase in cyclic GMP and bronchoconstriction.

GENERAL SCHEME
OF NERVOUS CONTROL IN LUNG

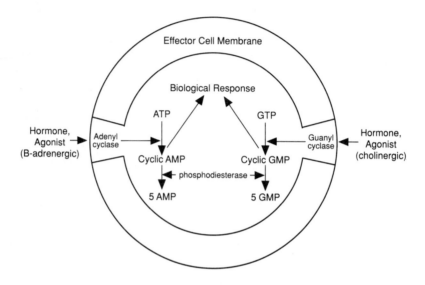

Cyclic AMP — biologic response = bronchodilation
Cyclic GMP — biologic response = bronchoconstriction

FIG 4–14. Comprehensive view of autonomic effects mediated through the intracellular nucleotides cyclic AMP and cyclic GMP. (From Rau JL: Autonomic airway pharmacology, *Respir Care* 22:263, 1977.)

Beta-Receptor Stimulation: results in increased cyclic AMP and bronchodilation.

Alpha-Receptor Stimulation: results in decreased cyclic AMP and vaso- or bronchoconstriction.

Pharmacological Control of Bronchoconstriction

This view offers a unified mechanism of bronchoconstriction, whether due to pollution, dust, aerosols, exercise, anxiety, or allergy. Rather than a simple beta-blockade theory to explain an intrinsic irritability or hypersensitivity of the bronchi such as with asthma, a more comprehensive theory of biochemical balance at the cellular level and opposing autonomic effects could be operative. Patients with hyperreactive airways (e.g., those with asthma or bronchitis) are usually characterized as such by their increased sensitivity to bronchoconstricting or irritating agents. For example, methacholine (cholinergic) stimulation or beta-blockade will typically produce greater constriction in an asthmatic patient than in a healthy subject. There is evidence that some asthmatic patients suffer from parasympathetic or alpha-sympathetic overactivity, whereas others may have decreased responsiveness of beta receptors to circulating epinephrine (Cropp, 1975; Gross et al., 1974; Nelson, 1975; Szentivanyi, 1968).

In addition to illuminating the pathologic condition of bronchoconstriction, this view has offered alternatives in drug therapy. To reverse bronchoconstriction, use the following types of drugs.

Beta Sympathomimetics. Beta sympathomimetics are the traditional class of drugs (e.g., terbutaline), many of which are used in respiratory care. EFFECT: increased cyclic AMP.

Alpha Sympatholytics. If alpha stimulation decreases cyclic AMP, blocking alpha receptors should prevent such a decrease. This has been attempted by using phentolamine (alpha blocker) with some success in a few asthmatic patients. EFFECT: blocks decrease of cyclic AMP.

Parasympatholytics. This class of drugs (e.g., atropine) should block any increase in cyclic GMP, allowing a relative rise in cyclic AMP to cause bronchodilatation. EFFECT: blocks the rise of cyclic GMP.

These three types of drugs, used singly or in combination, have given new possibilities in treatment, as well as new understanding of the causes of pulmonary disease.

BIBLIOGRAPHY

Adolphson RL, Abern SB, Townley RG: Human and guinea pig respiratory smooth muscle: demonstration of alpha adrenergic receptors, J Allergy 47:110, 1971 (abstract).

Ahlquist RP: Study of adrenotropic receptors, Am J Physiol 153:586, 1948.

Badr-El-Din MK et al: A study on beta-adrenergic receptors in children with asthmatic bronchitis, Ann Allergy 46:336, 1981.

Barnes PJ: Autonomic control of airway function in asthma, Chest 91(May suppl):45S, 1987.

Conolly ME, Greenacre JK: The lymphocyte β-adrenoreceptor in normal subjects and patients with bronchial asthma, J Clin Invest 58:1307, 1976.

Cropp GJA: The role of the parasympathetic nervous system in the maintenance of chronic airway obstruction in asthmatic children, Am Rev Respir Dis 112:599, 1975.

Darin J: The mode of action of cyclic AMP, Respir Care 26:228, 1981.

Falliers CJ, Tinkelman DG: Alternative drug therapy for asthma, Clin Chest Med 7:383, 1986.

Fleish JH, Kent KM, Cooper T: Drug receptors in smooth muscle. In Austen KF, Lichtenstein LM, eds: Asthma: physiology, immuno-pharmacology and treatment, New York, 1973, Academic Press.

Fraser CM, Venter JC: Beta-adrenergic receptors. Relationship of primary structure, receptor function, and regulation, Am Rev Respir Dis 141:S22, 1990.

Gaddie J et al: The effect of alpha-adrenergic receptor blocking drug on histamine sensitivity in bronchial asthma, Brit J Dis Chest 66:141, 1972.

Gross GN, Souhadra JF, Farr RS: The long term treatment of an asthmatic patient using phentolamine, Chest 66:397, 1974.

Hardman JG et al: The formation and metabolism of cyclic GMP, Ann NY Acad Sci 185:27, 1971.

Iversen LL: The uptake of catecholamines at high perfusion concentrations in the rat isolated heart: a novel catecholamine uptake process, Br J Pharmacol 25:18, 1965.

Iversen LL: Role of transmitter uptake mechanisms in synaptic neurotransmission, Br J Pharmacol 41:571, 1971.

Iversen LL, Salt PJ: Inhibition of catecholamine uptake$_2$ by steroids in the isolated rat heart, Br J Pharmacol Chemother 40:528, 1970.

Kaliner M, Orange RP, Austen KF: Immunological release of histamine and slow reacting substance of anaphylaxis in lung. IV. Enhancement by cholinergic and alpha adrenergic stimulation, J Exp Med 136:556, 1972.

Kolata GB: Cyclic GMP: cellular regulatory agent? Science 182:149, 1973.

Lands AM et al: Differentiation of receptor systems activated by sympathomimetic amines, Nature (London) 214:597, 1967.

Langer SZ: Presynaptic regulation of the release of catecholamines,Pharmacol Rev 32:337, 1980.

Lefkowitz RJ: β-adrenergic receptors: recognition and regulation, N Engl J Med 295:323, 1976.

Lemanske RF Jr et al: Impaired *in vitro* β-adrenergic granulocyte response in chronic obstructive pulmonary disease, Am Rev Respir Dis 122:213, 1980.

Logsdon PJ et al: The effect of phentolamine on adenylate cyclase and on isoproterenol stimulation in leukocytes from asthmatic and nonasthmatic subjects, J Allergy Clin Immunol 52:148, 1973.

Middleton E Jr: The biochemical basis for the modulation of allergic reaction by drugs, Ped Clin North Am 22:111, 1975.

Modell W, Schild HO, Wilson A: Applied pharmacology, ed 11, Philadelphia, 1976, WB Saunders.

Nelson HS: The beta adrenergic theory of bronchial asthma, Ped Clin North Am 22:53, 1975.

Parker CD, Bilbo RE, Reed CE: Methacholine aerosol as test for bronchial asthma, Arch Intern Med 115:452, 1965.

Patel KR, Kerr JW: The airways response to phenylephrine after blockade of alpha and beta receptors in extrinsic bronchial asthma, Clin Allergy 3:439, 1973.

Porcelli RJ et al: Relation between hypoxic pulmonary vasoconstriction, its humoral mediators and alpha-beta adrenergic receptors, Chest 71(suppl):249, 1977.

Rau JL: Autonomic airway pharmacology, Respir Care 22:263, 1977.

Richardson JB: Nerve supply to the lungs. Am Rev Respir Dis 119:785, 1979.

Richardson JB: The innervation of the lung, Eur J Respir Dis 117(suppl):13, 1982.

Richardson JB, Beland J: Nonadrenergic inhibitory nervous system in human airways, J Appl Physiol 41:764, 1976.

Rosenthal RR et al: The role of α-adrenergic receptors in allergic asthma, J Allergy Clin Immunol 57:223, 1976 (abstract).

Sahyoun N et al: Topographic separation of adenylate cyclase and hormone receptors in the plasma membrane of toad erythrocyte ghosts, Proc Natl Acad Sci U S A 74:2860, 1977.

Said SI: The lung in relation to vasoactive hormones, Fed Proc 32:1972, 1973.

Shiner RJ, Molho MI: Comparison between an α-adrenergic antagonist and a β_2-adrenergic agonist in bronchial asthma, Chest 83:602, 1983.

Simonsson NG et al: *In vivo* and *in vitro* studies on α-receptors in human airways, Scand J Respir Dis 53:227, 1972.

Steer ML, Atlas D, Levitzki A: Inter-relations between β-adrenergic receptors, adenylate cyclase and calcium, N Engl J Med 292:409, 1975.

Szentivanyi A: The beta adrenergic theory of the atopic abnormality in bronchial asthma, J Allergy 42:203, 1968.

Walden SM et al: Effect of alpha-adrenergic blockade on exercise-induced asthma and conditioned cold air, Am Rev Respir Dis 130:357, 1984.

5

Sympathomimetic Bronchodilators

Chapter 5 presents information on the adrenergic bronchodilator group. These drugs relax bronchial smooth muscle by stimulating β_2 receptors, to treat asthma and chronic obstructive pulmonary disease. The drug agents in this group are as follows:

Epinephrine
Isoproterenol
Isoetharine
Bitolterol
Metaproterenol
Terbutaline
Albuterol
Pirbuterol

The following topics are presented:

- History and development
- Structure-activity relations (how the chemical structure of these agents affects their activity)
- Mode of action
- Specific adrenergic agents
- Routes of administration (differences among inhalation, oral, and parenteral administration)
- Adverse side effects
- Conclusions and recommendations

Sympathomimetic (adrenergic) bronchodilators comprise one of the most useful and potent groups of respiratory care drugs, and this class contains more specific drug agents administered by respiratory therapists than any other single class.

The primary clinical application of this drug class is to relax bronchial smooth muscle and to dilate the airways. Since airway diameter is the most important determinant of airway resistance, the effect of these drugs is to lower airway resistance in asthma, bronchitis, and reversible airway obstruction of chronic obstructive pulmonary disease. A secondary effect is to facilitate mucociliary transport of secretions and thereby promote expectoration. Bronchodilatation and secretion clearance are the desired effects when these drugs are used in cases of pneumonia, bronchiectasis, cystic fibrosis, and other respiratory infections. A drug such as epinephrine is also used to relieve mucosal edema or upper airway congestion through its effect on alpha receptors. A variety of epinephrine brands and other sympathomimetics are used as nasal decongestants.

The direction of development of sympathomimetic bronchodilators has been toward agents that are more β_2 specific (fewer cardiac effects) and longer acting.

HISTORY AND DEVELOPMENT

The subcutaneous use of epinephrine was reported as early as 1903, and the use of epinephrine as an aerosol dates to at least 1910, making this one of the oldest sympathomimetic agents in current use. It was not until 1940 that isoproterenol was reported as a "broncholytic" agent. Another commonly used bronchodilator, isoetharine, was synthesized in 1936, and its use in asthma was reported in 1951. Interestingly, until the mid-1970s, when several other sympathomimetic bronchodilators were approved for use in the United States, epinephrine (natural and racemic), isoproterenol, isoetharine, and ephedrine were the only commonly used, approved bronchodilators in this class.

Ephedrine is a very old bronchodilator in the sympathomimetic group, dating back to the ancient Chinese herb ma huang *(Ephedra vulgaris)*, in which ephedrine is the active ingredient. The Chinese used this herb for approximately 5000 years for a variety of disorders, not all respiratory. After the active ingredient was isolated in 1885, the name *ephedrin* was coined. The epinephrine-like effects of ephedrine were demonstrated as early as 1915 by Japanese investigators. Ephedrine was introduced for use in the United States in 1926, and its use in asthma was reported in 1927. Pseudoephedrine, found in many preparations, is an isomer of ephedrine that exhibits less peripheral vasoconstriction. The bronchodilator effect of ephedrine is relatively weak, its duration of action is less than 4 hours, and it has greater stimulatory effects on the central nervous system than the other bronchodilators cited. As discussed in Chapter 4, ephedrine has a longer clinical effect than the catecholamines because it is not broken down by catechol-O-methyltransferase (COMT) or monoamine oxidase (MAO). Ephedrine and its isomers are often used in over-the-counter cold remedies, but the advent of the newer β_2 bronchodilators combined with controlled serum levels of theophylline have rendered ephedrine obsolete for control of reversible bronchospasm. A good review of ephedrine is offered by Weinberger (1975).

In 1964, after Lands reported that certain changes in catecholamine structure would increase bronchial activity, the way was indicated for laboratory development of a number of β_2-specific sympathomimetics. Metaproterenol was known to exist since the late 1930s and was reported for the treatment of asthma as early as 1961. Boehringer Ingelheim, Inc released this drug for general clinical use in the United States in metered-dose inhaler (MDI) form in 1973. In January 1981 a solution for nebulization was marketed. Terbutaline was synthesized in 1966 and its use in asthma reported in 1970. It has been available in injectable and oral forms for use in the United States since the mid-1970s, and an MDI aerosol was released in the mid-1980s. Albuterol, known as salbutamol in Europe, was released for general clinical use in the United States in the early 1980s as an MDI aerosol and in oral (tablet) form. In 1987, a solution for aerosolization was marketed. In 1985, a new drug bitolterol was released as an MDI aerosol. This agent is actually a pro-drug that is converted to its active form, colterol, in the body. In the late 1980s, pirbuterol was released in MDI form as Maxair (3M Pharmaceuticals) and is a β_2-selective agent similar to albuterol.

The trend in future development of beta-adrenergic bronchodilators seems to be toward preservation of β_2 specificity and even longer duration of action. This is seen in the release of an extended-action tablet of albuterol, termed *Repetab*, and in several β_2 agents with an 8- to 24-hour effect. These are formoterol, salmeterol, and bambuterol, which are under investigation at this time in the United States. Salmeterol is currently available in the United Kingdom as Serevent, in both dry-powder inhaler (DPI) and MDI formulations. Other potential β_2 agents (e.g., procaterol, hexoprenaline, and fenoterol) do not seem to offer advantages over currently available agents.

A good overview of the clinical pharmacology and metabolism of beta-adrenergic drugs, along with detailed references on experimental research findings, can be found in the following sources, which are cited in the Bibliography: Fernandez (1987), McFadden (1981), Popa (1986), Popa (1984), Reed (1985). One of the most comprehensive presentations of adrenergic agents in the literature is given by Venter et al. (1983).

STRUCTURE-ACTIVITY RELATIONS

The evaluation of the chemical structure of this class of bronchodilators provides a good example of structure-activity relations cited in Chapter 1. Minor changes in drug structure have led to important clinical differences. The two major effects resulting from development of the newer beta bronchodilators are greater β_2 specificity and longer duration of action.

Catecholamines

The sympathomimetic bronchodilators are all either catecholamines or derivatives of catecholamines. In Figure 5–1 the basic catecholamine structure is seen to be composed of a benzene ring with hydroxyl groups at the third and fourth carbon sites and an amine side chain attached at the first carbon position.

Catecholamine: One of a group of similar compounds having a sympathomimetic action, the aromatic portion of whose molecule is catechol and the diphatic portion an amine.

Examples of catecholamines are dopamine, epinephrine, norepinephrine, and isoproterenol. The first three occur naturally in the body. Catecholamines, or sympathomimetic amines, mimic the actions of epinephrine more or less precisely, causing tachycardia, elevated blood pressure, smooth muscle relaxation of bronchioles and skeletal muscle blood vessels, glycogenolysis, skeletal muscle tremor, and central nervous system stimulation. Sympathomimetic bronchodilators should be used with caution in the presence of exist-

Catecholamines { benzene ring / 2 hydroxyl groups / amine side chain

Structure:

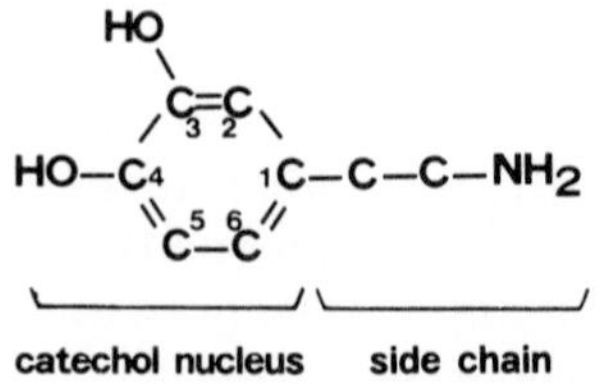

catechol nucleus   side chain

FIG 5–1. Basic catecholamine structure shows the catechol nucleus (benzene ring and two hydroxyl groups) connected to the amine side chain.

ing congestive heart failure, to avoid further cardiac stimulation producing ineffective cardiac pumping. Existing glaucoma could be adversely affected by a mydriatic (dilating) effect on the pupil of the eye.

Keyhole Theory of β_2 Specificity

Figure 5–2 gives the chemical structures of norepinephrine, epinephrine, isoproterenol, and isoetharine. The basic catecholamine structure is seen in all four agents. The order of the four agents, starting with norepinephrine and going to isoetharine, is associated with activity ranging from alpha effects (norepinephrine), through alpha *and* beta (epinephrine), to beta nonspecific (isoproterenol), and finally to β_2 specific (isoetharine). The theory that explains the shift from alpha activity to β_2 specificity has been termed the *keyhole theory* of beta sympathomimetic receptors: The larger the side-chain attachment to a catechol base, the greater is the β_2 specificity. If the catecholamine

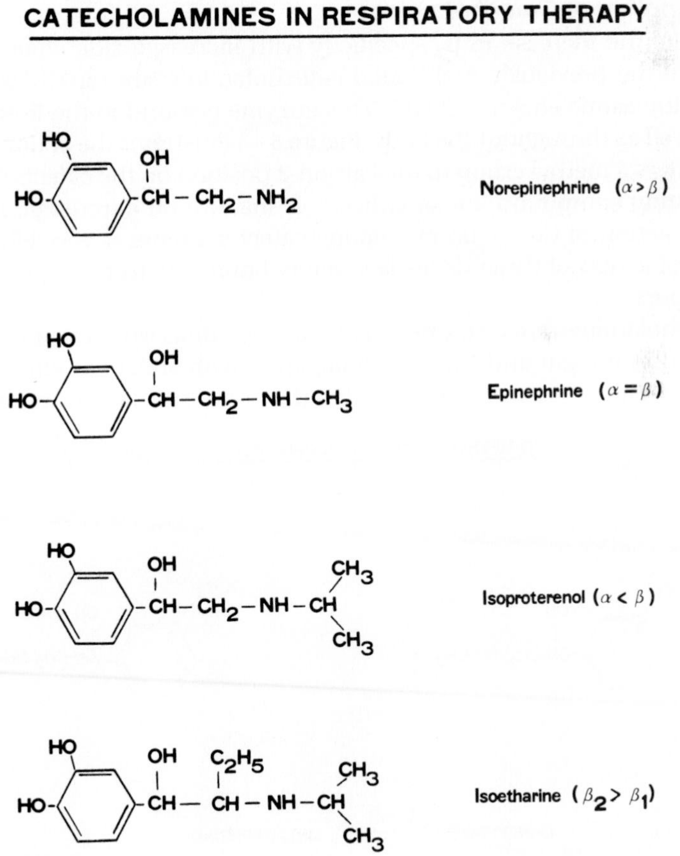

CATECHOLAMINES IN RESPIRATORY THERAPY

FIG 5–2. Structural formulas for norepinephrine, epinephrine, isoproterenol, and isoetharine. The direction of activity is toward a specific β_2 stimulation.

structural pattern is seen as a keylike shape, then the larger the "key" (side chain) the more β_2 specific is the drug. The vertical arrangement of the chemical structures in Figure 5–2 allows this to be seen. The relative degree of stimulation of alpha, β_1, and β_2 receptors is indicated.

Epinephrine substitutes a methyl group for hydrogen attached to the side chain of norepinephrine, making the former an equal activator of alpha and beta receptors. As the bulk of the substitution on the side chain increases, the beta stimulation is increased and alpha activation is lessened. **Isoproterenol** is the best example of this, with strong beta stimulation and very little alpha stimulation. **Isoetharine** (Dilabron) further increases the bulk of the amine side chain and adds an ethyl group (Fig 5–2), modifying the structure of isoproterenol and producing β_2-preferential activity. Actually, bronchodilator activity is reduced by an approximate factor of 10 compared with that of isoproterenol, but cardiovascular stimulation is less by a factor of 300.

Metabolism of Catecholamines

Despite the increase in β_2 specificity with increased side chain substituents, all of the previously mentioned catecholamines are rapidly inactivated by the cytoplasmic enzyme COMT. This enzyme is found in the liver and kidneys, as well as throughout the body. Figure 5–3 illustrates the action of COMT as it transfers a methyl group to the carbon-3 position on the catechol nucleus. The resulting compound, metanephrine, is inactive on adrenergic receptors. Since the action of COMT on circulating catecholamines is very efficient, the *duration* of action of these drugs is severely limited, with a range of 1½ to at most 3 hours.

Catecholamines are also unsuitable for *oral* administration since they are inactivated in the gut and liver by conjugation with sulfate or glucuronide at the carbon-4 site. Because of this action, they have no effect taken by mouth,

O-METHYLATION OF CATECHOLAMINE

EPINEPHRINE $\xrightarrow{\text{COMT}}$ METANEPHRINE

FIG 5–3. Inactivation of the catecholamine epinephrine by the enzyme COMT.

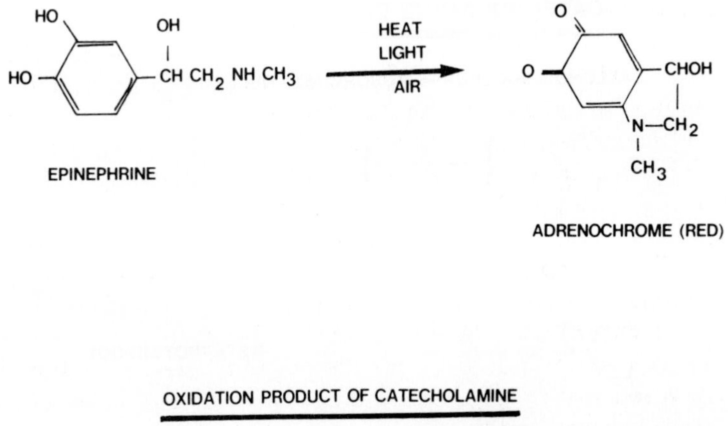

OXIDATION PRODUCT OF CATECHOLAMINE
_____

FIG 5−4. Conversion of the catecholamine epinephrine to an adrenochrome.

limiting their route of administration to inhalation or injection. Catecholamines are also readily inactivated to inert adrenochromes by heat, light, or air (Fig 5−4). For this reason, racemic epinephrine, isoetharine, and isoproterenol are stored in amber bottles. The residue from nebulizer rain-out in tubing may appear pinkish after treatment, and a patient's sputum may even appear pink tinged after using aerosols of catecholamines.

The sympathomimetic bronchodilator ephedrine, discussed previously in Chapter 4, is not a catecholamine and is not metabolized by COMT. Because ephedrine does not have the catechol nucleus, it can be taken orally.

Resorcinol Agents

Because the limited duration of action with catecholamines is hardly suitable for maintenance therapy of bronchospastic airways, drug researchers sought to modify the catechol nucleus, which is so vulnerable to inactivation by COMT. As a result, the hydroxyl attachment at the carbon-4 site was shifted to the carbon-5 position, producing a resorcinol nucleus (Fig 5−5). This change resulted in **metaproterenol** (named for the 3, 5-attachments in the meta position) and **terbutaline** (for the tertiary butyl group). Since neither drug is acted upon by COMT, both have a significantly longer duration of action of up to 6 hours compared with the short-acting catecholamine bronchodilators. Because of the bulky side chain, they are β_2 preferential in their receptor affinity, thus possessing minimal cardiac (β_1) effects. Finally, they can be taken orally since they resist inactivation by the sulfatase enzymes in the gastrointestinal (GI) tract and liver. For these reasons, the newer generation of resorcinols are much better suited to maintenance therapy on a long-term basis.

CATECHOLAMINE DERIVATIVES

CATECHOL NUCLEUS → RESORCINOL NUCLEUS

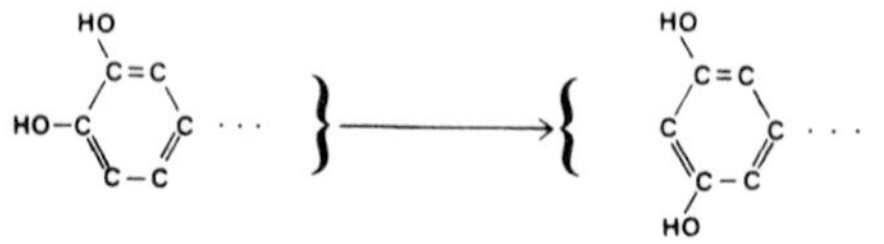

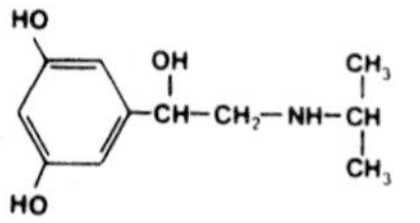

METAPROTERENOL

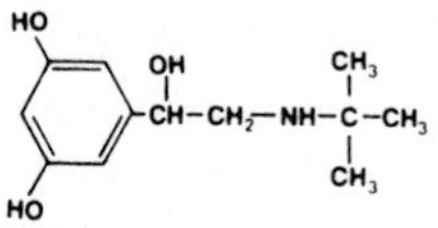

TERBUTALINE

FIG 5–5. Modification of the benzene ring attachments produces the resorcinol nucleus seen in the β_2 agonists metaproterenol and terbutaline sulfate.

Saligenin Agents

A different modification of the catechol nucleus at the carbon-3 site resulted in the saligenin **albuterol,** called salbutamol in Europe (Fig 5–6). Albuterol is available in a variety of pharmaceutical vehicles in the United States. These include oral tablets, a syrup, a nebulizer solution, MDI, extended-release tablets, and a DPI capsule. As with the resorcinol bronchodilators, this

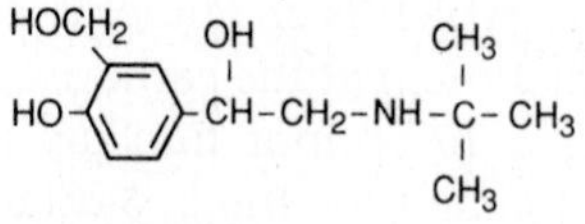

ALBUTEROL

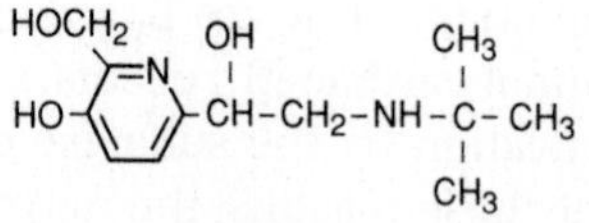

PIRBUTEROL

FIG 5–6. Additional modifications of the catechol nucleus show production of the saligenin albuterol and of pirbuterol, with β_2-specific effects.

drug has a β_2-preferential effect, is effective by mouth, and has a duration of up to 6 hours.

Pirbuterol

Pirbuterol is another noncatecholamine adrenergic agent. The drug is currently available as pirbuterol acetate (Maxair) in only an MDI formulation in the United States; the strength is 0.2 mg per puff, and the usual dose is two puffs. The MDI canister contains 300 inhalations and is produced by 3M Pharmaceuticals. Pirbuterol is structurally similar to albuterol except for a pyridine ring in place of the benzene ring (Fig 5–6). The onset of activity by aerosol is 5 to 8 minutes, with a peak effect at 30 minutes and a duration of action of approximately 5 hours. When pirbuterol is given orally, the pharmacokinetics differ, with onset of action within 1 hour, time to peak activity around 2 hours, and duration of 5 to 6 hours. Aerosol inhalation results in undetectable plasma concentrations with a maximum dose of 0.8 mg. The drug has a plasma half-life of 2 to 3 hours, measured with oral doses, and is primarily metabolized by sulfate conjugation. Around 60% of an oral dose is excreted in urine. Pirbuterol is said to be less potent on a weight basis than albuterol and similar in both efficacy and toxicity to metaproterenol (Richards and Brogden, 1985). The side effect profile is the same as with other β_2 agonists. An oral dose of 10 to 15 mg has effectively produced bronchodilatation in asthmatic patients, and a syrup of 7.5 mg/5 ml has been used in pediatric patients.

Relative Potency

The order of potency for these agents is as follows, from lowest to greatest (Ahrens, 1991; Richards and Brogden, 1985):

Metaproterenol
Pirbuterol
Terbutaline
Albuterol

Of the noncatecholamine bronchodilators, terbutaline and albuterol have the greatest β_2 selectivity and minimal cardiac effects. Metaproterenol has less β_2 selectivity (Weinberger et al., 1980), minimal cardiac effect, and is a less-potent drug. For example, the oral dose of metaproterenol is 10 to 20 mg, compared with 2.5 to 5 mg for terbutaline or 2 to 4 mg for albuterol.

A Pro-drug: Bitolterol

Bitolterol (Tornalate) differs from the previous agents discussed in that the administered form must be converted in the body to the active drug. Because of this, bitolterol is referred to as a *pro-drug*. The sequence of activation is seen in Figure 5–7.

The bitolterol molecule consists of two toluate ester groups on the aromatic ring at the carbon-3 and carbon-4 positions. These attachments protect the molecule from degradation by COMT. The large *N*-tertiary butyl substituent on the amine side chain prevents oxidation by MAO. Bitolterol is administered by inhalation using an MDI, and once in the body, the bitolterol molecule is hydrolyzed by esterase enzymes in the tissue and blood to the active bronchodilator colterol. The process of activation begins when the drug is administered and gradually continues over time. This results in a prolonged duration or sustained-release effect of up to 8 hours. The active form, colterol, is a catecholamine and will be inactivated by COMT like any catecholamine. The speed of this inactivation is offset by the gradual hydrolysis of bitolterol, to provide the prolonged duration of activity. The bulky side chain gives a preferential β_2 effect.

In animal studies, bitolterol given orally or intravenously selectively distributed to the lungs. The inhalation route in humans seems preferable to treat the lungs locally, and the hydrolysis of bitolterol to colterol proceeds faster in the lungs than elsewhere, giving a selective effect and accumulating in the lungs. When given orally to humans, any activated colterol will be conjugated by the GI tract during absorption, as with other catecholamines. Unchanged

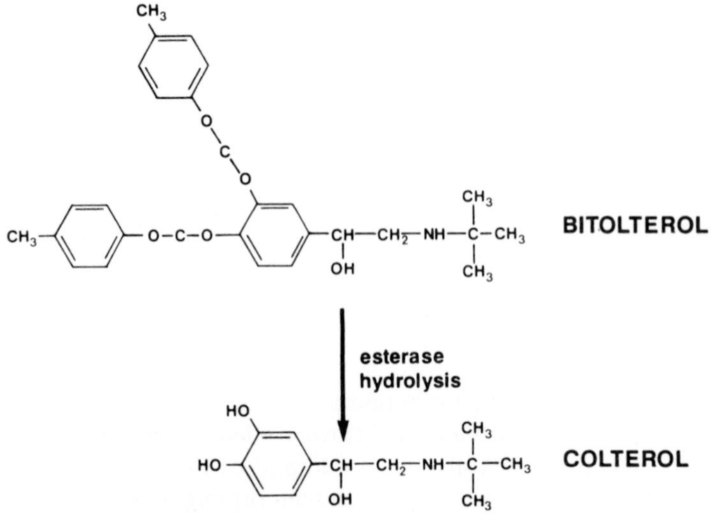

FIG 5–7. Conversion of the pro-drug bitolterol (Tornalate) by esterase enzymes to the active catecholamine colterol.

bitolterol will avoid such inactivation and enter the bloodstream, to be converted in plasma and tissues to the active colterol. Colterol is excreted in urine and feces as free and conjugated colterol and metabolites of colterol.

Potential Beta-Adrenergic Bronchodilators

In addition to those agents previously mentioned, there are a number of beta-adrenergic drugs not currently approved for general clinical use in the United States at the time of this edition. Some of these agents under investigation are shown in Figure 5–8. This group includes examples of catecholamines, resorcinols, saligenins, and other catecholamine derivatives.

Potential Beta-Adrenergic Bronchodilators

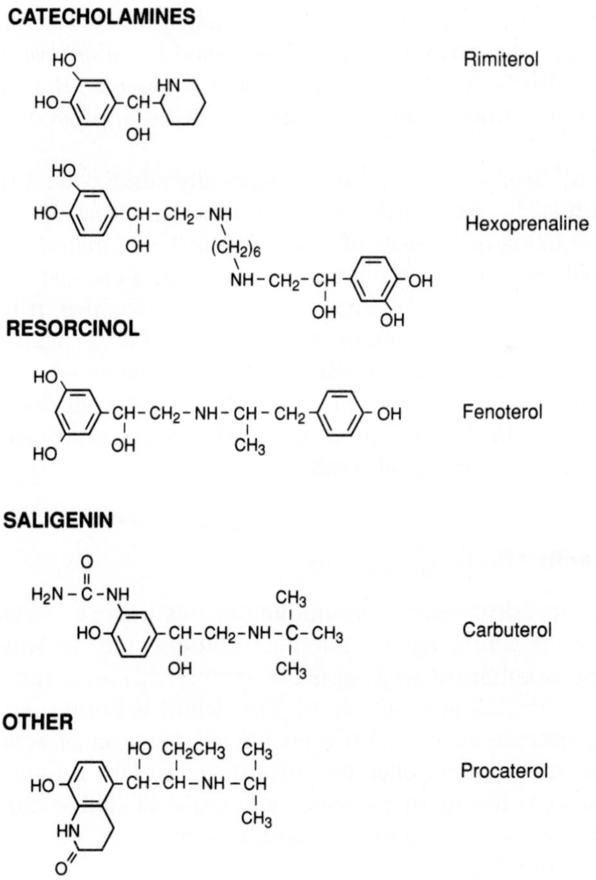

FIG 5–8. Potential beta-adrenergic bronchodilators.

Rimiterol (Pulmadil) and **hexoprenaline** (Ipradol) are short acting, because they are metabolized by COMT as catecholamines. Because of the bulk of their side chains, they have β_2-preferential activity and are similar in action to isoetharine.

Fenoterol (Berotec), with a metered dose of 0.2 mg per puff and an oral dose of 5 to 10 mg 3 times daily, is similar in action to terbutaline and albuterol (Svedmyr, 1985). It is β_2 selective, has prolonged action of 4 to 6 hours, and can be taken orally since it is a resorcinol. This drug has been investigated as a nebulized solution, with 0.5 mg found to be equipotent to 0.4 mg inhaled with an MDI (Watanabe et al., 1981). It is marketed in Europe as a compound with ipratropium, which is termed *Duovent*.

Fenoterol has been implicated in the question of increased mortality from asthma with beta agonist use (Sears et al., 1990). Although the issue of risk with beta-adrenergic agents is still unresolved, fenoterol may differ from other beta agonists.

The 200 mg per puff dose of fenoterol in use in other countries may have greater stimulant properties than the doses used for albuterol or terbutaline. Fenoterol may also be shorter acting and less β_2 specific than terbutaline. It is not clear at this time whether fenoterol will be approved for use in the United States.

Carbuterol (Bronsecur) is pharmacologically similar to albuterol, being a saligenin, but it is shorter acting (around 4 hours) and less potent. It has been investigated by using oral doses of 2 to 4 mg and an inhaled dose of 200 µg.

Procaterol replaces the catechol portion with a carbostyril and in addition has a bulky side chain, making this agent β_2 selective. It is not metabolized by COMT, and the side chain is resistant to MAO. Procaterol was evaluated for oral and inhalational use and was found to be an effective bronchodilator with a prolonged duration of action. Investigational doses of 0.01 and 0.02 mg by inhalation have resulted in 4 and 8 hours of improvement in expiratory flow rates (Storms et al, 1985).

Long-Acting Beta-Adrenergic Agents

The trend in adrenergic bronchodilators has been a development from nonspecific, short-acting agents such as epinephrine, to more β_2-specific agents such as isoetharine, to β_2-specific agents with an action lasting 4 to 6 hours such as terbutaline or albuterol. This trend is continued in the development of β_2-specific agents with even longer duration of action between 8 and 24 hours. Such agents offer the advantages of less frequent dosing and protection through the night for asthmatic patients. These agents include a sustained-release form of albuterol and newer drugs such as salmeterol, formoterol, and bambuterol.

Sustained-Release Albuterol

A sustained-release form of albuterol is available as Proventil Repetabs (Schering). This is a 4-mg tablet taken orally with extended activity up to 12 hours. The extended activity is achieved with a tablet formulation that contains 2 mg of drug in the coating for immediate release and 2 mg in the core for release after several hours. Thus the 6-hour duration can be extended for 8 to 12 hours and mimics the effect of taking two doses of 2 mg each. Terbutaline has also been marketed in Europe by AB Draco as a 10-mg, sustained-release tablet Bricanyl depot. This is not currently available in the United States.

Investigational Long-Acting Beta-Adrenergic Agents

In addition to sustained-release pharmaceutical preparations such as albuterol (Proventil Repetabs), attempts have been made to develop drugs with augmented duration of action. This has involved three general approaches: first, increase the number and size of lipid-soluble groups on the drug molecule to enhance receptor binding; second, lengthen the molecule's side chain to promote drug attachment to sites next to the beta receptor; and third, develop a pro-drug such as bitolterol for sustained activation of the agonist moiety. These three approaches are each exemplified by formoterol, salmeterol, and bambuterol, respectively, and are illustrated in Figure 5–9. A concise but clear review of these and other investigational bronchodilators is given by Mathewson (1991).

Formoterol is a catecholamine analogue with β_2-selective action. A 12-μg dose by MDI was shown to be effective for up to 12 hours, maintaining FEV_1 (forced expiratory volume in 1 second) values 20% above baseline in patients with stable asthma (Maesen et al., 1990). The drug can be used on a twice-daily schedule with a 24-μg dose, and with p.r.n. added doses in stable asthmatic patients (Midgren et al., 1992). This simplifies dosing demands on the patients and can provide longer duration of activity during the night for asthmatic patients. The longer duration of activity seen with formoterol may be due to increased lipid solubility, which enhances beta-receptor binding (Fig 5–9). Formoterol is 5 to 15 times as potent as albuterol (Midgren et al., 1992) and has been marketed in an oral preparation in Japan (Malo et al., 1990).

Salmeterol is another β_2-specific, long-acting agent that is a modification of albuterol (Fig 5–9). The drug has been investigated in 50-, 100-, and 200-μg doses by aerosol, and its effect on pulmonary function persists for up to 12 hours (Ullman et al., 1988). Salmeterol xinafoate is marketed as Serevent in the United Kingdom and is delivered both by DPI (50 μg per blister in the Diskhaler) and by MDI (25 μg per puff, two puffs twice daily). The drug's longer duration of action may be due to increased exoreceptor binding with its lengthened side chain (Fig 5–9). Alternatively, the airway epithelium may act

FORMOTEROL

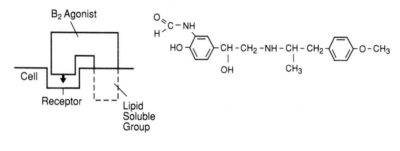

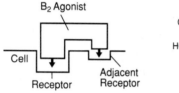

SALMETEROL

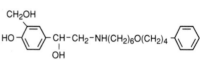

BAMBUTEROL

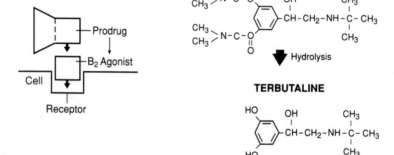

TERBUTALINE

FIG 5–9. Illustration of three mechanisms explored for increasing the duration of action with beta-adrenergic bronchodilators.

as a reservoir for the drug as it diffuses through to the β_2 receptor site (Ullman et al., 1988).

Bambuterol is a terbutaline pro-drug and as a pro-drug is similar in mechanism to bitolterol-colterol. A 20-mg dose by oral tablet improved peak flow rates for up to 24 hours with few side effects in adult patients with asthma (Vilsvik et al., 1991). The structure of this drug is pictured in Figure 5–9. When taken orally, the terbutaline moiety is protected from first-pass metabolism. The active terbutaline part is formed by oxidation and hydrolysis. Bambuterol also inhibits cholinesterase hydrolysis action, and this slows down the rate at which terbutaline is generated, contributing to the long action of the drug. The 24-hour duration allows once-daily dosing each evening, a definite advantage for patient compliance.

MODE OF ACTION

Drugs included in the sympathomimetic bronchodilator group stimulate one or more of the following receptors, with the effects given:

Alpha Adrenergic: vasoconstriction and vasopressor effect; nasal and upper airway decongestion.

β_1 **Adrenergic:**   increased myocardial conductivity and heart rate, and increased force of contraction.

β_2 **Adrenergic:**   bronchial dilatation and vasodilatation.

The adrenergic receptors have been identified and discussed previously in Chapter 4. Although ephedrine and epinephrine have stronger alpha (decongestant) effects and are used for such purpose, most of the agents in this group are applied for their β_2 effects. β_2 stimulation has the following clinical effects:

- Relaxation of bronchial smooth muscle (bronchodilatation)
- Inhibition of inflammatory mediator release
- Stimulation of mucociliary clearance

These effects of β_2 stimulation are mediated by activation of the enzyme adenyl cyclase, which in turn leads to an increase in the production of cellular cyclic adenosine 3', 5',-monophosphate (cyclic AMP). The metabolic pathway by which this occurs was illustrated in Chapter 4. Cyclic AMP causes relaxation of smooth muscle by decreasing intracellular calcium concentrations. Mycoplasmic calcium concentrations are reduced as cyclic AMP stimulates the binding of calcium ions to the cell membrane and the cytoplasmic reticulum (Fig 5–10). This inhibitory effect of cyclic AMP on cellular calcium is probably the same mechanism by which beta-adrenergic drugs retard release of mediators of inflammation from mast cells, a process that is known to require free calcium. The blocking of the contractile process of smooth muscle and mediator-containing cells is detailed in Popa (1986) and Tashkin and Jenne (1985).

SPECIFIC ADRENERGIC AGENTS

Table 5–1 lists the major sympathomimetic bronchodilators currently approved for general clinical use in the United States. Also listed are receptor

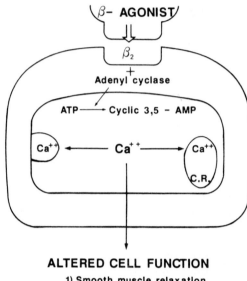

ALTERED CELL FUNCTION

1) Smooth muscle relaxation

2) ⁺Mast cell histamine release

FIG 5–10. Mode of action of beta-adrenergic agonists to increase cyclic AMP, decrease intracellular calcium, and modify bronchial smooth muscle and mast cell function.

preference and the time course of the drug's action by the routes of administration indicated.

Ephedrine has already been discussed in the historical perspective at the beginning of this chapter and in chapter 4. It is a noncatecholamine and a weak bronchodilator. Because of its alpha-receptor stimulation, it is used more as a decongestant in cold medications than as a bronchodilator. Structurally, it is not metabolized by COMT, and it combines with MAO to inhibit this enzyme, without being inactivated. Ephedrine directly stimulates both alpha and beta (β_1 and β_2) receptors and has an indirect effect on such receptors by competitively inhibiting MAO to allow endogenous norepinephrine and epinephrine to act. Because ephedrine lacks the hydroxyl groups on its ring structure, the drug crosses the blood-brain barrier (see Chapter 1) to cause central nervous system stimulation, resulting in insomnia and amphetamine-like effects.

Epinephrine is a potent catecholamine bronchodilator that stimulates both alpha and beta receptors. It is naturally occurring in the adrenal medulla and has a rapid onset but a short duration due to metabolism by COMT. It is used both by inhalation and subcutaneously to treat patients with acute asthmatic episodes. It is also used as a cardiac stimulant, based on its strong β_1 effects. Self-administered, intramuscular injectable doses of 0.3 and 0.15 mg

TABLE 5-1.

Receptor Preference and Basic Pharmacokinetics of the Beta-Adrenergic Bronchodilators

Drug	Receptor	Onset (min)	Route*	Peak (min)	Duration (hr)
Noncatecholamine	$\alpha + \beta$†	15–60	PO	2‡	3–5
Ephedrine					
Catecholamines					
Epinephrine	$\alpha + \beta$	3–5	INH	5–20	1–3
		6–15	SC		
Isoproterenol	β	2–5	INH	5–30	½–2
Isoetharine	β_2	1–6	INH	15–60	1–3
Bitolterol	β_2	3–4	INH	30–60	5–8
Resorcinol					
Metaproterenol	β_2	1–5	INH	60	2–6
		15–30	PO		
Terbutaline	β_2	5–30	INH	30–60	3–6
		6–15	SC	30–60	1½–4
		30	PO	2–4‡	4–8
Saligenin					
Albuterol	β_2	15	INH	30–60	3–8
		30	PO	1–2‡	4–6
Other					
Pirbuterol	β_2	5	INH	30	5

*PO, orally; *INH*, inhalation; *SC*, subcutaneously.
†β, beta nonspecific, β_1, and β_2 receptors.
‡Hours.

are marketed to control systemic hypersensitivity (anaphylactoid) reactions. This drug is more useful for management of acute asthma rather than for daily maintenance therapy because of its pharmacokinetics.

Racemic epinephrine is a synthetic form of naturally occurring epinephrine and is most often used for nebulization administration as MicroNefrin or Vaponefrin. The mode of action of racemic epinephrine is the same as with natural epinephrine, giving both alpha and beta stimulation. However, there is approximately one half the vasopressor effect of natural epinephrine, because the racemic mixture is composed of two stereoisomers. The body normally manufactures mainly *l*-epinephrine, which is one of the stereoisomers and which is the only active form of epinephrine physiologically. The synthetic mixture is comprised of 50% *d*-epinephrine and 50% *l*-epinephrine. The *d*-epinephrine is inactive. Thus the result is a 50% diluted solution in terms of physiological effect, and so a 2.25% solution is administered by inhalation instead of a 1% strength. The presence of the stereoisomers is indicated by the optical inactivity of the mixture since a stereoisomer is identified by its ability to polarize light; racemic epinephrine is optically inactive because the two stereoisomers are mutually canceling. The concept of stereoisomers is illustrated in Figure 5–11 by a simple chemical structure.

CONCEPT OF A STEREOISOMER

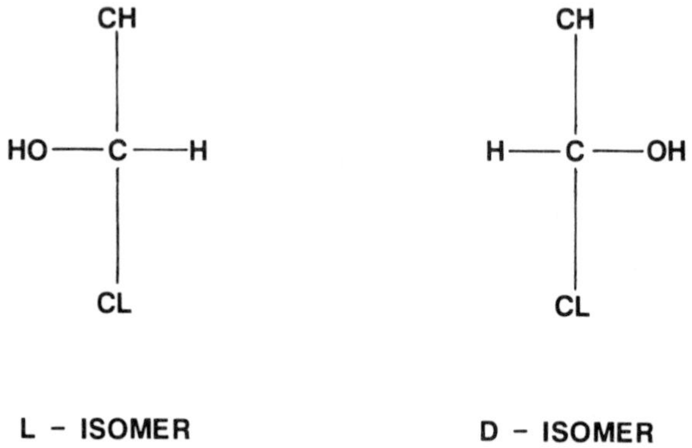

CH   CH

HO—C—H   H—C—OH

CL   CL

L – ISOMER   D – ISOMER

FIG 5–11.   Simple representation of a left- and right-handed stereoisomer.

Isoproterenol is another potent catecholamine bronchodilator that was widely used for nebulization until the advent of the more β_2-specific agents such as isoetharine and later the resorcinols, saligenins, and others. The main disadvantages of isoproterenol are its short duration due to COMT breakdown and its strong cardiac (β_1) effects, causing tachycardia. Isoproterenol is metabolized to a weak beta blocker, 3-methoxyisoproterenol, which has been thought to cause resistance to its bronchodilating effects. This is probably not clinically important as a cause of reduced response to the drug (Patterson et al., 1968).

Isoetharine was one of the first β_2-specific adrenergic bronchodilators in the United States. As a catecholamine, it has a short duration of action, but its rapid onset and minimal cardiac (β_1) stimulation make it ideal for before-and-after bronchodilator studies or to prevent bronchospasm from other inhaled drugs. Originally the brand of isoetharine was marketed with two other active ingredients: thenyldiamine, which is an antihistamine, and phenylephrine, a strong alpha stimulant for reducing mucosal swelling. Both have been deleted for lack of efficacy. Theoretically, alpha stimulation may antagonize the relaxing effect of β_2 stimulation if alpha receptors are present in human airways.

Metaproterenol, terbutaline, albuterol, and **pirbuterol** are all noncatecholamines with a relatively long duration of 4 to 6 hours and β_2 specificity to reduce cardiac stimulation. They are available in a variety of administration forms for inhalation, oral use, or injection. These features make them the first sympathomimetic bronchodilators suitable for maintenance therapy of airway hyperreactivity. By the same reasoning, they are not well used for short-term preventive bronchodilatation or bronchodilator studies. Their slowness to peak (30 to 60 minutes) may cause before-and-after pulmonary function studies to be unreasonably lengthy or to miss effects, and they may not act in time to prevent drug-induced bronchospasm unless given well in advance.

Bitolterol is unique in its sequence of activation among the beta-adrenergic agents discussed. It is essentially a β_2-preferential catecholamine with the pharmacokinetics (onset, peak, and duration) of the noncatecholamines. Although this drug is relatively new, it has compared favorably with albuterol in one study (Orgel et al., 1985). The annoying side effect of muscle tremor occurs in about 15% of subjects despite aerosol administration. The drug was originally marketed in MDI form, and most recently, a nebulizer solution has been released.

Table 5–2 lists the currently available beta-adrenergic bronchodilators used in the United States and gives some pharmaceutical detail on each. Although each drug has been characterized briefly with regard to clinical phar-

TABLE 5–2.

Dosages and Strengths Used for Various Methods of Administering Beta-Adrenergic Bronchodilators

Drug	Brand Names	Administration Method	Strength	Dosage
Epinephrine	Adrenalin	Nebulizer	1:100 (1%)	0.25–0.5 ml qid
Racemic epinephrine	MicroNefrin Vaponefrin AsthmaNefrin	Nebulizer	2.25%	0.25–0.5 ml qid
Isoproterenol	Isuprel	Nebulizer	1:200 (0.5%)	0.25–0.5 ml qid
	Isuprel Mistometer	MDI	131 µg/puff	1–2 puffs qid
Isoetharine	Bronkosol	Nebulizer	1%	0.25–0.5 ml qid
	Bronkometer	MDI	340 µg/spray	1–2 puffs qid
Metaproterenol	Alupent	Nebulizer	5%	0.3 ml tid, qid
	Metaprel	MDI	0.65 mg/puff	2–3 puffs q4h
		Tablets	10, 20 mg	20 mg tid, qid
		Syrup	10 mg/5 ml	10 mg tid, qid
Terbutaline	Brethaire	MDI	0.2 mg/puff	2 puffs q4–6h
	Brethine	Injection	1 mg/ml	0.25 mg SC
	Bricanyl	Tablets	2.5, 5 mg	2.5 or 5 mg tid
Albuterol	Proventil	Nebulizer	0.5%	0.5 ml tid, qid
	Ventolin	MDI	90 µg/puff	2 puffs tid, qid
		DPI	200 µg/caps.	1 caps. q4–6h
		Tablets	2, 4 mg	2 or 4 mg tid, qid
		Extended-release tablet	4 mg	q12h
		Syrup	2 mg/5 ml	2 or 4 mg tid, qid
Bitolterol (colterol)	Tornalate	MDI	0.37 mg/puff	2 puffs q8h
		Nebulizer	0.2%	1.25 ml tid or as ordered
Pirbuterol	Maxair	MDI	0.2 mg/puff	2 puffs q4–6h

macology, practitioners are urged to read package inserts on a drug before administration. Such inserts give details of dosage strengths and frequencies, adverse effects, shelf life, and storage requirements, all of which are needed for safe application. Table 5–2 is not intended to replace more detailed information supplied by the manufacturer on each of the bronchodilator agents.

ROUTES OF ADMINISTRATION

Beta-adrenergic bronchodilators are currently available in inhaled form (MDI, nebulizer solution, or DPI), orally (tablets or syrup), and parenterally, although not all agents are found in each form. Regardless of the route of administration, there are two general patterns to the time course of bronchodilation with drugs in this group. The *catecholamines* show a rapid onset of 1 to 3 minutes, a peak effect around 15 to 20 minutes, and a rapid decline in effect after 1 hour. The *noncatecholamines* (resorcinols, saligenins) have a slower onset of 3 to 6 minutes, a delayed peak effect of 30 to 60 minutes, and a prolonged effect of 4 to 6 hours (Popa, 1986, 1984). Aside from this general difference, which depends on the type of drug used, the route of administration will further affect the time course of a drug. Inhaled and injected adrenergic bronchodilators have a quicker onset than orally administered agents.

Inhalation Route

All of the beta-adrenergic bronchodilators marketed in the United States are available for inhalational delivery, either using an MDI, a nebulizer (including intermittent positive pressure breathing nebulization), or a DPI. Catecholamines must be given by inhalation since they are ineffective by mouth (orally). Inhalation is the preferred route for administering beta-adrenergic drugs for all of the following reasons:

1. Onset is rapid.
2. Smaller doses are needed compared with that of oral use.
3. Side effects such as tremor and tachycardia are reduced.
4. Drug is delivered directly to the target organ (i.e., lung).
5. Inhalation is painless and safe.

There is some controversy concerning use of the aerosol delivery *during* an acute attack of airway obstruction. However, several studies have failed to show substantial differences between inhaled and parenteral beta-adrenergic agents in acute severe asthma (McFadden, 1985; Robertson and Levison, 1985). There is no reason to avoid nebulizing these bronchodilators during acute episodes (Tinkelman et al., 1983). In fact, combining the oral delivery with additional inhalation has been shown to produce good additive effects with albuterol (Fernandez, 1987).

The major difficulties with aerosol administration are the time needed for nebulization (5 to 10 minutes), the possible embarrassment of using an MDI in public or at school, and inability to use an MDI correctly. Difficulty in correctly using an MDI can be remedied by using spacer devices or, alternatively, by using a gas-powered hand-held nebulizer. A DPI eliminates problems associated with both nebulizers and MDIs, although only one beta-adrenergic agent (albuterol) is currently available in DPI form in the United States.

Continuous Nebulization

One particular form of administering inhaled adrenergic agents is by continuous nebulization. The clinical use of this method of administration has been for management of severe asthma, in an effort to avoid respiratory failure, intubation, and mechanical ventilation. The *Guidelines for the Diagnosis and Management of Asthma* released by the National Heart, Lung, and Blood Institute panel of experts also refers to both frequent (every 20 minutes) and continuous nebulization of beta agonists (Part VIII, Management of Acute Exacerbations of Asthma). Portnoy and associates (1992) give a succinct review of continuously nebulized β_2 agonists in status asthmaticus. The following is a summary of published experience on this topic.

Delivery Methods.   A number of delivery methods to accomplish continuous nebulization have been tried and reported. These include the following:

- Measured refilling of a small-volume nebulizer (SVN)
- Volumetric infusion pump with an SVN (Moler et al., 1988)
- Small-particle aerosol generator (SPAG)-2 unit
- Large-reservoir, Vortran, high-output nebulizer

Dosages and Agents Reported.   Portnoy and associates (1992) reported continuous nebulization of both terbutaline and albuterol. The following data were given:

1. Continuous terbutaline.
    a. Average dosage: 6.9 mg/hr.
    b. Range of dosages: 1 to 12 mg/hr.
    c. Average duration: 8.63 hours.
    d. Range of duration: 1 to 24 hours.
2. Continuous albuterol.
    a. Average dosage: 12.1 mg/hr.
    b. Range of dosages: 10 to 20 mg/hr
    c. Average duration: 3.9 hours
    d. Range of duration: 1 to 10 hours

With delivery using the SPAG unit, a mixture of 16 ml of 0.5% albuterol in 96 ml of preservative-free saline was administered by face mask to pediatric patients. Moler and others (1988) used 4 mg/hr of continuously nebulized terbutaline with a volumetric pump infusion system connected to an SVN.

Toxicity and Monitoring.   Continuous nebulization of β_2 agonists is not standard therapy, and patients receiving this treatment are in serious condition. Potential complications include cardiac arrhythmias, hypokalemia, or hyperglycemia. Unifocal premature ventricular contractions were reported in one patient by Portnoy et al. (1992). Significant tremor may also occur. Subsensitivity to continuous therapy was not observed by Portnoy. Close monitoring of patients receiving continuous beta agonists is necessary and includes observation and cardiac monitoring. Selective β_2 agonists, such as terbutaline and albuterol, should be used to reduce side effects. With these stipulations, continuously nebulized beta agonists in status asthmaticus can be safe and effective, with little difference between terbutaline and albuterol.

Oral Route

The oral route has the advantages of ease, simplicity, short time required for administration, and exact reproducibility and control of dosage. However, in terms of clinical effects, this is not the preferred route. The time course of oral beta agonists differs from the inhaled route. Onset of action begins in about ½ hour, with a peak effect reached after 1 to 2 hours and a duration of action between 3 and 6 hours (Popa, 1986). Larger doses are required than with inhalation, and the frequency and degree of unwanted side effects increase substantially. The catecholamines are ineffective by mouth, as previously discussed. Noncatecholamine bronchodilators in the adrenergic group seem to lose their β_2 specificity with oral use, possibly due to reduction of the side chain bulk in a first pass through the liver (Leifer and Wittig, 1975). Patient compliance on a 3 or 4 times a day schedule may be better than with a nebulizer. If this is the case with an individual patient, and the side effects are tolerable, then oral use may be indicated for bronchodilator therapy. The introduction of an oral tablet of albuterol with extended-action properties (Repetabs) offers the possibility of protection from bronchoconstriction for longer than 8 hours. This is advantageous in preventing nocturnal asthma and deterioration of flow rates in the morning.

Parenteral Administration

Beta-adrenergic bronchodilators have been given subcutaneously as well as intravenously, usually in the emergency management of acute asthma. Subcutaneously, epinephrine 0.3 mg (0.3 ml of 1:1000 strength) every 15 to 20 minutes up to 1 mg in 2 hours and terbutaline 0.25 mg (0.25 ml of a 1-mg/ml solution) repeated in 15 to 30 minutes, not exceeding 0.5 mg in 4 hours, have been used. Shim (1984) suggests that for practical purposes both aerosolized and subcutaneous routes should be used to manage acute obstruction, although there may be little difference in effect with the two routes. No difference in effect between epinephrine and terbutaline has been found when given subcutaneously.

The intravenous route has been used most commonly with isoproterenol and also with albuterol. Intravenous administration of these agents was thought useful during severe obstruction because these agents would be distributed throughout the lungs, whereas aerosol delivery would not allow them to penetrate the periphery. This is questionable for both subcutaneous and intravenous bronchodilator therapy since aerosols do exert an effect with obstruction. Intravenous isoproterenol is not clearly advantageous as a bronchodilator, although this route is used for cardiac stimulation in shock and bradycardia. The dose-limiting factor is tachycardia. Intravenous therapy is a last resort and requires an infusion pump, cardiac monitor, and close attention. Children's dosages range from 0.1 to 0.8 μg/kg per minute, and adult dosages range from 0.03 to 0.2 μg/kg per minute, until bronchial relaxation or side effects occur (Shim, 1984). Albuterol has been given intravenously as a bolus between 100 and 500 μg or by perfusion between 4 and 25 μg/min (Popa, 1984). Although albuterol is more β_2 specific by aerosol than is isoproterenol, the usefulness of intravenous administration compared with oral, aerosol, or subcutaneous is not clearly established.

ADVERSE SIDE EFFECTS

Just as the adrenergic bronchodilators exert a therapeutic effect by stimulation of alpha-, β_1-, or β_2-adrenergic receptors, they can likewise cause unwanted effects due to stimulation of these receptors. Generally, the term *side effect* indicates any effect other than the intended therapeutic effect. The most common clinically observed side effects of adrenergic bronchodilators are listed below:

Tremor
Palpitations and tachycardia
Headache
Rise in blood pressure
Nervousness
Dizziness
Nausea
Worsening ventilation-perfusion ratio (decrease in Pao_2)

It must be remembered that the later adrenergic agents (isoetharine, terbutaline, metaproterenol, albuterol, bitolterol, and pirbuterol) are much more β_2 specific than previous agents such as ephedrine, epinephrine, or isoproterenol. Because of this, there is greater likelihood of cardiac stimulation causing tachycardia and blood pressure increases with the last three agents than with the newer drugs. The more recent agents are safe, and the side effects listed are more of a nuisance than a danger and are easily monitored by clinicians.

Tremor

The annoying effect of muscle tremor with beta agonists is due to stimulation of β_2 receptors in skeletal muscle, is dose related, and is the dose-limiting side effect of the β_2-specific agents, especially with oral administration. The adrenergic receptors mediating muscle tremor have been shown to be of the β_2 type (Larsson and Svedmyr, 1974; Marsden et al., 1967). As stated previously, this side effect is much more noticeable with oral delivery, which provides a rationale for aerosol administration of these agents. Tolerance to the side effect of tremor usually develops after a period of days to weeks with the oral route, and patients should be reassured of this when beginning to use these drugs.

Cardiac Effects

The older adrenergic agents with strong β_1 and alpha-stimulating effects were considered dangerous in the presence of congestive heart failure. The dose-limiting side effect with these agents was tachycardia. They increase cardiac output and oxygen consumption by stimulating β_1 receptors leading to a decrease in cardiac efficiency, which is the work relative to the oxygen consumption. Newer agents have a preferential β_2 effect to avoid cardiac stimulation. However, tachycardia may also follow use of the newer agents, and there is evidence that this is due to the presence of β_2 receptors even in the heart (Brown et al., 1983). β_2 agonists cause vasodilatation, and this can also cause a reflex tachycardia. Despite this effect, agents such as terbutaline or albuterol can actually improve cardiac performance. Albuterol and terbutaline can cause peripheral vasodilatation and increase myocardial contractility without increasing oxygen demand by the heart (McFadden, 1985). The net effect is to reduce afterload and improve cardiac output with no oxygen cost. These agents are therefore attractive for use with airway obstruction combined with congestive heart failure.

Tolerance

Drug tolerance is defined as a decreased response to a drug occurring with continuous therapy (Plummer, 1978). With beta-adrenergic bronchodilators, there is a decrease of sensitivity to the relaxing effect, with maximal loss of response occurring within the first 2 weeks of therapy. The loss of response is due to a decrease in the density of beta receptors on the cell surface that occurs in the presence of beta stimulants (Reed, 1985). Full response will return in approximately 2 weeks with cessation of the drug, and response can also be restored at least partially by concomitant use of glucocorticoids. A 2-week washout period is important in comparative drug studies or studies of tolerance with beta agonists. Although peak and duration of activity decline after repeated use of beta-adrenergic bronchodilators, this is not generally considered to be clinically important and does not contraindicate use of these agents. This same phenomenon of tolerance is responsible for the diminished muscle tremor once patients are on regular dosages of bronchodilators.

Central Nervous System Effects

Commonly reported side effects of the adrenergic bronchodilators include headache, nervousness, irritability, anxiety, and insomnia, which are caused by central nervous system stimulation. Feelings of nervousness or anxiety may be due to the muscle tremor seen with these drugs, rather than to direct central nervous system stimulation. This is not true in the case of ephedrine, which does cross the blood-brain barrier. Excessive stimulation of the central nervous system, or at least symptoms of such, should be noted by clinicians and can warrant evaluation of the dosage used.

Fall in Pao$_2$

A fall in Pao$_2$ has been noted with isoproterenol administration during asthmatic bronchospasm, as the ventilation improves and the attack is relieved. The mechanism for this seems to be an increase in perfusion of poorly ventilated portions of the lung. It is known that regional alveolar hypoxia produces regional pulmonary vasoconstriction in an effort to shunt perfusion to lung areas of higher oxygen tension. This vasoconstriction is probably accomplished by alpha-sympathetic receptors (Hales and Kazemi, 1974; Porcelli et al., 1977).

There are several possible pulmonary mechanisms by which arterial Po$_2$ could drop with bronchodilator administration:

1. Reversal of hypoxic pulmonary vasoconstriction by beta stimulation increases perfusion to underventilated lung regions (Chick and Nicholson, 1973).

2. Preferential delivery of aerosol to better ventilated lung regions increases the ventilation-perfusion mismatch.
3. Lung units with the most hyperinflation have the highest vascular resistance and the lowest perfusion.
4. Isoproterenol may only allow the trapped air to escape, without immediately promoting good *exchange* of air. The ventilation-perfusion ratio will remain very low in these units.

Sharp (1978) has noted that Pao_2 drops are statistically significant but physiologically may be negligible. He observed that O_2 tension falls most in subjects with the highest initial Pao_2. Decreases in arterial Po_2 rarely exceed 10 mm Hg, and the Pao_2 values tend to be on the flat portion of the oxyhemoglobin curve, so that drops in saturation (Sao_2) are minimized. Oxygen tensions usually return to baseline within 30 minutes.

Metabolic Disturbances

Adrenergic bronchodilators can increase blood glucose and insulin levels, as well as decrease serum potassium levels. This is a normal effect of sympathomimetics. In diabetic patients, clinicians should be aware of a possible effect on glucose and insulin levels. Hypokalemia has also been reported after parenteral administration of albuterol and epinephrine (Kung, 1986). The clinical importance of this is controversial and would mainly be of concern in patients with cardiac disease or in interpreting serum potassium levels obtained shortly after use of adrenergic bronchodilators. The mechanism of the effect on potassium is probably due to activation of the sodium-potassium pump by the beta receptor, with enhanced transport of potassium from the extracellular to the intracellular compartment. Such metabolic effects are minimized with inhaled aerosols of beta-adrenergic agents, since plasma levels remain low.

In addition to the common clinical side effects seen with adrenergic bronchodilators, there has been concern over other possible hazards to the use of these agents. These hazards include propellant toxicity of MDI aerosols, sulfite sensitivity in asthmatic patients, and increased mortality from asthma.

Propellant Toxicity

MDIs contain supposedly inert propellants that are generally termed *freon propellants*. The specific propellants used are the following fluorinated hydrocarbons:

Trichloromonofluoromethane (propellant 11)
Dichlorodifluoromethane (propellant 12)
Dichlorotetrafluoromethane (propellant 114)

Although in the United States these propellants have been banned from a wide variety of sprays (deodorants, hair sprays, fresheners), they continue to be used in aerosolized drugs.

There is concern over possible adverse effects in patients with use of hydrocarbon propellants (Belej and Aviado, 1975; Des Jardins, 1980). Several events have contributed to this concern. There were reports of sudden sniffing deaths among nonasthmatic youths who discharged commercial aerosols into bags and then inhaled the freon for a "high" (Bass, 1970). There have also been studies indicating cardiotoxicity of freon propellants (Taylor and Harris, 1970) and bronchospasm after MDI use (Yarbrough et al., 1985).

The net result is that freon propellants should not be considered inert. In the case of sniffing deaths and MDI-induced bronchospasm, it does seem likely that hydrocarbon propellants played a role. Freon propellants may have precipitated cardiac arrhythmias in the case of substance abuse with sprays by adding to the effects of endogenous catecholamines, especially if hypoxia or hypercapnea was present. These conditions could easily occur when rebreathing from a plastic bag. In asthma, the effect on the heart from MDI use is unlikely except with extreme overuse, since arterial plasma concentrations of freon after MDI use are low, and peaks occur in 20 seconds and then decrease (Dollery et al., 1974). If a person inhaled 12 to 24 actuations of a canister in rapid succession, propellant levels in the blood could be sufficient to combine with the effect of a drug such as epinephrine and cause cardiac arrhythmias.

The conclusion currently is that cardiotoxicity of freon propellants in bronchodilator MDI aerosols is unlikely unless there is definite overuse. This overuse would have to be in a very short period of time to build toxic plasma levels given the time course of these levels. It would not occur using an MDI once every hour. Of course repeated use of an MDI without seeking medical help can lead to serious obstruction or death because of progressive worsening of inflammation.

The more likely hazard in use of freon-powered MDIs is bronchospasm from hyperreactive airways. This reaction to the propellant was shown by Yarbrough et al. (1985). They found that 7% of 175 subjects who used placebo MDI with propellant only experienced a decrease of 10% or more in their FEV_1. The incidence was about 4% using an MDI with metaproterenol and propellant, probably due to the bronchodilating effect overcoming the propellant effect. In most cases, bronchospasm lasts less than 3 minutes. A dry-powder formulation is an ideal alternative formulation to an MDI if sensitivity to propellants exists. Use of a nebulizer instead of an MDI can also be considered if bronchospasm occurs with a patient. Finally, the oral route offers an alternative to the inhalation route of administration.

Sulfite Sensitivity

An increasingly publicized problem for those with hyperreactive airways is sensitivity to sulfite preservatives, with resulting bronchospasm. Sulfiting agents are used as preservatives for food but are also used as antioxidants for bronchodilator solutions to prevent degradation and inactivation. Sulfites include sodium or potassium sulfite, bisulfite, and metabisulfite. When a sulfite is placed in solution, at warm temperature in an acid pH such as saliva, it converts to sulfurous acid and sulfur dioxide. Sulfur dioxide is known to cause bronchoconstriction in asthmatic patients. Solutions of Bronkosol, Isuprel, Vaponefrin, MicroNefrin, and Alupent all contain sulfites. Unit-dose vials, ampules, and MDIs, as well as the multidose bottle of Proventil 0.5% solution (Schering), are all sulfite free. There have been reports of coughing and wheezing, as well as pruritus, following use of sulfite-containing bronchodilators. These are reviewed by Simon (1986), with references for more detailed information. The lack of response to a bronchodilator may also be due to the canceling effect of a sulfite in some cases. To avoid sulfites, unit-dose solutions or sulfite-free multidose solutions should be used. If multidose bottles are used, clinicians should check for sulfites and monitor patients' reactions.

Increased Deterioration in Asthma from Beta Agonists?

A troublesome paradox has emerged with asthma: Although the theoretical understanding and treatment options for asthma have steadily increased, so has the mortality from asthma. Most importantly, the increased use of beta agonists has been correlated with increased deaths from asthma worldwide. This was shown as early as 1969 by Inman and Adelstein who correlated increasing use of beta-adrenergic agents by MDI with increasing mortality from asthma. In 1992, Spitzer and associates reported a similar correlation in a Canadian study. Sears and colleagues (1990) demonstrated that more patients (70%) exhibited better asthma control with adrenergic agents used only as needed and not on a regular daily basis.

The findings can be summarized as follows: (1) An association has been shown between use of beta agonists and mortality from asthma, and (2) worldwide mortality from asthma has increased. Two broad interpretations of these data are possible: (1) Use of beta agonists in asthma can somehow cause a deterioration and increased risk of death, or there is some other cause of death such as undertreatment with definitive medical intervention in acute asthma or underuse of steroids and antiinflammatory agents in maintenance therapy. Increased beta-agonist use is necessitated by more severe asthma, where there is also increased risk of death. If the second alternative is the case, then the association between beta agonist use and mortality from asthma is simply coincidental, not causative.

To demonstrate that mortality from asthma actually is an effect of beta-agonist use would require data showing a cause-effect relation through some physiological or metabolic pathway. Several hypothetical explanations for such an effect from beta-agonist use have been proposed:

1. Protection from beta agonists declines with continuous use, possibly through subsensitivity (down-regulation) of beta receptors (Vathenen et al., 1988).
2. Beta agonists actually inhibit natural antiinflammatory mechanisms usually triggered by mast cell degranulation (Page, 1991).
3. Some deaths from asthma are cardiac related, caused by effects of beta-adrenergic agonists (Robin and McCauley, 1992).

CONCLUSIONS AND RECOMMENDATIONS

Overall, the beta-adrenergic bronchodilators are effective and safe especially by aerosol. Aerosol abuse or overuse is not a problem with the newer agents from the point of view of hazardous side effects. The entire contents of an albuterol or terbutaline canister is only slightly more than the usual 24-hour oral dose. Clinicians should be aware of the Position Statement of the American Academy of Allergy and Immunology (1985) regarding the adverse effects with this group of drugs, which points out that the complications cited do not pose a threat to their proper clinical use.

General recommendations for use of these drugs are the following:

1. Beta-adrenergic agents should be prescribed in the inhaled form whenever possible. This route gives rapid onset, minimal dose, and minimal side effects.
2. Patients should be monitored for adverse cardiac effects when using beta-adrenergic agents. In some situations, especially with patients at risk for arrhythmias, this may involve continuous cardiac monitoring.
3. Patients should be well instructed in the use of nebulizers, MDI devices, or DPI devices. Verbal and written instructions, practice, and a return demonstration are needed. Correct breathing pattern should be repeatedly emphasized.
4. Over-the-counter agents should not be used as an alternative to seeking medical help during an asthmatic episode.

BIBLIOGRAPHY

Ahrens RC: On comparing inhaled beta adrenergic agonists, Ann Allergy 67:296, 1991 (editorial).

The American Academy of Allergy and Immunology—Committee on Drugs: Position statement: adverse effects and complications of treatment with beta-adrenergic agonist drugs, J Allergy Clin Immunol 75:443, 1985.

Bass MJ: Sudden sniffing death, JAMA 212:2075, 1970.

Belej MA, Aviado DM: Cardiopulmonary toxicity of propellants for aerosols, J Clin Pharmacol 15:105, 1975.

Brown JE, McLeod AA, Shand DG: Evidence for cardiac adrenoreceptors in man, Clin Pharmacol Ther 33:424, 1983.

Chick TW et al: Effects of bronchodilators on the distribution of ventilation and perfusion in asthma, Chest 63:11S, 1973.

DesJardins T: Freon-propelled bronchodilator use as a potential hazard to asthmatic patients, Respir Care 25:50, 1980.

Dollery CT et al: Arterial blood levels of fluorocarbons in asthmatic patients following use of pressurized aerosols, Clin Pharmacol Ther 15:59, 1974.

Fernandez E: Beta-adrenergic agonists, Semin Respir Med 8:353, 1987.

Hales CA, Kazemi H: Hypoxic vascular response of the lung: effect of aminophylline and epinephrine, Am Rev Respir Dis 110:126, 1974.

Inman WHW, Adelstein AM: Rise and fall of asthma mortality in England and Wales in relation to use of pressurized aerosols, Lancet 2:279, 1969.

Kemp JP et al: Comparison of bronchodilator responses with bitolterol mesylate solution with the use of two different nebulizer systems in asthma, J Allergy Clin Immunol 77:509, 1986.

Kung M: Parenteral adrenergic bronchodilators and potassium, Chest 89:322, 1986.

Larsson S, Svedmyr N: Studies of muscle tremor induced by beta-adrenostimulating drugs, Scand J Respir Dis 88(suppl):54, 1974.

Leifer KN, Wittig HJ: The beta-2 sympathomimetic aerosols in the treatment of asthma, Ann Allergy 35:69, 1975.

Maesen FPV et al: Bronchodilator effect of inhaled formoterol vs salbutamol over 12 hours, Chest 97:590, 1990.

Malo J et al: Formoterol, a new inhaled beta-2 adrenergic agonist, has a longer blocking effect than albuterol on hyperventilation-induced bronchoconstriction, Am Rev Respir Dis 142:1147, 1990.

Mathewson HS: Adrenergic bronchodilators: trends in drug design, Respir Care 36:861, 1991.

McFadden ER Jr: Clinical use of B-adrenergic agonists: metabolism and pharmacology, J Allergy Clin Immunol 68:91, 1981.

McFadden ER, Jr: Clinical use of B-adrenergic agonists, J Allergy Clin Immunol 76:352, 1985.

Marsden CD et al: Peripheral beta-adrenergic receptors concerned with tremor, Clin Sci 33:53, 1967.

Midgren B, Melander B, Persson G: Formoterol, a new long-acting B2 agonist, inhaled twice daily in stable asthmatic subjects, Chest 101:1019, 1992.

Moler F, Hurwitz M, Custer J: Improvement of clinical asthma scores and Paco$_2$ in children with severe asthma treated with continuously nebulized terbutaline, J Allergy Clin Immunol 81:1101, 1988.

Nelson HS, Szefler SJ, Martin RJ: Regular inhaled beta-adrenergic agonists in the treatment of bronchial asthma: beneficial or detrimental? Am Rev Respir Dis 144:249, 1991.

Orgel HA et al: Bitolterol and albuterol metered-dose aerosols: comparison of two long-acting beta-2-adrenergic bronchodilators for treatment of asthma, J Allergy Clin Immunol 75:55, 1985.

Page CP: One explanation of the asthma paradox: inhibition of natural anti-inflammatory mechanism by B2-agonists. Lancet 337:717, 1991.

Patterson JW et al: Isoprenaline resistance and the use of pressurized aerosols in asthma, Lancet 2:426, 1968.

Plummer AL: The development of drug tolerance to beta$_2$ adrenergic agents, Chest 73(suppl):949, 1978.

Popa V: Beta-adrenergic drugs, Clin Chest Med 7:313, 1986.

Popa V: Clinical pharmacology of adrenergic drugs. J Asthma 21:183, 1984.

Porcelli RJ et al: Relation between hypoxic pulmonary vasoconstriction, its humoral mediators and alpha-beta adrenergic receptors, Chest 71(suppl):249, 1977.

Portnoy J et al: Continuous nebulization for status asthmaticus, Ann Allergy 69:71, 1992.

Reed CE: Adrenergic bronchodilators: pharmacology and toxicology. J Allergy Clin Immunol 76:335, 1985.

Richards DM, Brogden RN: Pirbuterol: a preliminary review of its pharmacological properties and therapeutic efficacy in reversible bronchospastic disease, Drugs 30:7, 1985.

Robertson C, Levison H: Bronchodilators in asthma, Chest 87:64S, 1985.

Robin ED, McCauley R: Sudden cardiac death in bronchial asthma, and inhaled beta-adrenergic agonists: Chest 101:1699, 1992.

Sears MR et al: Regular inhaled beta-agonist treatment in bronchial asthma, Lancet 336:1391, 1990.

Sharp JT: Workshop No. 2: bronchodilator therapy and arterial blood gases, Chest 73(suppl):980, 1978.

Shim C: Adrenergic agonists and bronchodilator aerosol therapy in asthma, Clin Chest Med 5:659, 1984.

Simon RA: Sulfite sensitivity, Ann Allergy 56:281, 1986.

Spitzer WO et al: The use of B-agonists and the risk of death and near death from asthma, N Engl J Med 326:501, 1992.

Storms WW et al: Procaterol metered-dose inhaler in adults with asthma, Ann Allergy 55:476, 1985.

Svedmyr N: Fenoterol: a beta-2-adrenergic agonist for use in asthma. Pharmacology, pharmacokinetics, clinical efficacy and adverse effects, Pharmacotherapy 5:109, 1985.

Tashkin DP, Jenne JW: Alpha and beta adrenergic agents. In Weiss EB, Segal MS, Stein M, eds: Bronchial asthma. Mechanisms and therapeutics, Boston, 1985, Little, Brown & Co.

Taylor GJ, Harris WS: Cardiac toxicity of aerosol propellants, JAMA 214:81, 1970.

Tinkelman DG et al: Comparison of nebulized terbutaline and subcutaneous epinephrine in the treatment of acute asthma, Ann Allergy 50:398, 1983.

Ullman A, Svedmyr N: Salmeterol, a new long-acting inhaled B2 adrenoceptor agonist: comparison with salbutamol in adult asthmatic patients, Thorax 43:674, 1988.

Vathenen AS et al: Rebound increase in bronchial responsiveness after treatment with inhaled terbutaline, Lancet 1:554, 1988.

Venter JC et al: Adrenergic agents. In Middleton E Jr, Reed CE, Ellis EF, eds: Allergy: principles and practice, ed 2, St. Louis, 1983, CV Mosby.

Vilsvik JS et al: Bambuterol: a new long-acting bronchodilating prodrug, Ann Allergy 66:315, 1991.

Watanabe S et al: Bronchodilator effects of nebulized fenoterol: a comparison with isoproterenol. Chest 80:292, 1981.

Weinberger MM: Use of ephedrine in bronchodilator therapy, Ped Clin North Am 22:121, 1975.

Weinberger M, Hendeles L, Ahrens R: Pharmacologic management of reversible obstructive airways disease, Med Clin North Am 65:579, 1980.

Yarbrough J, Mansfield LE, Ting S: Metered dose inhaler induced bronchospasm in asthmatic patients, Ann Allergy 55:25, 1985.

Ziment I: Infrequent cardiac deaths occur in bronchial asthma, Chest 101:1703, 1992.

6

Parasympatholytic (Anticholinergic) Bronchodilators

In Chapter 6, aerosolized anticholinergic bronchodilators are discussed. This class of drugs is used to decrease bronchoconstriction in bronchitis-emphysema patients, and is also used in asthma. Ipratropium bromide (Atrovent) is the only currently approved aerosol agent, although atropine and glycopyrrolate have been aerosolized. The following topics are reviewed:

- History and development of this class of drug
- Mode of action
- Clinical pharmacological properties
- Clinical application

INTRODUCTION

The potential for bronchodilatation by parasympatholytic agents is based on the effect of bronchoconstriction caused by parasympathetic stimulation. To the extent that the parasympathetic branch causes airway constriction in disease, agents that block parasympathetic receptors will provide airway relaxation. Ipratropium bromide (Atrovent) is the only anticholinergic bronchodilator currently approved in the United States for inhalation and is available in a metered-dose inhaler (MDI) form. A solution for nebulization is available in countries other than the United States. Injectable solutions of atropine sulfate and glycopyrrolate (Robinul) have been nebulized for bronchodilator effect. An agent under investigation is oxitropium, which is available as Oxivent in the United Kingdom. Parasympatholytic (or anticholinergic) agents are used for bronchial relaxation in chronic obstructive pulmonary disease (COPD) and asthma.

HISTORY AND DEVELOPMENT

The prototype parasympatholytic agent is atropine, which is an alkaloid found naturally in the plants *Atropa belladonna* (the nightshade plant) and *Datura* species *(D. stramonium, D. metel,* and *D. innoxa).* Scopolamine (hyoscine) is also extracted from the belladonna plant, and both atropine and scopolamine are therefore referred to as belladonna alkaloids.

There is evidence that these alkaloid ingredients have been ingested in one form or another for thousands of years for their effects on the central nervous system. An excellent historical review of these agents is given by Gandevia (1975). Of interest for respiratory care is the fact that fumes from burning the *Datura* species of plants were inhaled as a treatment for respiratory disorders as early as the seventeenth century in India. The earliest documentation of this was in the Ayurvedic literature, where *Datura* was mentioned specifically for asthma or for cough with dyspnea! By 1802, inhalation of *Datura* fumes to treat asthma had reached Britain, brought from India by British medical officers. In the mid-nineteenth century, inhalational therapy with alkaloids was advocated in America. Cigars, cigarettes, and pipes of various design were employed to smoke a preparation of *Datura* leaves. In Australia, severe patients were placed inside a tent of sheets, inside of which stramonium leaves were burned.

Even aerosols of liquid with *Datura* were noted in the nineteenth century, and the respiratory route for delivery of medications began to be appreciated. A variety of inhalational devices appeared for delivering liquids and gases, far predating the incorporation of respiratory therapy as a profession. In 1833, the previously named alkaloid "daturine" was identified as atropine by Geiger and Hesse. Controversy surrounded the inhalational use of parasympatholytic agents. Many physicians attacked their use in Britain and America in the nineteenth century as quackery, but use of *Datura* was widely accepted by patients who often obtained the ingredient without their physician's knowledge. Physician disagreement on the use of *Datura* probably rested on several issues: (1) difficulty in accurate dosage with smoking or aerosol therapy (a familiar contention); (2) irritant effects of smoke especially when other ingredients were added to the *Datura;* and (3) probably most of all, confusion over diagnosing and clinically differentiating asthma, bronchitis, emphysema, occupational diseases, and mediastinal gland dysfunction in the nineteenth and early twentieth centuries. The last factor led to inappropriate use of the *Datura* alkaloids.

By the 1930s, adrenaline and ephedrine, both sympathomimetics, had been introduced and largely replaced stramonium and belladonna extracts for treatment of asthma. However, parasympatholytic (anticholinergic) agents never completely disappeared in treatment of asthma and other obstructive diseases. Anticholinergics were used as an adjunct to the beta-adrenergic drugs, and in the 1980s interest in anticholinergic drugs was renewed, based on two factors: (1) new understanding of the role of the parasympatholytic system in airway obstruction, and (2) introduction of atropine derivatives with fewer obnoxious side effects. In 1987, ipratropium bromide, previously known by the code name SCH 1000, was released by Boehringer Ingelheim, Inc. in the United States as an aerosol with the brand name Atrovent.

A comprehensive review of anticholinergic bronchodilators with almost 250 references is provided by Gross and Skorodin (1984). Additional reviews of this class of agents can be found in the following sources: Boushey and Gold, 1983; Mathewson, 1983; Ziment and Au, 1986.

MODE OF ACTION

The potential of bronchodilatation offered by parasympatholytic agents is based on the premise that the parasympathetic branch of the autonomic nervous system maintains a basal tone in bronchial smooth muscle, and possibly exerts an abnormally active role in hyperreactive airway diseases, such as asthma and COPD, to produce constriction. Parasympatholytic agents such as atropine and its derivatives are antimuscarinic—that is, they block the action of acetylcholine at parasympathetic postganglionic effector cell receptors by competitively occupying the receptor sites. A conceptual illustration of the action produced by anticholinergic bronchodilators is given in Figure 6–1. The result is blockade of cholinergic-induced bronchoconstriction, smooth muscle relaxation, and inhibition of mast cell mediator release.

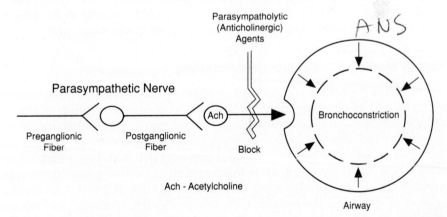

FIG 6–1. Conceptual illustration of the action of parasympatholytic (anticholinergic) bronchodilating agents.

Parasympathetic Innervation in the Lung

In Chapter 4 the autonomic innervation of the airway was outlined. This consists of the traditional sympathetic and the parasympathetic branches, as well as a possible third system termed *purinergic* or *peptidergic*. This last system is inhibitory (or relaxing) and is not part of the sympathetic branch; its influence is still largely unexplored in humans.

The sympathetic branch does not actually extend its fibers beyond the peribronchial ganglia or plexa to the airway, although adrenergic receptors are present throughout the airway, especially in the periphery. Parasympathetic nerves do enter the lung, deriving from the vagus, and travel along the airways. Parasympathetic postganglionic fibers terminate on or near airway epithelium, submucosal mucous glands, smooth muscle, and probably mast cells. Parasympathetic innervation is greatest in midsized airways of 3 to 8 mm, although present from the trachea to the respiratory bronchioles.

In the normal airway, a basal level of bronchomotor tone is caused by parasympathetic activity. This basal level of tone can be abolished by anticholinergic agents such as atropine, indicating it is mediated by acetylcholine. Administration of parasympathomimetics (cholinergic) agents such as methacholine (e.g., in bronchial provocation testing) can intensify the level of bronchial tone to the point of constriction in healthy subjects and more so in asthmatic patients.

An important point to realize with use of a blocking agent, such as an anticholinergic bronchodilator, is that the effect seen will depend on the degree of tone present that can be blocked. In healthy subjects, there will be minimal airway dilatation with an anticholinergic agent because there is only a basal or resting level of tone to be blocked. Variation in the clinical effect of such drugs will be partially due to variation in the degree of parasympathetic activity. One particular mechanism for parasympathetic activity in the lung is vagally mediated reflex bronchoconstriction, which is discussed next.

Vagally Mediated Reflex Bronchoconstriction

In Figure 6–2 the basic concept of vagally mediated reflex bronchoconstriction, and its parasympatholytic blockade, is sketched. A variety of immunologic (allergens) and nonimmunologic stimuli can activate subepithelial receptors in the airways. Impulses from these receptors travel via *afferent* branches of the vagus and lead to reflex *efferent* vagal impulses, which cause release of acetylcholine *(Ach)* at neuroeffector sites, including smooth muscle, mucous glands, and probably mucosal mast cells. Stimulation of such cholinergic receptors causes bronchoconstriction, production of mucus, and release of potent chemical mediators of inflammation from the mast cell. Activation of the subepithelial receptors also induces coughing, and these receptors have

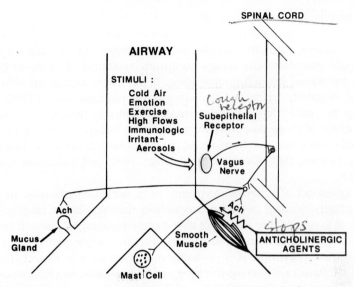

FIG 6–2. Illustration of the vagal reflex arc, with blockade of bronchial cholinergic receptors by anticholinergic bronchodilators.

been termed *cough receptors.* The stimuli that can trigger this reflex pathway are numerous.

Allergens result in antigen-antibody reactions that not only cause reflex bronchoconstriction but initiate other pathways of inflammation as well. Non-immunologic stimuli (no antigen-antibody reaction) include exercise, with air-way cooling and drying; cold air and high-velocity flow rates; hypo- and hypertonic aerosols; sulfer dioxide; cigarette smoke; dust; and even hair spray. This mechanism of vagal reflex is thought to be at least part of the reason that hypertonic aerosols are effective for sputum induction and in general for mobilization of secretions. Production of mucus and coughing both result from irritation of the subepithelial receptors. Asthmatic patients and those with hyperreactive airways are much more sensitive to such stimuli. In fact, airway hyperresponsiveness is defined by a lower threshold of reaction to bronchoconstrictor agents than occurs in healthy subjects.

Since atropine or its derivatives are competitive inhibitors of acetylcho-line at the neuroeffector junction, such antagonists should block parasympathetic reflex bronchoconstriction. Atropine has been shown to inhibit exercise-induced asthma and psychogenic bronchospasm, as well as bronchoconstric-tion caused by beta-blockade or cholinergic agents. Use of a topical anesthetic such as 4% lidocaine by aerosol to the large airways has also inhibited reflex bronchoconstriction, by blocking the sensory irritant receptors in the epithe-lial lining.

Changes in the airway may also sensitize the subepithelial cough receptors, making them more responsive to lower thresholds of stimulation. This is often seen during colds that involve lung congestion. Lung inflation during a deep breath stimulates the cough receptors, resulting not only in coughing but also increased bronchomotor tone. It has been suggested that greater bronchial reactivity in asthmatic patients or patients with COPD may be caused by mucosal edema and deformation of airway tissue, which increases the sensitivity of these receptors in response to irritants. References and discussion of cholinergic mechanisms of airway obstruction can be found in the following: Barnes, 1987; Bleecker, 1986; Hogg, 1982; Leff, 1982; and Simonsson et al., 1967.

The question of whether atropine, or a parasympatholytic in general, blocks antigen-induced bronchoconstriction during allergic reactions is not clear-cut. It is reasonable to expect that parasympatholytics would only block the cholinergic component of bronchospasm in allergic (extrinsic) and non-allergic (intrinsic) asthma. It is probably not reasonable to expect that the effects of an inhaled antigen on the lung are *all* mediated by cholinergic receptors or by the neurotransmitter acetylcholine. For instance, histamine is known to have local effects on surrounding tissue at the site of its release. Injection of histamine under the skin to produce a local wheal and flare reaction demonstrates this. Also, a parasympatholytic will not prevent the antigen-antibody reaction itself. Parasympatholytics *can* block the parasympathetic mediation of allergic lung responses, which is variable among asthmatic patients and which may be only *secondary* to the primary inflammatory reaction deforming epithelial sensory receptors in the airways. References to a discussion of this question by Fish et al. (1977) and Orehek and Gayrard (1977) are given.

Intracellular Mechanism of Cyclic GMP

Research indicates that smooth muscle relaxation and contraction is mediated at the cellular level through the intracellular nucleotides cyclic AMP and cyclic GMP (see Chapter 4). Beta sympathomimetics have been seen to increase cyclic AMP through interaction with the receptor enzyme adenyl cyclase (see Chapter 5). This results in the relaxation of smooth muscle in bronchioles or blood vessels. Conversely, a beta blocker such as propranolol (Inderal) might decrease cyclic AMP, causing contraction of the smooth muscle. Effects of parasympathetic stimulation of cholinergic receptors are thought to be followed by an increase in the intracellular nucleotide cyclic $3',5'$-guanosine monophosphate, or cyclic $3',5'$-GMP. The intracellular pathway and its blockade by anticholinergic agents are illustrated in Figure 6–3. Cyclic $3',5'$-GMP causes smooth muscle contraction and enhances release of inflammatory chemicals from mast cells. Therefore parasympathetic blockade by a cho-

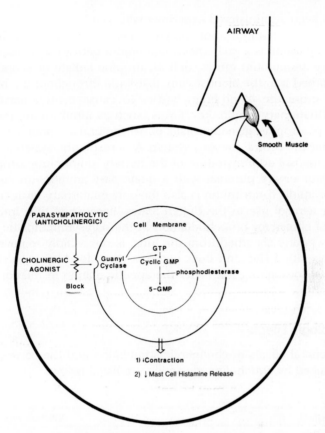

FIG 6–3.   Intracellular pathway for cholinergically induced bronchoconstriction by cyclic GMP, and its blockade by parasympatholytic bronchodilators.

linergic antagonist such as atropine ultimately results in a decrease in intracellular cyclic 3′,5′-GMP. This decrease reduces bronchoconstriction or mast cell release of mediators caused by cyclic GMP.

CLINICAL PHARMACOLOGICAL PROPERTIES

Chemical structures of the two naturally occurring belladonna alkaloids, atropine and scopolamine (also called hyoscine), are pictured in Figure 6–4. Atropine, including its sulfate (atropine sulfate), and scopolamine are both tertiary ammonium compounds that differ from each other only by an oxygen bridging the carbon-6 and carbon-7 positions. Quaternary ammonium derivatives of atropine include atropine methylnitrate (not available in the United States) and ipratropium bromide. Another quaternary atropine derivative, which has been administered experimentally as a bronchodilator by aerosol, is glycopyrrolate (Robinul) (not shown in Fig 6–4). Oxitropium bromide, an experimental agent, is a quaternary ammonium derivative of scopolamine.

Tertiary ammonium forms such as atropine sulfate or scopolamine are easily absorbed into the bloodstream, distribute throughout the body, and in particular cross the blood-brain barrier to cause central nervous system changes. Quaternary ammonium forms (such as ipratropium, the methylnitrate form of atropine, glycopyrrolate, or oxitropium) are poorly absorbed and do not enter the central nervous system. As a result, the systemic side effects seen with aerosol administration of the tertiary ammonium atropine sulfate do not occur or are minimal with a quaternary ammonium such as ipratropium bromide. Ipratropium is also the only quaternary form currently approved for aerosol use in the United States. Because of this, ipratropium is the drug of choice for bronchodilation in the parasympatholytic class. Ipratropium is poorly absorbed from the lung, is not rapidly removed from the aerosol deposition site, and does not cross the blood-brain barrier, as atropine sulfate does, giving it a wider therapeutic margin in relation to side effects.

Pharmacologic Effects

The general effects of cholinergic stimulation and the corresponding effects produced by anticholinergic action are listed below:

Cholinergic Effect	Anticholinergic Effect
Decreased heart rate	Increased heart rate
Miosis (contraction of iris, eye)	Mydriasis (pupil dilatation)
Contraction (thickening) of lens, eye	Cycloplegia (lens flattened)
Salivation	Dries upper airway
Lacrimation	Inhibits tear formation
Urination	Urinary retention
Defecation	Antidiarrheal or constipation
Secretion of mucus	Mucociliary slowing
Bronchoconstriction	Inhibition of constriction

Anticholinergic effects will differ with specific agents, depending on their absorption and distribution, which is determined by drug structure as well as route of administration. Since parasympathetic stimulation can cause bronchoconstriction, whether directly or through a vagal reflex, the desired therapeutic effect of aerosolized parasympatholytics is blockade of bronchoconstriction. To the extent that parasympathetic activity is present, parasympathetic blockade will produce bronchial relaxation.

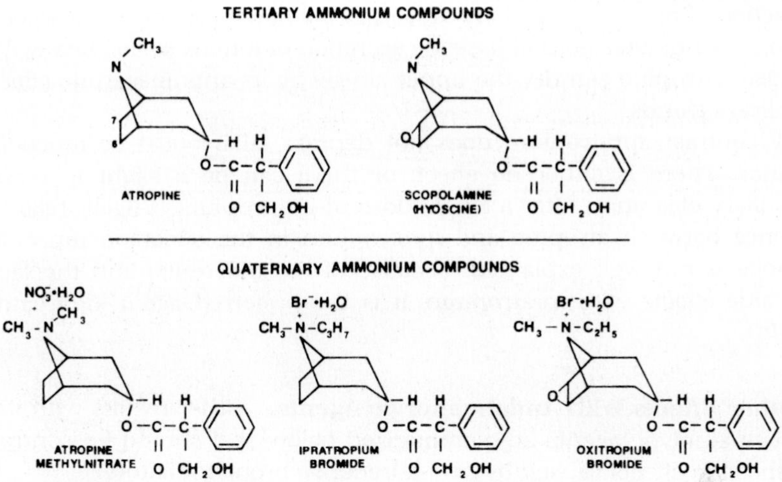

FIG 6–4. Chemical structures of atropine and scopolamine derivatives used as parasympatholytic (anticholinergic) bronchodilators.

Side Effects

There is a difference in side effects between tertiary and quaternary forms of an aerosolized parasympatholytic drug because of the difference in absorption, as previously discussed. Atropine sulfate, a tertiary ammonium form, is well absorbed and distributed throughout the bloodstream, producing numerous side effects. For the tertiary ammonium, atropine sulfate, the side effects are dose related:

At 0.5 mg: dryness of the mouth and skin.

At 2.0 mg: tachycardia, blurred vision, and pupillary dilatation.

At 5.0 mg: difficulty with speech, swallowing, and micturition; flushing of skin.

Higher doses: mental confusion or excitement, possible ganglionic and neuromuscular blockade.

Because of these side effects, patients with glaucoma or bladder obstruction are at risk with atropine as a bronchodilator. Because the smallest inhaled dose of atropine sulfate that produces bronchodilatation in adults is 0.4 mg and usually a 1- to 2-mg dose is used by aerosol, the first two groups of side effects can be seen. In contrast a quaternary ammonium compound such as ipratropium, which is poorly absorbed from the lung, rarely causes any side effect other than dry mouth, even in patients with glaucoma.

Effect on Mucociliary Function.   Atropine can depress ciliary action and overall mucociliary clearance in the airway. Atropine can also block the production of mucous secretions caused by cholinergic agonists. However, atropine does not alter normal baseline secretion of mucus in the airway (Wanner, 1986). Atropine can dry the upper airway by its antimuscarinic effect on the salivary glands.

By contrast, ipratropium does not depress ciliary beat or mucociliary clearance. There is either no effect, or there can be a slight increase in mucociliary clearance, after a single dose of ipratropium (Cugell, 1986). The difference between atropine and ipratropium in the effect on mucociliary clearance is not well explained. Because of the difference and the lack of other side effects with ipratropium, it is the preferred agent for treatment in COPD.

Other Effects With Anticholinergic Agents.   Other results with use of parasympatholytic agents are summarized below and should be contrasted with the side effects caused by beta-adrenergic bronchodilators:

1. Tremor is not produced.
2. Tolerance, if present at all, is very slight.
3. Reports indicate that there is a trivial and inconsistent effect on arterial Po_2 with anticholinergic aerosols.
4. Unfavorable interactions between anticholinergic and either beta-adrenergic or xanthine bronchodilators have not been noted in the literature.

Site of Action

Beta-adrenergic agents act on receptors in the peripheral, smaller airways. By contrast, anticholinergic agents given by inhalation seem to have more effect on receptors in the central, larger airways. Intravenous atropine, however, has a uniform effect throughout the airways. This would imply that the two types of agents would be additive and more effective given together than alone, which has been found to be the case. However, the type of lung disease must be considered. This is discussed under Clinical Application in this chapter.

Specific Parasympatholytic Agents

Parasympatholytic agents given by aerosol include atropine sulfate, ipratropium bromide, glycopyrrolate, and the investigational drug oxitropium bromide. Pharmaceutical details on each agent are given in Table 6–1.

Atropine sulfate has been administered as a nebulized solution, using either the injectable solution or preferably solutions marketed for aerosolization such as Dey-Dose. Both duration of bronchodilatation and the incidence of side effects are dose dependent. Dosages for children and adults are given

TABLE 6–1.
Strengths, Dosages, and Duration of Action for Aerosolized Anticholinergic Bronchodilat†

Drug	Brand Name	Strength	Dosage	Onset (min)	Peak (hr)	Duration (hr)
Atropine sulfate	Dey-Dose Atropine Sulfate					
Adult		0.2% (1 mg/0.5 ml)	0.025 mg/kg tid, qid	15	½–1	3–4
Child		0.5% (2.5 mg/0.5 ml)	0.05 mg/kg tid, qid			3–4
Ipratropium bromide	Atrovent	18 µg/puff	2 puffs qid	15	1–2	4–6
Glycopyrrolate	Robinul*	0.2 mg/ml	1.0 mg tid, qid	15–30	½–1	6
Oxitropium bromide	Experimental agent	100 µg/puff	2 puffs	15	2	6–8

*Available in injectable solution; used experimentally by aerosol (Gal, Suratt, Lu, 1984).

in Table 6–1. Although greater bronchodilatation and duration are seen with dosage schedules of 0.05 or 0.1 mg/kg for adults, the side effects of dry mouth, blurred vision, and tachycardia become unacceptable. Dosages in Table 6–1 are based on maximal benefit with minimal side effects (Cavanaugh and Cooper, 1976, Pak et al., 1982). Because it is a tertiary ammonium compound, atropine is readily absorbed by aerosol, and side effects are seen in doses required for effective bronchodilatation.

Ipratropium bromide (Atrovent) is currently the only approved anticholinergic bronchodilator for use as an inhaled aerosol in the United States. Ipratropium bromide is available in an MDI, and being a quaternary ammonium compound, has a wider therapeutic margin than atropine. This agent is an *N*-isopropyl derivative of atropine. Dryness of the mouth is the main side effect usually noticed. Optimal dose per administration for bronchodilatation has been found in the range of 40 to 80 μg. Systemic side effects have not occurred at higher doses of 500 μg. There is no substantial effect on cardiovascular function with inhaled ipratropium. There was no effect on urinary flow in elderly men, nor on intraocular pressure and pupillary size, including use with glaucoma patients. Accidental spraying of the eye must be avoided to prevent lens paralysis and pupillary dilatation with blurred vision. Pending release of other quaternary compounds for aerosol use, this agent remains the drug of choice as an inhaled anticholinergic bronchodilator. Ipratropium has also been investigated intranasally to treat vasomotor rhinitis. Cugell (1986) gives a brief but clear review of the clinical pharmacology and toxicology of ipratropium.

A combination product of ipratropium bromide (0.04 mg per puff) and fenoterol (0.1 mg per puff) is marketed in Great Britain as Duovent (Boehringer Ingelheim, Inc.) to provide the additive effect of anticholinergic and beta-adrenergic activity.

Glycopyrrolate, which is a quaternary ammonium derivative of atropine, is usually administered parenterally as an antimuscarinic agent during reversal of neuromuscular blockade, as an alternative to atropine, with fewer ocular or central nervous system side effects. For the same reason, the injectable solution has been nebulized in a 1-mg dose for bronchodilatation. Gal et al. (1984) reported a comparison of glycopyrrolate with atropine and established dose-response curves.

Oxitropium bromide (Ba 235) is a quaternary derivative of scopolamine and has been investigated as an aerosolized anticholinergic bronchodilator in subjects with obstructive airway disease. A 200-μg dose by MDI provided a peak effect on FEV_1 (forced expiratory volume in 1 second) within 1 to 2 hours, with a duration of 6 to 8 hours. Side effects were minimal and consisted of dry mouth and a mildly unpleasant taste. Several references are given on oxitropium: Flohr and Bischoff, 1979; Frith et al., 1986; Skorodin et al., 1986.

CLINICAL APPLICATION

Anticholinergic aerosols have been investigated for use with asthma and with COPD of the bronchitis-emphysema variety. General discussions of the clinical application of anticholinergic agents in asthma and COPD are found in Gross (1987), Gross and Skorodin (1984), and Rebuck et al. (1982).

Use in COPD

Anticholinergic agents were found to be more potent bronchodilators than are beta-adrenergic agents in bronchitis-emphysema, and this is likely to be their primary clinical application. This difference is illustrated in the data from Tashkin et al. (1986) seen in Figure 6–5. In that 90-day, multicenter study, the investigation compared 40 μg of ipratropium with 1.5 mg of metaproterenol, both given by MDI, in a population of patients with COPD. Explanations for the superiority of anticholinergic action in COPD are debated but may relate to the complicated, inflammatory, noncholinergic pathways seen in asthma, especially with antigen-antibody reactions mentioned previously in the section on the vagal reflex mechanism. Conversely, the pathology of COPD may reveal the reason for the superior effect of anticholinergic over beta-adrenergic drugs.

Ipratropium bromide has approval by the Food and Drug Administration

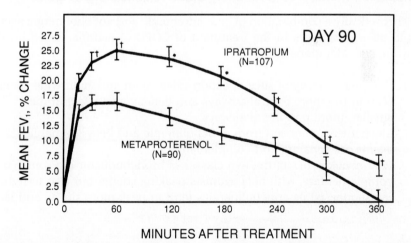

FIG 6–5. The effect of the beta agonist metaproterenol and the anticholinergic ipratropium on FEV_1 in patients with COPD after 90 days of treatment (*,$P < 0.01$; ±, $P < 0.05$). (From Tashkin et al: Comparison of the anticholinergic bronchodilator ipratropium bromide with metaproterenol in chronic obstructive pulmonary disease, Am J Med 1986, 81(suppl 5A):59. Used with permission.)

specifically for use in the treatment of COPD, although the drug is also prescribed for treatment of asthma.

Use in Asthma

Anticholinergic agents such as ipratropium are not clearly superior to beta-adrenergic agents in treating asthma. Anticholinergic and beta-adrenergic agents have an approximately equal effect on flow rates in many patients. The anticholinergic agents offer an additional avenue of pharmacological management in asthma. These agents may be especially useful in the following applications when prescribed for asthmatic patients (Weber, 1990):

1. Nocturnal asthma, where the slightly longer duration of action may protect against nocturnal deterioration of flow rates (Cox et al., 1984).
2. Psychogenic asthma, which may be mediated through vagal parasympathetic fibers.
3. Asthmatic patients with glaucoma, angina, or hypertension who require treatment with beta-blocking agents.
4. As an alternative to theophylline in patients with notable side effects from that drug.

Combination Therapy: Beta-Adrenergic and Anticholinergic Agents

Theoretically a combination of beta-adrenergic and anticholinergic agents should offer advantages in the treatment of COPD or asthma, based on the following considerations:

1. Complementarity of sites of action exists, with anticholinergic effect seen in the more central airways and beta-agonist effect in the smaller, more peripheral airways.
2. Mechanisms of action from anticholinergic and beta-adrenergic agents are separate and complementary.
3. Pharmacokinetics of the two classes of bronchodilator are somewhat complementary, with beta agonists peaking sooner but also terminating sooner, while anticholinergics tend to peak more slowly and last longer.

The last characteristic can result in a more even control of airflow obstruction in COPD or asthma. Other advantages of combined beta-agonist and anticholinergic therapy include a possibly additive effect, reduced individual drug doses, and avoidance of systemic steroid therapy.

Additive Effect of Beta Agonists and Anticholinergic Agents

There are conflicting results on the question of whether the bronchodilator effect of beta agonists is increased by adding an anticholinergic agent. Rebuck and co-workers, in 1987, published the results of a large-sample study on 148 patients with acute asthma and 51 patients with acute COPD in which a combination of nebulized ipratropium (0.5 mg) and fenoterol (1.25 mg) was investigated. In acute asthma, combination therapy was more effective than therapy with either type of agent alone. In acute COPD exacerbation, either agent alone provided bronchodilatation, but there was no added benefit with combination therapy.

Owens and George (1991) found no additional effect when atropine sulfate (2.5 mg nebulized) was combined with metaproterenol (0.3 ml of 5% strength) in 37 patients with acute asthma. This is in conflict with Rebuck's findings with acute asthma. Karpel (1991) also studied the combination of ipratropium and metaproterenol in acute and stable COPD. Her study showed no additional improvement when the second agent was added, regardless of which agent was given first, in both the acute and stable phases. These results agree with Rebuck's findings in acute COPD.

Lightbody and co-workers (1978) found that combined salbutamol (albuterol, 200 µg) and ipratropium (40 µg), both by MDI, gave a greater effect on FEV_1 than either agent alone in 11 patients with stable asthma and 10 patients with COPD. However, Petrie and Palmer (1975) found no increase in effect on FEV_1 with combined salbutamol (200 µg, MDI) and ipratropium (40 µg, MDI) in patients with stable asthma or COPD.

Reasons for Conflicting Results

Assuming that the reported results are valid, several reasons may exist to explain differences in findings with combined beta-adrenergic and anticholinergic therapy.

1. Patients can vary in their responses.
2. Different types of asthma (exercise-induced vs. atopic) may differ in response to these agents.
3. Perhaps there are differences among the anticholinergic agents.

Specifically, in mild asthma, there could be a ceiling effect, with a beta agonist producing near-maximal bronchodilatation and little effect being produced by adding an anticholinergic agent.

Conclusion

Despite conflicting results, the use of anticholinergic agents in combination with beta agonists is theoretically sensible. Empirical trials with appropriate evaluation of effect in individual patients with asthma or COPD is reasonable.

BIBLIOGRAPHY

Barnes PJ: Autonomic control of airway function in asthma, Chest 91(suppl):45S, 1987.

Bleecker ER: Cholinergic and neurogenic mechanisms in obstructive airways disease, Am J Med 81(suppl 5A):2, 1986.

Boushey HA, Gold WM: Anticholinergic drugs. In Middleton E Jr, Reed CE, Ellis EF, eds: Allergy: principles and practice, ed 2, St. Louis, 1983, CV Mosby.

Cavanaugh MJ, Cooper DM: Inhaled atropine sulfate: dose response characteristics, Am Rev Respir Dis 114:517, 1976.

Cox ID, Hughes DTD, McDonnell KA: Ipratropium bromide in patients with nocturnal asthma, Postgrad Med J 60:526, 1984.

Cugell DW: Clinical pharmacology and toxicology of ipratropium bromide, Am J Med 81(suppl 5A):27, 1986.

Fish JE et al: The effect of atropine on acute antigen-mediated airway constriction in subjects with allergic asthma, Am Rev Respir Dis 115:371, 1977.

Flohr E, Bischoff KO: Oxitropium bromide, a new anticholinergic drug, in a dose-response and placebo comparison in obstructive airway diseases, Respiration 38:98, 1979.

Frith PA et al: Oxitropium bromide: dose-response and time-response study of a new anticholinergic bronchodilator drug, Chest 89:249, 1986.

Gal TJ, Suratt PM, Lu J: Glycopyrrolate and atropine inhalation: comparative effects on normal airway function, Am Rev Respir Dis 129:871, 1984.

Gandevia B: Historical review of the use of parasympatholytic agents in the treatment of respiratory disorders. Postgrad Med J 51(suppl 7):13, 1975.

Gross NJ: Anticholinergic agents in COPD, Chest 91(suppl):52S, 1987.

Gross NJ, Skorodin MS: Anticholinergic, antimuscarinic bronchodilators. Am Rev Respir Dis 129:856, 1984.

Hogg JC: The pathophysiology of asthma, Chest 82(suppl):8S, 1982.

Idell S, Kronenberg RS: Drug therapy for chronic obstructive pulmonary disease, Semin Respir Med 8:129, Oct 1986.

Karpel JP: Bronchodilator responses to anticholinergic and beta-adrenergic agents in acute and stable COPD, Chest 99:871, 1991.

Leff A: Pathophysiology of asthmatic bronchoconstriction, Chest 82(suppl):13S, 1982.

Lightbody IM et al: Ipratropium bromide, salbutamol and prednisolone in bronchial asthma and chronic bronchitis, Br J Dis Chest 72:181, 1978.

Mathewson HS: Anticholinergic aerosols, Respir Care 28:467, 1983.

Orehek J, Gayrard P: Atropine effects on antigen-mediated airway constriction, Am Rev Respir Dis 116:792, 1977.

Owens MW, George RB: Nebulized atropine sulfate in the treatment of acute asthma, Chest 99:1084, 1991.

Pak CCF et al: Inhaled atropine sulfate: dose-response characteristics in adult patients with chronic airflow obstruction, Am Rev Respir Dis 125:331, 1982.

Petrie GR, Palmer KNV: Comparison of aerosol ipratropium bromide and salbutamol in chronic bronchitis and asthma, Br Med J 1:430, 1975.

Rebuck AS, Chapman KR, Braude AC: Anticholinergic therapy of asthma, Chest 82(suppl):55S, 1982.

Rebuck AS et al: Nebulized anticholinergic and sympathomimetic treatment of asthma and chronic obstructive airways disease in the emergency room, Am J Med 82:59, 1987.

Simonsson BG, Jacobs FM, Nadel JA: Role of autonomic nervous system and the cough reflex in the increased responsiveness of airways in patients with obstructive airway disease, J Clin Invest 46:1812, 1967.

Skorodin MS et al: Oxitropium bromide: a new anticholinergic bronchodilator, Ann Allergy 56:229, 1986.

Wanner A: Effect of iprotropium bromide on airway mucociliary function, Am J Med 81(suppl 5A):32, 1986.

Weber RW: Role of anticholinergics in asthma, Ann Allergy 65:348, 1990 (editorial).

Ziment I, Au JP: Anticholinergic agents, Clin Chest Med 7:355, 1986.

7

Xanthines

In Chapter 7, xanthine bronchodilators are presented. The drug theophylline and its salt, aminophylline, are found in this class. The following topics are discussed:

- Identification of the xanthine drug group
- General pharmacological properties
- Clinical uses
- Mode of action
- Titration of theophylline doses
- Toxicity and side effects
- Factors affecting theophylline activity
- Clinical application of theophylline
- Summary

In addition to the beta-adrenergic and anticholinergic bronchodilators, there is a third class of bronchodilator—the xanthines. For clinical use, there is only one agent in this class, and that is theophylline. Aminophylline is a salt form of theophylline, which has greater aqueous solubility and can be given intravenously.

IDENTIFICATION

Theophylline is related chemically to the natural metabolite xanthine, which is a precursor of uric acid. Figure 7–1 gives the general xanthine structure, along with that of theophylline (1,3-dimethylxanthine) and caffeine (1,3,7-trimethylxanthine). Because of their methyl attachments, these agents are often referred to as *methylxanthines*. Another xanthine is theobromine. All three agents are found as alkaloids in plant species. Caffeine is found in coffee beans and in colas. Caffeine and theophylline are contained in tea leaves, and caf-

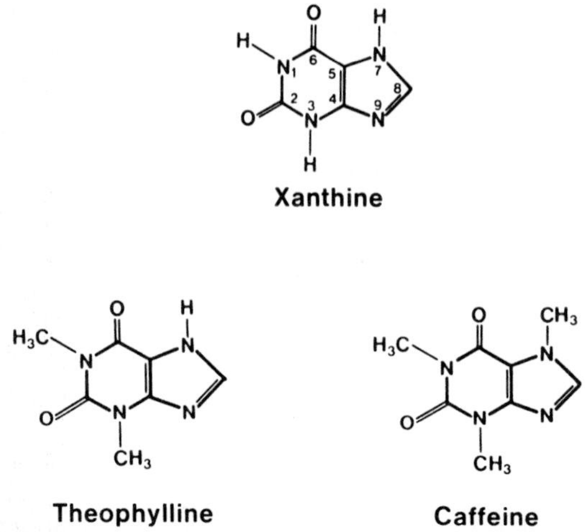

Xanthine

Theophylline   **Caffeine**

FIG 7–1. Chemical structure of xanthine and its methylated derivatives theophylline and caffeine.

feine and theobromine are in cocoa. Historically, these natural plant substances have all been used as brews for their stimulant effect.

Xanthine Derivatives

There are several synthetic modifications to the naturally occurring methylxanthines. These include dyphylline [7-(2,3-dihydroxypropyl theophylline)], proxyphylline [7-(2-hydroxypropyl)-theophylline], and enprofylline (3-propylxanthine).

A comprehensive review of methylxanthines can be found in Hendeles and Weinberger (1983) and Miech and Stein (1986).

GENERAL PHARMACOLOGICAL PROPERTIES

The xanthine group has the following general physiological effects in humans:

- Central nervous system stimulation
- Cardiac muscle stimulation
- Diuresis
- Bronchial, uterine, and vascular smooth muscle relaxation
- Peripheral and coronary vasodilatation
- Cerebral vasoconstriction

Some of the effects seen with xanthines are well known to those who drink caffeinated beverages (coffee, colas, tea). Coffee in particular can be taken for the central nervous system stimulatory effect to remain awake. The diuretic effect after drinking coffee or cola is also well known. Caffeine or theophylline can also cause tachycardia, and the cerebral vasoconstricting effect has been used to treat migraine headaches. A specific agent intended for this use is Cafergot, which contains 100 mg of caffeine and 1 mg of ergotamine tartrate.

Caffeine and theophylline differ in the intensity of the effects listed previously. These differences are summarized below:

Effect	Caffeine	Theophylline
Central nervous system stimulation	+++	++
Cardiac stimulation	+	+++
Smooth muscle relaxation	+	+++
Skeletal muscle stimulation	+++	++
Diuresis	+	+++

Caffeine has more central nervous system stimulating effect than theophylline, and this includes ventilatory stimulation. In clinical use, theophylline is generally classified as a bronchodilator, because of the relaxing effect on bronchial smooth muscle.

CLINICAL USES

Theophylline has traditionally been used in the management of asthma and chronic obstructive pulmonary disease (COPD). Theophylline and caffeine have been used to treat apnea of prematurity, and theophylline is biotransformed to caffeine in neonates (Yeh, 1985). A now-obsolete use of theophylline was as a diuretic.

Theophylline is available in a variety of formulations, including sustained-release oral forms, powder to be sprinkled on food for pediatric use, as aminophylline for intravenous administration, and in rectal suppository forms.

Although theophylline is usually classified as a bronchodilator, it actually has a relatively weak bronchodilating effect compared with the beta agonists. Its therapeutic action in asthma and COPD may occur by other means, such as stimulation of the ventilatory drive or direct strengthening of the diaphragm. Any of these actions could result in the clinical outcome of improved ventilatory flow rates. This is further discussed in the section on clinical application in this chapter.

MODE OF ACTION

Structure-Activity Relations

Figure 7–2 illustrates the general xanthine structure and the effect of attachments at various sites on the molecule. Also, the chemical structure of theophylline is shown in comparison with that of the theophylline derivatives dyphylline and enprofylline. The methyl attachments at the nitrogen-1 and nitrogen-3 positions for theophylline enhance its bronchodilating effect, as well as its toxic side effects, which will be discussed later in this chapter. In contrast, the structure of caffeine (Fig 7–1) has an additional methyl group at the nitrogen-7 position, thereby decreasing its bronchodilator effect in relation to theophylline. Dyphylline has the same methyl attachments at the nitrogen-1 and nitrogen-3 positions as theophylline but also has a large attachment at the nitrogen-7 position that decreases its bronchodilator potential. Enprofylline, which is not clinically available in the United States at this time, has potent bronchodilating effects probably due to the large substitution at the nitrogen-3 position.

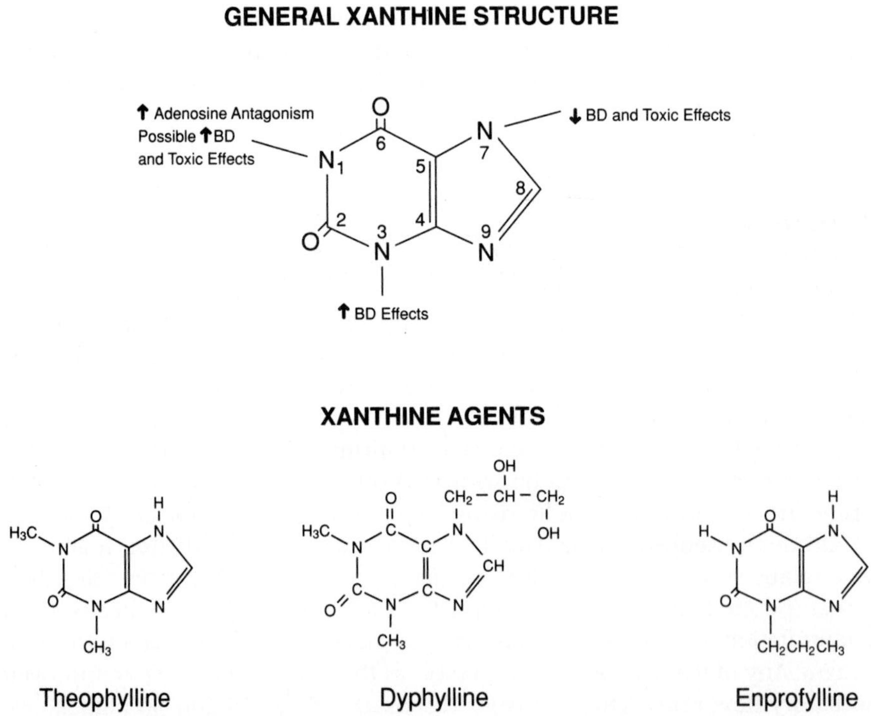

GENERAL XANTHINE STRUCTURE

XANTHINE AGENTS

| Theophylline | Dyphylline | Enprofylline |

FIG 7–2.   Effect of attachments at different sites on the xanthine molecule and comparative illustration of the structures of theophylline, dyphylline, and enprofylline.

Theories of Activity

The exact mechanism of action of the xanthines, and theophylline in particular, is not known. For some years, it was thought that xanthines caused smooth muscle relaxation by inhibition of phosphodiesterase, leading to an increase in intracellular cyclic AMP. An increase in cyclic AMP causes relaxation of bronchial smooth muscle. The effect of increased cyclic AMP was previously described in Chapter 5 when discussing beta-adrenergic agents. However, this explanation is no longer generally accepted to account for therapeutic xanthine actions.

Several alternative theories of action for xanthines have been proposed in addition to phosphodiesterase inhibition. Each of the modes of action proposed for xanthines is briefly described and commented on in the following sections.

Inhibition of Phosphodiesterase.   Theophylline has the capability of inhibiting phosphodiesterase. The pathway by which this inhibition can lead to an increase in intracellular cyclic AMP, with consequent bronchial relaxation, is illustrated in Figure 7–3, *A*. However, at the dosage levels used clinically in humans, theophylline is a poor inhibitor of the enzyme (Persson and Karlsson, 1987). As a result, this is not considered to be an acceptable explanation of how xanthines exert a therapeutic effect.

Antagonism of Adenosine.   An alternative explanation is that theophylline acts by blocking the action of adenosine. This mechanism is illustrated in Figure 7–3, *B*. Adenosine is a purine nucleoside that can stimulate A_1 and A_2 receptors. A_1-Receptor stimulation inhibits cyclic AMP, while A_2-receptor stimulation increases cyclic AMP. Inhaled adenosine has produced bronchoconstriction in asthmatic patients. Theophylline is a potent inhibitor of both A_1 and A_2 receptors and could block smooth muscle contraction mediated by A_1 receptors.

This explanation is contradicted by the action of enprofylline, which is about 5 times more potent than theophylline for relaxing smooth muscle, yet lacks a sufficient attachment at the nitrogen-1 position to provide adenosine antagonism (Jenne, 1987a). This can be seen in Figure 7–2 by comparing the structures of theophylline and enprofylline. In addition, A_1 receptors are sparse in smooth muscle, and isolated animal tissue preparations have actually shown smooth muscle relaxation through adenosine stimulation of the A_2 receptors.

Catecholamine Release.   A third explanation of xanthine action is that these agents cause the production and release of endogenous catecholamines, which in turn could cause muscle tremor, tachycardia, and bronchial relaxation. Studies on plasma levels of catecholamines such as epinephrine have

THEOPHYLLINE: MODES OF ACTION

A

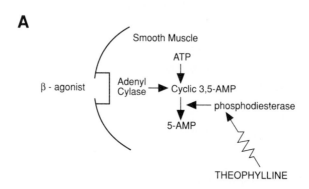

B

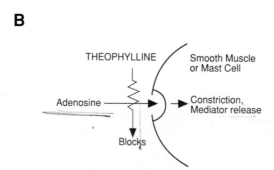

FIG 7–3. Proposed mechanisms of action by which theophylline reverses airway obstruction. **A,** Inhibition of phosphodiesterase. **B,** Antagonism of adenosine.

reported conflicting results, with both an increase and no change reported (Svedmyr, 1987).

Conclusion

There are other theories proposed for how xanthines exert their effects in addition to those just described. Caffeine and theophylline may inhibit calcium uptake by the sarcoplasmic reticulum, thereby relaxing smooth muscle. Xanthines may also antagonize the effects of prostaglandins such as prostaglandin E_2 and prostaglandin $F_{2\alpha}$.

There is no accepted definitive explanation for the action of xanthines to date. It is possible that there are multiple mechanisms involved with the specific agents in this class. For example, theophylline may cause its effect on smooth muscle by antagonism of adenosine receptors (specifically A_1), while enprofylline does so by a different mechanism.

TITRATING THEOPHYLLINE DOSES

In the past, clinical use of the xanthine theophylline, in its many forms, was questioned because of wide variability in its therapeutic effect. It was subsequently found that individuals metabolize theophylline at differing rates, which makes it difficult to determine therapeutic doses. This is complicated further by the fact that different forms of the drug are not always equivalent.

Equivalent Doses of Theophylline Salts

The standard with which salts of theophylline are compared is anhydrous theophylline. Anhydrous theophylline is 100% theophylline. By contrast, salts of theophylline such as oxtriphylline (Choledyl) are not pure theophylline by weight. A 200-mg dose of Choledyl (brand of theophylline) contains approximately 130 mg of theophylline, whereas Theo-Dur (brand of theophylline) is 100% anhydrous theophylline. A 200-mg dose of Choledyl will not give the same amount of theophylline as a 200-mg dose of Theo-Dur.

Outlined below is a partial listing of brands of anhydrous theophylline, its salts and derivatives, and the anhydrous theophylline equivalents (i.e., the equivalent dose of pure theophylline provided by the salts, such as oxtriphylline or aminophylline).

1. Theophylline anhydrous (100% theophylline).
   a. Bronkodyl (Winthrop-Breon).
   b. Elixophyllin (Berlex).
   c. Somophyllin-T (Fisons).
   d. Slo-Phyllin (Rorer).
   e. Theolair (Riker).
   f. Theo-Dur (Key).
   g. Theo-Dur Sprinkle (Key).
   h. Constant-T (Geigy).
   i. Quibron-T/SR (Mead Johnson).
   j. Respbid (Boehringer Ingelheim).
2. Theophylline sodium glycinate (46% theophylline).
   a. Synophylate (Central).
3. Oxtriphylline (choline theophyllinate; 64% theophylline).
   a. Choledyl (Parke-Davis).
4. Aminophylline (theophylline ethylenediamine; 79% theophylline).
   a. Aminophylline (various).
   b. Phyllocontin (Purdue Frederick).

5. Dyphylline (dihydroxypropyl theophylline; not a theophylline).

   a. Lufyllin (Wallace)

Since oxtriphylline is 64% theophylline, a dose equivalent to 100 mg of theophylline anhydrous would be 156 mg of oxtriphylline (100 mg/0.64 = 156 mg). Similarly 127 mg of aminophylline (theophylline ethylenediamine) would be required for equivalency to 100 mg of theophylline anhydrous. It should be noted the dyphylline is not a theophylline but a derivative of theophylline. It does not form theophylline in the body and is about one tenth as potent as theophylline. This is consistent with its structure-activity relation described previously.

Serum Levels of Theophylline

In 1972, Jenne et al. indicated that the optimum serum theophylline level for maximal bronchodilatation in adults was between 10 and 20 μg/ml. The effects associated with a range of serum levels are as follows:

<5 μg/ml: no effects seen.

10–20 μg/ml: therapeutic range.

>20 μg/ml: nausea.

>30 μg/ml: cardiac arrhythmias.

40–45 μg/ml: seizures.

Some prefer a slightly broader range of 8 to 20 μg/ml for the therapeutic range. It is stressed that the ranges listed for toxic effects are general. It is possible for an individual to bypass the nauseous phase of toxicity and immediately enter the seizure phase.

Although there is a dose-related response to higher serum levels of theophylline, there is evidence that the response does not continue at the same rate of increase as levels rise. This is illustrated in Figure 7–4. The improvement in FEV$_1$ (forced expiratory volume in 1 second) tends to flatten above a serum level of 10 to 12 μg/ml, while the toxic effects of theophylline (to be discussed subsequently) tend to increase even within the therapeutic range of 10 to 20 μg/ml (Tashkin, 1987).

Dosage Schedules

Because of the variability in the rate at which individuals metabolize theophylline and the other factors that affect theophylline metabolism and clearance rates, dosage schedules are used to titrate the drug. These schedules are found in the product literature, in references such as *Drug Facts and Comparisons* and the *Physicians' Desk Reference,* and in general pharmacology texts.

Dosage schedules are complicated by the age of the patient, whether previous theophylline doses were taken, whether the situation is acute or chronic, and whether the dose is a loading dose or for maintenance of serum levels.

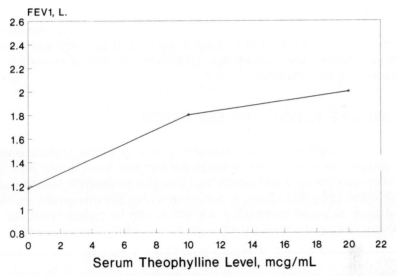

FIG 7–4. Illustration of the decreasing rate of improvement with theophylline levels above 10 μg/ml, even though levels may be in the therapeutic range of 10 to 20 μg/ml. (Based on Tashkin DP: Measurement and significance of the bronchodilator response. In Jenne JW, Murphy S, eds: Drug therapy for asthma. Research and clinical practice, New York, 1987, Marcel Dikker.)

To rapidly metabolize theophylline, the patient may be given an oral loading dose of 5 mg/kg, **provided** the patient was not previously receiving theophylline. This dose is based on anhydrous theophylline. Lean body weight should be used in calculating theophylline doses, since theophylline does not distribute into fatty tissue. In titrating the dose, each 0.5 mg/kg dose of theophylline given as a loading dose will result in a serum level of approximately 1 μg/ml. If theophylline was taken previously by the patient, a serum theophylline level should be measured if at all possible.

For chronic therapy, a slow titration is helpful, with an initial dose of 16 mg/kg per 24 hours or 400 mg/24 hr, whichever is less. These dosages may need to be modified in the presence of factors such as age (younger children vs. the elderly), congestive heart disease, or liver disease. The effect of these factors on serum theophylline levels and on dosage will be discussed subsequently.

Dosage of theophylline can be guided by the clinical reaction of the patient, or better, by measurement of serum drug levels. Without a serum drug level, the dose of theophylline should be based on the benefit provided and should be reduced if the patient experiences toxic side effects.

When monitoring serum theophylline levels, take the sample at the time of peak absorption of the drug, that is, 1 to 2 hours after administration for immediate-release forms and 5 to 9 hours following the morning dose for sustained-release forms.

The previous examples of dosage schedules are by no means complete for all situations; they are intended only as an example of such schedules and of the complexity involved in treating patients with theophylline. Complete tables for different ages and clinical applications should be consulted when administering theophylline.

THEOPHYLLINE TOXICITY AND SIDE EFFECTS

An unfortunate and important problem with use of theophylline is its narrow therapeutic margin. This refers to the fact that there is very little difference between the dose and serum level that give therapeutic benefit and that which cause toxic side effects. In fact, even within the therapeutic serum levels of 10 to 20 μg/ml, distressing side effects can be experienced. The most common adverse reactions usually seen with theophylline are listed below:

Central Nervous System	Gastrointestinal	Respiratory	Cardiovascular	Renal
Headache	Nausea	Tachypnea	Palpitations	Diuresis
Anxiety	Vomiting		Supraventricular	
Restlessness	Anorexia		tachycardia	
Isomnia	Abdominal pain		Ventricular	
Tremor	Diarrhea		arrhythmias	
Convulsions	Hematemesis		Hypotension	
	Gastroesophageal reflux			

Gastric upset, headache, anxiety, and nervousness are not unusual as less toxic side effects of theophylline and can result in loss of schooltime or workdays. The diuretic effect should be noted in patients with excess airway secretions (e.g., patients with bronchitis or cystic fibrosis), with adequate fluid replacement when necessary to prevent dehydration and thickening of secretions.

Reactions to levels of theophylline can also be unpredictable from patient to patient. In a review by Kelly (1987) on theophylline toxicity, studies were cited in which the reported serum levels of 78.5 and 104.8 μg/ml caused only gastrointestinal symptoms, while mean levels of 35 μg/ml caused cardiac arrhythmias or seizures. Also, there may be little warning from minor side effects before serious toxic effects such as arrhythmias or seizures occur.

FACTORS AFFECTING THEOPHYLLINE ACTIVITY

Theophylline is metabolized in the liver and eliminated by the kidneys. Any condition that affects these organs can affect theophylline levels in the body. There are also a number of interactions between other drugs and theophylline that can affect serum levels of the drug. Some of the common drugs and conditions that increase or decrease theophylline levels are listed below:

Increase	Decrease
Beta-blocking agents	Barbiturates
Calcium channel blockers	Beta agonists
Cimetidine, ranitidine	Rifampin
Corticosteroids	Phenytoin
Ephedrine	Cigarette smoking
Influenza virus vaccine	
Mexilitine	
Quinolones	
Hepatitis	
Cirrhosis	
Congestive heart failure	
Pneumonia	
Renal failure	

Viral hepatitis or left ventricular failure can cause elevated serum levels of theophylline for a given dose because of decreased liver metabolism of the drug. An opposite effect of decreased serum levels is caused by cigarette smoking, which stimulates the production of liver enzymes that inactivate the methylxanthines (Powell et al., 1978). This necessitates higher theophylline doses. Some drugs used for treatment of tuberculosis, such as isoniazid, and the loop diuretics, such as furosemide (Lasix) or bumetanide (Bumex), are unpredictable in their effect and may either increase or decrease theophylline levels. Measurement of serum levels is extremely important when using these agents with theophylline.

The beta agonists and theophylline have an additive effect and are often combined when treating patients with asthma or COPD. Theophylline may antagonize the sedative effect of the benzodiazepines (Valium and others). Theophylline can also reverse the paralyzing effect of the nondepolarizing neuromuscular blocking agents (pancuronium, atracurium) in a dose-dependent manner. This is important to realize when paralyzing patients with severe asthma to facilitate ventilatory support and when intravenous administration of aminophylline is used.

CLINICAL APPLICATION

Theophylline, together with beta-sympathomimetic agents, has provided a first-line drug treatment for asthma in the United States. Aminophylline by aerosol has been tried unsuccessfully in asthmatic subjects (Stewart and

Block, 1976). The aerosol is irritating to the pharynx, has a bitter taste, and can cause coughing and wheezing. The oral form of aminophylline, usually in sustained-release preparations, is prescribed for maintenance therapy in chronic, moderate asthma, and intravenous aminophylline is given during acute episodes. Corticosteroids are added to the drug regimen in severe asthma. The use of theophylline (or aminophylline) during acute, severe asthmatic episodes is not usually questioned. However, in mild asthma, theophylline may not be a wise choice for daily maintenance because of its narrow therapeutic margin and side effects. Aerosolized corticosteroids and cromolyn sodium are becoming more acceptable in the United States as first-line drugs for maintenance therapy because of safety and efficacy. A critical viewpoint on the discontinuation of theophylline as a first-line maintenance drug in asthma is well discussed by Marks (1987).

The symptoms of exercise-induced asthma may be controlled better with inhaled sympathomimetic agents before activity, on a p.r.n. basis, than with continual theophylline. Alternatively, cromolyn sodium offers freedom from side effects, if it is effective for a patient.

Theophylline has been combined with expectorants, such as potassium iodide and glyceryl guaiacolate (an emollient), with possible mucolytic and expectorant side effects.

Because of side effects in the gastrointestinal system, xanthines are contraindicated in subjects with active peptic ulcer or acute gastritis. Suppositories should not be used if the rectum or lower colon is irritated. If stomach upset occurs with theophylline, the drug may be taken with food. Ingestion of large amounts of caffeine from other sources such as tea or coffee may precipitate side effects when taking theophylline.

Discussions of the clinical use of theophylline in disease states can be found in Idell and Kronenberg, 1986; Isles et al, 1982; Jenne, 1987b; and Webb-Johnson and Andrews, 1977.

Nonbronchodilating Effects of Theophylline

The use of theophylline in COPD is debated since many patients with COPD do not demonstrate reversibility of obstruction. However, a simple screening pulmonary function test for reversibility of obstruction in patients with COPD provides a rational basis for using theophylline. In addition, the nonbronchodilating effects of theophylline may be helpful in both COPD and asthma. Although theophylline is classified as a bronchodilator, it actually has a relatively weak bronchodilating action. The efficacy of theophylline in obstructive lung disease may be due to its nonbronchodilating effects on ventilation. This concept of the effectiveness of theophylline is consistent with the finding of significant clinical improvement despite little increase in expiratory flow rates in asthmatic patients (Supinski, 1987). Mahler et al. (1985) documented the effect of theophylline in reducing dyspnea in COPD subjects, when there was no reversibility of obstruction and no objective improvement in lung function, gas exchange, or exercise performance capability. The non-bronchodilating effects of theophylline include the following:

Respiratory Muscle Strength. Theophylline can increase the force of respiratory muscle contractility, and this effect is thought to inhibit or even reverse muscle fatigue and subsequent ventilatory failure. Theophylline can have the same effect on limb skeletal muscle. Aubier and coworkers (1981) demonstrated increased diaphragmatic strength and transdiaphragmatic pressure generation by using electromyographic stimuli before and after theophylline administration.

Respiratory Muscle Endurance. Methylxanthines also show evidence of increasing respiratory muscle endurance, as well as strength. This can prevent fatigue of the respiratory muscles, especially with an increased resistance. Xanthines have been shown to increase the time that an external inspiratory load could be sustained (Supinski, 1987).

Central Ventilatory Drive. The methylxanthines have also been shown to increase ventilatory drive at the level of the central nervous system. In particular, theophylline can increase phrenic nerve activity for a given level of chemical stimulus (Aubier, 1981). This effect on ventilatory drive seems to occur at the level of the midbrain and may involve the neurotransmitter dopamine.

SUMMARY

The effects on respiratory muscle function and the ventilatory stimulus response could be as important or even more important than the bronchodilating action of xanthines. Such effects would be complementary to the bronchodilating action of beta agonists and anticholinergic bronchodilators in managing COPD and asthma. As the structure-activity relations of the xanthines are better understood, it is hoped that new analogues may prove effective in preserving ventilatory function, while eliminating the troublesome side effects and the narrow therapeutic margin associated with current forms.

BIBLIOGRAPHY

Aubier M et al: Aminophylline improves diaphragmatic contractility, N Engl J Med 305:249, 1981.

Becker AB et al: The bronchodilator effects and pharmacokinetics of caffeine in asthma, N Engl J Med 310:743, 1984.

Bleecker ER: Cholinergic and neurogenic mechanisms in obstructive airways disease, Am J Med 81(suppl 5A):2, 1986.

Hendeles L, Weinberger M: Theophylline. In Middleton E, Reed CE, Ellis EF, eds: Allergy: principles and practice, vol 1, St Louis, 1983, CV Mosby.

Holgate ST, Mann JS, Cushley MJ: Adenosine as a bronchoconstrictor mediator in asthma and its antagonism by methylxanthines, J Allergy Clin Immunol 74:302, 1984.

Idell S, Kronenberg RS: Drug therapy for chronic obstructive pulmonary disease, Semin Respir Med 8:129, Oct 1986.

Isles AF, MacLeod SM, Levison H: Theophylline: new thoughts about an old drug, Chest 82(suppl):49S, 1982.

Jenne JW: Physiology and pharmacodynamics of the xanthines. In Jenne JW, Murphy S, eds: Drug therapy for asthma. Research and clinical practice, New York, 1987a, Marcel Dikker.

Jenne JW: Theophylline as a bronchodilator in COPD and its combination with inhaled β-adrenergic drugs, Chest 92(suppl):7S, 1987b.

Jenne JW, Murphy S, eds: Drug therapy for asthma. Research and Clinical Practice, New York, 1987, Marcel Dikker.

Jenne JW et al: Pharmacokinetics of theophylline: application to adjustment of the clinical dose of aminophylline, Clin Pharmacol Ther 13:349, 1972.

Kelly HW: Theophylline toxicity. In Jenne JW, Murphy S, eds: Drug therapy for asthma. Research and clinical practice, New York, 1987, Marcel Dikker.

Mahler DA et al: Sustained-release theophylline reduces dyspnea in nonreversible obstructive airway disease, Am Rev Respir Dis 131:22, 1985.

Marks HB: Theophylline: primary or tertiary drug? A brief review. Ann Allergy 59:85, 1987.

Miech RP, Stein M: Methylxanthines, Clin Chest Med 7:331, 1986.

Persson CGA, Karlsson J: In vitro responses to bronchodilator drugs, In Jenne JW, Murphy S, eds: Drug therapy for asthma. Research and clinical practice, New York: 1987, Marcel Dikker.

Powell JR et al: Theophylline disposition in acutely ill hospitalized patients: the effect of smoking, heart failure, severe airway obstruction and pneumonia. Am Rev Respir Dis 118:229, 1978.

Stewart BN, Block AJ: A trial of aerosolized theophylline in relieving bronchospasm, Chest 69:718, 1976.

Supinski GS: Effects of methylxanthines on respiratory skeletal muscle and neural drive. In Jenne JW, Murphy S, eds: Drug therapy for asthma. Research and clinical practice, New York, 1987, Marcel Dikker.

Svedmyr N: Theophylline. Am Rev Respir Dis 136(suppl):568, Oct 1987.

Tashkin DP: Measurement and significance of the bronchodilator response. In Jenne JW, Murphy S, eds: Drug therapy for asthma. Research and clinical practice, New York, 1987, Marcel Dikker.

Webb-Johnson DC, Andrews JL Jr: Bronchodilator therapy. II. N Engl J Med 297:758, 1977.

Yeh TF: Drug therapy in the neonate and small infant, Chicago, 1985, Year Book Medical Publishers.

Ziment I, Au JP: Anticholinergic agents, Clin Chest Med 7:355, 1986.

8

Mucus-Controlling Agents

Chapter 8 considers drugs intended to affect the secretion of respiratory mucus. The agent approved for general aerosol administration in this class is acetylcysteine (Mucomyst). Recombinant human deoxyribonuclease (rhDNase) is under investigation for aerosol use. The clinical use of these agents is to treat diseases involving mucus hypersecretion. The major topics presented are the following:

- Perspective on drug control of mucus
- Physiological characteristics of mucus production
- Nature of mucus secretion
- Mucus-controlling agents

INTRODUCTION

One of the themes of respiratory care pharmacology is airway patency, accomplished through smooth muscle relaxation, control of pulmonary secretions, and decongestion. The sympathomimetic (beta-adrenergic), parasympatholytic (anticholinergic), and xanthine agents previously considered have all been targeted at relaxation of bronchial smooth muscle. Dysfunctional mucus production and regulation of mucus in the respiratory tract play a major part in the pathogenesis of diseases such as chronic and acute bronchitis, asthma, bronchiectasis, and cystic fibrosis. In this chapter, agents that affect respiratory mucus will be considered.

DRUG CONTROL OF MUCUS: A PERSPECTIVE

One of the major defense mechanisms of the lung is the self-renewing, self-cleansing mucociliary escalator. Failure of this system results in mechanical obstruction of the airway, often with thickened, adhesive secretions. In many diseases associated with abnormal mucociliary function (e.g., bronchitis, asthma, and cystic fibrosis), a marked slowing of mucous transport is noted (Denton et al., 1968; Sackner, 1978). Whether such slowing is due to changes in the physical properties of mucus or to decreased ciliary activity, or both, is not clear. Recently, knowledge has been growing concerning the complex substance that is mucus, the physicochemical nature of mucus, and the physiological regulation of mucus in the body. Mucus is found in several areas of the body, including the lung, stomach, eye, and female genital tract. Regardless of its location, mucus seems to serve protective purposes, especially in the lungs: lubrication, waterproofing, and protection against osmotic changes.

Historically in respiratory care, drug therapy for secretions has been aimed at liquefying thick, viscous mucus to a thin, watery state. It is now recognized that mucus is a gel with complex physical properties of viscosity *and* elasticity. Drug therapy for mucous secretions in acute and chronic bronchitis, asthma, respiratory infections, and cystic fibrosis should optimize the physical state of the mucus gel for efficient ciliary transport. This can mean lowering viscosity without destroying elasticity in some cases. As a result, the term *mucolytic*, indicating breakdown of mucus, could better be replaced with *mucus-controlling agent*. Although acetylcysteine, which is a mucolytic, is the only drug in this group approved for aerosol administration, the development of mucus-controlling drugs is desired. The subsequent review of mucus physiology presents the concepts necessary for discussing the current and future pharmacological management of secretions. The amount of this chapter devoted to understanding the production, nature, and regulation of respiratory mucus reflects the current situation in which the knowledge of airway mucus has outstripped the development of therapies, including pharmacological, for control of secretion dysfunction.

PHYSIOLOGICAL CHARACTERISTICS OF MUCUS PRODUCTION

Source of Respiratory Mucus and Related Terminology

The conducting airways in the lung and the nasal cavity to the oropharynx are lined with a mucociliary system (Fig 8–1). Cell types responsible for secretion in the airway and the source of components found in respiratory mucus have been summarized by Basbaum and associates (1988). Although there are many cell types in the mammalian airway, the essential secretory structures of the mucociliary system are the following:
1. Surface epithelial cells.
   a. Pseudostratified, columnar, ciliated epithelial cells.
   b. Surface goblet (or surface secretory) cells.
   c. Clara cells.
2. Subepithelial cells.
   a. Submucosal gland, with serous and mucous cells.

CROSS-SECTION, BRONCHIOLE WALL

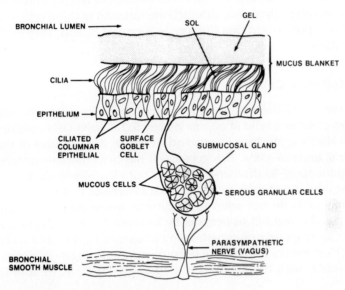

FIG 8-1. Mucociliary system in the lung.

The secretion lining the surface of the airway is termed *mucus* and consists of two physical phases: (1) a *gel* that is propelled upward toward the larynx by the cilia; and (2) a thin, watery, proteinaceous *sol* layer in which the cilia beat. The terminology of Reid and Clamp (1978) is used in referring to respiratory secretions.

Mucus: Total secretion from goblet cells and submucosal glands. The purified glycoprotein from mucus is termed *mucus glycoprotein* or *mucin* (Basbaum, 1991).

Sputum: Expectorated secretion that contains oropharyngeal and nasopharyngeal secretions in addition to the bronchial components mentioned. Saliva is also present in sputum. As a result, sputum and mucus do not represent the same secretion.

Gel: Portion of mucus that possesses a structure due to intermolecular attractions of its long glycoprotein chains and that possesses the physical properties of viscosity and elasticity.

Sol: That part of the mucous secretion in true solution. The sol layer has little elasticity but does possess viscosity.

The nature of mucus and the meaning of its physical properties will be presented subsequently.

Goblet cells and submucosal glands are found in cartilaginous airways, down to the terminal bronchioles. Beyond the distal airways, these mucus-producing cells are not found. Clara cells do exist in terminal bronchioles and possess a secretory structure, although the function of these cells is unknown. It has been hypothesized that Clara cells, reported in 1937, may be the source of the sol layer.

Surface Epithelial Cells

The surface of the trachea and bronchi includes primarily ciliated cells and goblet cells, in a ratio of approximately 5:1. Goblet cells contain granules of mucus that are electron lucent and resemble the granules of the submucosal gland mucous cells. The goblet cell has a membrane surface that dehisces (splits open) to discharge granules onto the airway surface. There are approximately 6,800 goblet cells per square millimeter of normal airway mucosa. Goblet cells do not seem to be directly innervated in human lung, although they do respond to irritants by increasing the production of mucus, and they may respond to sympathomimetic agents. Figures 8–2 and 8–3 show scanning electron micrographs of the mucous lining (Fig 8–2) and of the bronchiolar surface with the mucus stripped away (Fig 8–3). In addition to cili-

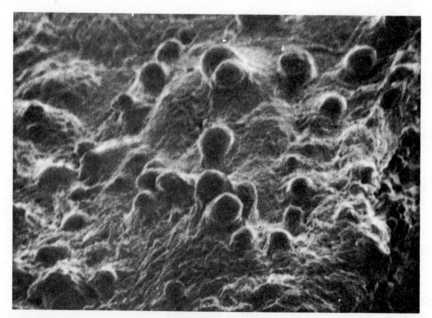

FIG 8–2.   Scanning electron micrograph of the mucous blanket in a bronchiole, prepared from hamster lung. (From Nowell JA and Tyler WS: Scanning electron microscopy of the surface morphology of mammalian lungs, Am Rev Respir Dis 103:313, 1971. Used by permission.)

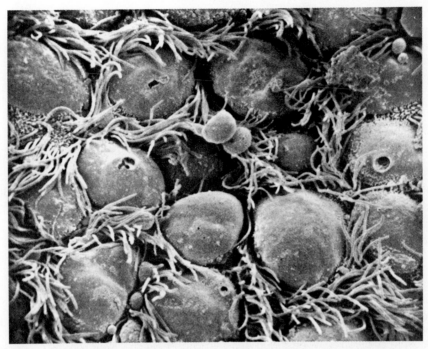

FIG 8–3. Scanning electron micrograph of the airway surface shows epithelial cells with cilia, possible surface goblet cells dehiscing, and some microvilli. (From Nowell JA and Tyler WS: Am Rev Respir Dis 103:313, 1971. Used by permission.)

ated and goblet cells, microvilli, which may have a reabsorptive function, can be seen in Figure 8–3.

Subepithelial Cells

Submucosal glands below the epithelial surface provide the majority of mucous secretion, having a total volume around 40 times greater than that of goblet cells. The submucosal gland is under parasympathetic (vagal) control and responds to cholinergic stimulation by increasing the amount of mucus secreted. There is also evidence suggesting that submucosal glands in the respiratory tract are innervated by sympathetic axons and the nonadrenergic-noncholinergic nerve system described previously in Chapter 4.

Two types of cells, mucous and serous, are found in the gland. Figure 8–4 shows an electron micrograph of human mucous cells, with electron-lucent granules *(mg)*. These granules contain an acid glycoprotein similar to that of the surface goblet cell. Serous cells in the submucosal gland are seen in Figure 8–5. This cell type contains electron-dense secretory granules *(sg)*, with a neutral glycoprotein. The secretions from the two cells mix in the sub-

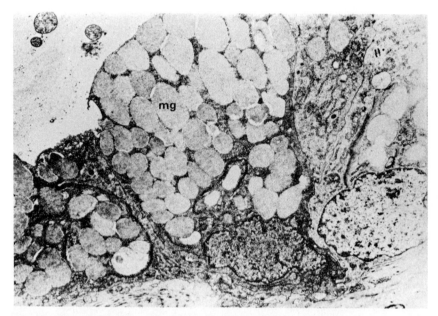

FIG 8–4. Mucus cells with electron-lucent granules *(mg)* from human bronchial submucosal gland. (From Jones R and Reid L: Br Med Bull 34:9, 1978; and Meyrick BE. In Elstein M and Parke DV, eds: *Mucus in health and disease.* New York, 1977, Plenum Press. Used by permission.)

mucosal gland and are transported through a ciliated duct onto the airway lumen.

Ciliary System

Droplets of mucus from the secretory cells described form plaques or "flakes" that coalesce into clumps to be transported by the cilia. It may be that the mucous flakes are stagnant for a short time before being propelled and that the watery sol layer separates from the upper viscoelastic layer. Regardless of the source of the sol layer, mucociliary transport results from the movement of the mucus gel by the beating cilia. There are approximately 200 cilia per cell, each cilium is 2 to 5 μm in length, and the cilia beat around 1200 to 1300 times per minute, allowing the mucus flakes to travel as much as a mile per week. Cilia beat in a metachronal fashion, referring to the property by which adjacent cilia beat in coordination to produce a wave of motion.

Factors Affecting Mucociliary Transport

The rate of mucociliary transport varies in the normal lung and has been estimated at around 1.5 mm/min in peripheral airways and 21.5 mm/min in

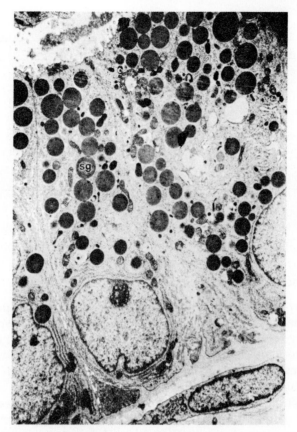

FIG 8−5. Serous cells with electron-dense granules *(sg)* from human bronchial submucosal gland. (From Jones R and Reid L: Br Med Bull 34:9, 1978; and Meyrick B and Reid L: J Cell Biol 67:320, 1975. Used by permission.)

the trachea. Transport rates are slower in the presence of the following conditions or substances:

- At age 56 or older
- In chronic obstructive pulmonary disease (COPD)
- General anesthetics
- Parasympatholytics (atropine)
- Narcotics
- Endotracheal suctioning and tracheostomy
- Cigarette smoke
- Atmospheric pollutants (SO2, NO2, ozone)
- Hyperoxia and hypoxia

TABLE 8-1.

Effects of Various Drug Groups on Mucociliary Clearance

Drug Group	Ciliary Beat	Mucous Production	Transport
Beta adrenergic	Increase	Possible increase*	Increase
Cholinergic	Increase	Increase	Increase
Methylxanthines	Increase	Increase	Increase
Cromolyn sodium	None	None	None
Corticosteroid (beclomethasone)	None	None	None
Prostaglandin E₁†	Variable	Increase plus lysis	Increase

*Wanner (1977)
†Iravani and Melville (1975)

Table 8-1 summarizes the effects of drug groups commonly used in respiratory care on ciliary beat, mucous output, and overall transport.

Milk Intake and Mucus Production

A common belief is that drinking dairy milk increases the production of mucus, or phlegm, and congestion in the respiratory tract. Respiratory care personnel may be asked for advice on withholding milk from children with colds, respiratory infections, or chronic respiratory conditions such as cystic fibrosis. Pinnock et al. (1990) innoculated 60 healthy subjects with rhinovirus-2 in a study designed to answer the question, Does milk make mucus? Milk intake ranged from 0 to 11 glasses a day. They reported no association between milk or dairy product intake and an increase in upper or lower respiratory tract symptoms of congestion or in nasal secretion weight. There was a trend for cough to be loose with increasing intake of milk, although this was not significant at a 5% level. None of the subjects was allergic to cow's milk. The authors concluded that the data do not support the withholding of milk or the belief that milk increases respiratory tract congestion.

NATURE OF MUCOUS SECRETION

A healthy person produces around 100 ml of mucus per 24 hours, and the secretion is clear, viscoelastic, and adhesive, with a variable thickness of 2 to 5 μm. Apparently most of this secretion is reabsorbed in the bronchial mucosa, with only 10 ml or so reaching the glottis. This amount is rarely noticed by the individual. During disease states, the volume of secretions can increase dramatically, and the secretions are expectorated or swallowed. One of the primary functions of respiratory tract mucus is thought to be transporting and removing trapped inhaled particles, cellular debris, or dead and aging cells.

Structure and Composition of Mucus

The structure and major constituents of the mucus secreted by the submucosal glands and surface goblet cells are pictured in Figure 8–6 and have been reviewed in Basbaum (1991). Basbaum et al. (1988) and Lundgren and Shelhamer (1990) also provide summaries of the composition and structure of mucus.

Mucus is actually a complex, high-molecular-weight macromolecule consisting of a polypeptide (protein) backbone formed by a string of amino acids to which carbohydrate (also termed *oligosaccharide*) side chains are attached. The carbohydrate content is 80% or more of the total weight of the macromolecule. This structure has been linked to a test tube brush in appearance. This general structure of protein and attached saccharide side chains is termed a *glycoprotein.* Mucus forms a flexible, threadlike strand, 200 to 1000

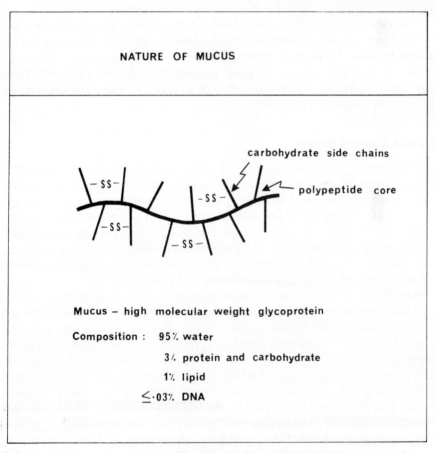

FIG 8–6. Basic structure and constituents of the mucous macromolecule.

nm in length, that is internally cross-linked with disulfide (—S—S—) bonds. Strands can be further cross-linked with each other by disulfide and hydrogen bonding. The result is a gel that consists of a high water content (approximately 95%) organized around the structural elements and that is intensely hydrophilic and spongelike (Lopez-Vidriero, 1981; Matthews et al, 1963). The final gelation of mucus is probably due to a combination of hydrogen, electrostatic and hydrophobic bonds, and the specific disulfide linkages.

Under normal circumstances, bonding within mucus produces low viscosity but high elasticity. Although mucus gel incorporates water during its formation, a gel is both a liquid and a solid, as will be discussed in a later section. A better analogy is Jell-O, which is mostly water but organizes into a semisolid by its chemical structure as the liquid "gels." It is important clinically to note that sufficient water must be available in the body to form mucus with normal physical properties, but once formed, mucus does not readily incorporate topically applied water (Dulfano et al., 1973).

In addition to the mucus gel secreted in the airway, bronchial secretions contain other substances such as serum proteins (albumin, secretory IgA immunoglobulins, alpha$_1$-antitrypsin, complement components), lysozyme, lactoferrin, and electrolytes (sodium, potassium, chloride, calcium). These electrolytes are important for hydration of mucus and water transport in the surface epithelium of the airway.

Mucus in Disease States

The normal clearance function of respiratory mucus can be altered by changes in the volume, hydration, or composition of the secretion (water, salts, protein, glycoconjugates). The volume is due to the production by surface goblet cells and submucosal gland cells. Water content is a function of transepithelial chloride secretion and osmosis. The composition of respiratory mucus is undergoing investigation by using molecular cloning techniques (Basbaum, 1991) that can reveal the structure of the varied mucin oligosaccharides, as well as the regulation of mucin synthesis and production.

Knowledge of these features of respiratory mucus may lead to a better understanding of the common diseases characterized by an abnormal production of mucus. The following diseases are characterized by mucus hypersecretion: chronic bronchitis, asthma, cystic fibrosis, and acute bronchitis. Acute bronchitis may be superimposed on any of the first three diseases. Mucus hypersecretion predisposes to bacterial infections in the bronchial tree in chronic bronchitis, asthma, or cystic fibrosis probably because of impaired clearance of mucus from the bronchi. During infection, deoxyribonucleic acid (DNA) from white cell debris changes mucus from clear to opaque. A green or yellow sputum is caused by the enzyme myeloperoxidase, seen with cellular breakdown, and indicates retained secretions (Hodgkin, 1979). In general, under pathologic conditions, these changes produce differences in the physical properties of mucus. Viscosity increases, ciliary motion is slowed or stopped, and stasis can result in mucus impaction. Bronchial obstruction by secretions can increase airflow resistance and lead to complete airway obstruction and atelectasis (Lundgren and Shelhamer, 1990).

Chronic Bronchitis

Chronic bronchitis is defined clinically by the amount of sputum produced, reflecting mucus hypersecretion. Histologic examination will show inflammatory changes in the airway, with hyperplasia of submucosal glands and goblet cells. The number of goblet cells increases, and there is hypertrophy of the submucosal glands, as measured by the Reid index of gland to airway wall thickness ratio (Reid, 1960). Submucosal glands from patients with chronic bronchitis produce excessive amounts of mucus when studied in vitro (Sturgen and Reid, 1972). Tobacco smoke is considered the most common predisposing factor to airway irritation and mucus hypersecretion, but other factors include viral infections, pollutants, and genetic predisposition such as immotile cilia syndrome (Lundgren and Shelhamer, 1990).

Asthma

Mucus hypersecretion can occur during an acute asthmatic episode or can be a chronic feature of asthma accompanying airway inflammation. In acute episodes, Shimura et al. (1988) estimated 8% of patients will have bronchorrhea, discharging more than 100 ml of sputum per day. As many as 80% of patients report sputum production (Turner-Warwick and Openshaw, 1987).

Cystic Fibrosis

Cystic fibrosis is characterized by impaired function of the exocrine glands, including airway glands and pancreas. The earlier term for cystic fibrosis was *mucoviscidosis*, describing well the hyperviscosity of airway secretions. The abnormal viscosity is caused by impaired chloride ion secretion from inside the airway epithelium to the lumen. Sodium is then drawn from secretions on the airway surface and into the epithelial cells, resulting in dehydration and viscous mucus. Impaired clearance predisposes to respiratory infections. Acute and chronic infections generate cycles of inflammatory changes, chronic mucus hypersecretion, secretion stasis, airway obstruction, and further infection.

Physical Properties of Mucus

As previously stated, the biochemical characteristics of mucus determine its physical properties, which influence the efficiency of the mucociliary interaction and resulting transport. In the mucociliary system, two general types of forces can occur: adhesive and cohesive.

Adhesive Forces.   Adhesion in general refers to forces between **unlike molecules.** In the airway, adhesive forces refer to the attractive and frictional forces between the gel phase and the aqueous sol or airway surface. The clinical importance of adhesive forces in affecting mucous transport is not clear. It is less clear how current mucolytics alter such forces.

Cohesive Forces.   Cohesion refers to forces between **like molecules.** Cohesive forces result from the cross-linking in the mucus macromolecule previously described and give the so-called rheologic properties of viscosity and elasticity seen with a gel. These terms are defined as follows:

Rheology: Study of the deformation and flow of matter. The rheologic behavior of mucus is the way it responds to forces by *deforming* and/or *flowing.*

Viscosity: Measure of the resistance of a fluid to flow. More specifically, viscosity is the proportionality constant (ratio) of applied force to rate of flow.

Elasticity: Measure of the ability of a deformed material to return to its original shape. Ideal elastic solids store all of the energy or force during deformation, and this energy is available when the force is removed.

Figure 8–7 illustrates the concept of viscosity (a property of fluids) and of elasticity (a property of solids). Denton et al. (1968) gives a clear discussion of such properties in their application to mucus.

VISCOSITY AND ELASTICITY

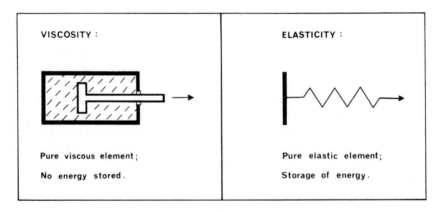

FIG 8–7.   Illustration of concepts of viscosity and elasticity.

Mucus as a Viscoelastic Material

The mucous gel is a viscoelastic material and therefore behaves partially as a fluid and partially as a solid. As a solid, gel has elastic deformation under applied force, and as a liquid, gel flows under applied force. Cilia supply the force. As the tips of the cilia contact the gel during the forward power stroke, the gel is stretched and its elastic recovery causes it to snap forward. At the same time, the mucus gel flows forward as a liquid under the forward beat of the cilia.

This model of gel transport is seen in Figure 8–8, using unvulcanized rub-

VISCOELASTIC SUBSTANCE (unvulcanized rubber)

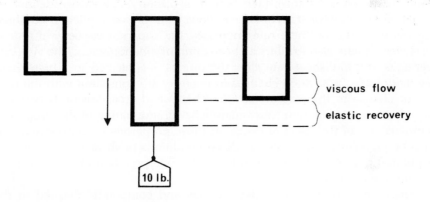

MUCUS : A VISCOELASTIC SUBSTANCE :

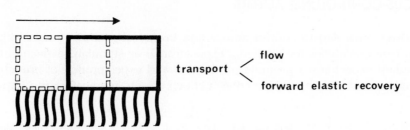

FIG 8–8. Illustration of the viscous and elastic properties affecting the movement of viscoelastic substances such as unvulcanized rubber and mucus.

ber as an example of a viscoelastic substance. If such a rubber strip is loaded on one end with a weight and allowed to hang, it would stretch instantaneously as an elastic solid. If the weight (applied force) remains, the strip will elongate very slowly due to its viscosity (i.e., the rubber would "flow"). After removing the weight, the rubber recovers the elastic elongation because of the stored energy, but will not recover the length due to flow. Mucus behaves similarly. Mucociliary transport results from both flow and forward elastic recovery. For this reason, the physical properties of viscosity and elasticity are extremely important for efficient and adequate transport of respiratory secretions. In general, normal mucus has a relatively low viscosity, and its elasticity is high enough to provide forward propulsive energy.

Non-Newtonian Nature of Mucus

Evaluation of the properties of mucus is complicated by the fact that mucus exhibits non-Newtonian viscosity. In an ideal Newtonian liquid, the proportion of applied force to rate of flow remains constant with changing force. A non-Newtonian substance, such as mucus, has *varying* viscosity (defined as the proportionality constant of force to flow) with varying applied force (shear rate). As the force, or shear rate, increases, the apparent viscosity of mucus decreases. Mucus also exhibits a shear-thinning phenomenon: The viscosity decreases at a low shear rate *after* the mucus is subjected to a high shear rate (Lourenco, 1973). Such changes in viscosity are consistent with the rupture or change in the macromolecular chains and cross-linking network of the gel. Because of its non-Newtonian behavior, evaluation of the properties of mucus and of the effect of drugs on those properties is complicated and must be performed under standardized conditions of shear rate. Otherwise, as pointed out by Dulfano and Adler (1975), interpretation of research findings on mucus viscosity is difficult.

There are a number of review articles and compendia devoted to the physiology of mucus secretion in the lung and the nature of mucus, and these references give more detailed research.*

MUCUS-CONTROLLING AGENTS

Drugs intended to control mucus and bronchial secretions have either been true mucolytics (or liquifying expectorants) or stimulant expectorants. Stimulant expectorants promote production and expectoration of bronchial secretions and will be considered as a cough or cold medication in Chapter 14.

*Basbaum (1991); Br Med Bull, vol 34, Jan 1978; Chest, vol 80, Dec 1981; Chest, vol 81, May 1982; Hirsch (1983) Chapter 20; Kaliner et al. (1984); Kilburn (1968); King (1983); King et al. (1974); Lundgren and Shelhamer (1990); Marin (1986).

Methods of Mucolysis

The action of the mucolytics is based on the previously described structure of mucus. Historically, each of the following methods of mucolysis has been used.

Proteolysis. Because mucus has a protein component, the proteolytic enzyme pancreatic dornase was used for lysis. This drug is no longer available because of its lack of selectivity in attacking lung protein and possible antibody stimulation. However, in principle, mucus can be broken down this way (Lieberman, 1968; Spier et al., 1961; Unger and Unger, 1953). A new DNase enzyme, operating on the same principle, is under investigation and is discussed subsequently.

pH Adjustment. Alteration of the environmental pH of mucus weakens the bonding of the saccharide side chains and reduces the viscosity of the gel. Bicarbonate solutions of 2% strength have been directly instilled in 2- to 5-ml amounts into the trachea or administered by aerosol for this purpose.

Disulfide Disruption. Acetylcysteine breaks the disulfide bond (—S—S—) of mucus by substituting a sulfhydril radical (—SH), thus reducing the viscosity and elasticity of the gel (Sheffner et al., 1964).

Of the three methods described, only acetylcysteine is currently approved for use as an aerosol. Bicarbonate solution is occasionally used when prescribed by a physician. The proteolytic enzyme rhDNase is in clinical trials at this time.

Mucolysis and Mucociliary Clearance

Unfortunately, these three methods of mucolysis destroy the elasticity of mucus while reducing the viscosity because the gel structure is broken down. Since elasticity is crucial for mucociliary transport, mucolytics have the potential for a negative effect on normal physiological mucus clearance. Reduction of mucus gel to a more liquid state *may* facilitate aspiration of secretions with use of suction catheters. However, it is undesirable to create the need for tracheal suctioning, with its attendant trauma to the airway and risk of infection and hypoxemia, by liquifying secretions unless a person is unable to cough adequately. Ideally the goal should be to facilitate physiological clearance by optimizing the viscoelasticity of mucus. A prophylactic method of doing this is by a sufficient intake of fluids systemically (orally or intravenously). Either over- or underhydration should be avoided, if normal mucus is to be achieved.

The status of mucolytic agents in pulmonary disease was well reviewed at the two conferences on the scientific basis of respiratory care (Barton, 1974; Wanner and Rao, 1980).

Until agents are developed to more specifically control the biochemical composition and viscoelastic properties of mucus, mucolytics such as acetyl-cysteine form part of a program aimed at optimal clearance of the airway and at preventing the cycle of obstruction and infection that causes further hy-persecretion. The therapeutic options for controlling mucous hypersecretion are outlined below:

1. Remove causative factors where possible.
   a. Stop smoking.
   b. Avoid pollution and allergens.
2. Optimize tracheobronchial clearance.
   a. Use a bronchodilator.
   b. Take bronchial hygiene measures.
       (1) Hydration.
       (2) Cough, deep breathing.
       (3) Postural drainage.
   c. Use mucolytics.
   d. Use expectorants.
3. Reduce inflammation.
   a. Treat infection (antibiotics).
   b. Use corticosteroids.

A mucolytic agent alone is not an effective program, given the nature of in-flammation in disease states of mucus hypersecretion.

Acetylcysteine (Mucomyst)

Indications for Use
As a mucolytic, acetylcysteine is used in the treatment of thick, viscous mucous secretions. Increased viscosity of secretions along with increased amount of secretions can occur in COPD especially chronic bronchitis, tuber-culosis, cystic fibrosis, and acute tracheobronchitis.

A second use of acetylcysteine is as an antidote to reduce hepatic injury with acetaminophen overdose. The drug is given orally, not by aerosol, for this use.

Dosage and Administration
Acetylcysteine is the N-acetyl derivative of the amino acid L-cysteine and is used as a solution for either aerosol administration or by direct instillation into the tracheobronchial tree. It is supplied in the following strengths and recommended dosages by the manufacturer Mead Johnson:

20% Solution: 3 to 5 ml t.i.d. or q.i.d.
10% Solution: 6 to 10 ml t.i.d. or q.i.d.
10% Acetylcysteine With 0.05% Isoproterenol: 3 to 5 ml q.i.d.
Direct Instillation: 1 to 2 ml of 10% or 20% solution.

It should be noted that the recommended amount of the 10% solution (6 to 10 ml) is not efficiently nebulized by the typical gas-powered, hand-held, disposable nebulizer (see Chapter 2), which requires an optimal filling volume of 3.0 to 5.0 ml for mechanical efficiency and for reasonable times of administration. When the mixture with isoproterenol is used, the upper limit on the dosage (5 ml) is determined by the amount of isoproterenol contained. A 0.05% strength solution contains 0.5 mg/ml, and therefore a total amount of 5 ml of solution would contain 2.5 mg of isoproterenol. This is the usual dose of isoproterenol in 0.5 ml of a 1:200 strength solution.

Mode of Action

Acetylcysteine disrupts the structure of the mucus molecule by substituting its own sulfhydril groups for the disulfide bonds in the mucus. This action is illustrated in Figure 8–9, which also shows the molecular structure of acetylcysteine. The substituted sulfhydril group in mucus does not provide a bond, or cross-linking, between strands, and as a result both the viscosity and the elasticity of the mucus are lowered. Acetylcysteine is active in mucolysis in the presence of DNA and cellular debris seen with purulent secretions. In physical contact with mucus, acetylcysteine begins to reduce viscosity immediately. Its mucolytic activity increases with higher pH and is optimal with a local pH of 7.0 to 9.0. The solution of acetylcysteine contains a chelating agent, ethylenediaminetetraacetic acid. A light-purple solution indicates metal ion

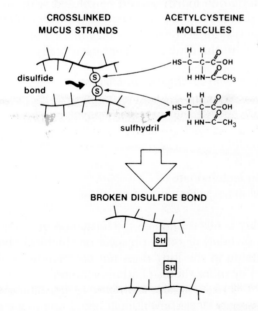

FIG 8–9. Mechanisms of action by which acetylcysteine reduces the viscosity of mucus. Acetylcysteine substitutes the sulfhydril for the disulfide bonds.

removal and does not change the safety or efficacy of the drug. It is suggested that opened vials of the drug be stored in a refrigerator and discarded after 96 hours to prevent contamination. Additional pharmaceutical and administration details in the manufacturer's package insert should be reviewed.

Hazards

The most serious potential complication with acetylcysteine is bronchospasm. This is more likely with hyperreactive airways, such as in asthmatic patients, and can be lessened by using the 10% solution instead of the 20%, or by use of the compound with isoproterenol. It is possible to use other bronchodilators either mixed with acetylcysteine or administered previously by nebulizer or MDI. If this is done, a bronchodilator with rapid onset and quick peak effect should be used, such as isoetharine. Noncatecholamine adrenergic bronchodilators (terbutaline, metaproterenol, albuterol) have a relatively slow time to peak effect and may not be as effective in preventing drug-induced bronchospasm.

Other complications can include stomatitis, nausea, and rhinorrhea. Mechanical obstruction of the airway can occur with rapid liquefaction of copious secretions, and suction should be available with artificial airways. The disagreeable odor of acetylcysteine is due to the release of hydrogen sulfide, and this may provoke nausea or vomiting. In prolonged nebulization, it has been suggested by the manufacturer that after three fourths of the solution is nebulized, the remaining one fourth should be diluted with an equal volume of sterile water to prevent a highly concentrated residue, which could irritate the airway. An aerosol of acetylcysteine may leave a sticky film on hands or face. Overdosage with the drug is unlikely, even orally.

Incompatibility with Antibiotics in Mixture

Acetylcysteine is incompatible in mixture with the following major antibiotics and should not be combined in physical solution:

- Sodium ampicillin
- Amphotericin B
- Erythromycin lactobionate
- Tetracyclines (tetracycline, oxytetracycline)

Incompatibility is taken to mean the formation of a precipitate; a change in color, clarity, or odor; or other physical or chemical change. The topical use of acetylcysteine in the lung does not contraindicate the simultaneous use of antibiotics by other routes of administration.

Acetylcysteine is reactive with a number of substances including rubber, copper, iron, and cork. Most conventional nebulizers made of plastic or glass are suitable for administering the drug. Aluminum, chromed metal, tantalum, sterling silver, or stainless steel are also safe to use, although silver may tarnish. This is not harmful to the patient. A complete list of incompatibilities for acetylcysteine can be found in the manufacturer's literature.

Use With Acetaminophen Overdose

Acetaminophen is normally metabolized in the liver, with about 2% excreted unchanged in urine. Of the 98% metabolized in the liver, approximately 4% enters a metabolic pathway termed the *cytochrome P-450 mixed-function-oxidase* pathway. The resulting metabolite is toxic to the liver. In normal doses, the metabolite reacts with glutathione in the liver, becomes nontoxic, and is excreted in the urine. In overdoses, the metabolite is in excess of the glutathione and binds to liver cells, causing liver necrosis. Giving glutathione intravenously does not prevent hepatotoxocity because it will not cross into the liver cells. Acetylcysteine is structurally similar to glutathione since both have a sulfhydril group free to react with the toxic metabolite. Acetylcysteine does cross the liver cell membrane and can be given orally in larger doses within 10 to 12 hours of acetaminophen ingestion to protect the liver (Macy, 1979).

Recombinant Human DNase

Identification

rhDNase is a mucolytic agent that can reduce the viscosity of respiratory secretions during infection by breaking down the DNA accumulated in the secretions. DNase is an enzyme produced in the pancreas that has been cloned, sequenced, and expressed as a recombinant product, or rhDNase.

Clinical Application

rhDNase is intended to reduce the viscosity of respiratory secretions that occurs with infection in the lungs. Thick, viscid mucus and impaired mucociliary clearance are commonly found in cystic fibrosis, as well as other forms of COPD associated with mucus hypersecretion, such as chronic bronchitis.

Use in Cystic Fibrosis

The general defect in cystic fibrosis results in an increased chloride ion concentration in airway epithelial cells. An increased number of sodium ions are then absorbed into the cells, presumably carrying the osmotic water equivalent from the mucus into the cells. This defective ion transport leads to dehydrated, viscous mucus, which in turn impairs mucociliary function and predisposes to bacterial infection. In the presence of infection, neutrophils congregate in the airway and release DNA, which further increases the viscosity of secretions. DNA is an extremely viscous polyanion that is present in infected, but not in uninfected, respiratory secretions (Aitken et al., 1992; Shak et al., 1990). DNA in secretions may also contribute to reduced effectiveness of aminoglycoside antibiotics such as gentamicin. This could be caused by binding of the antibiotic to the polyvalent anions of the DNA and would tend to lessen the effectiveness of aerosolized antibiotics in cystic fibrosis.

Respiratory infections are chronic in patients with cystic fibrosis and also pose a problem in patients on ventilators and in acute exacerbations of chronic bronchitis.

With use of recombinant molecular technology, human DNase I has been cloned and synthesized. rhDNase has been shown to be more effective in vitro than acetylcysteine in reducing the viscosity of infected sputum in cystic fibrosis (Shak et al., 1990). Acetylcysteine showed minimal effect in reducing the viscosity of sputum in cystic fibrosis, in the in vitro study of Shak and co-workers (1990).

Mode of Action

The mucolytic agent rhDNase is similar in action to the proteolytic enzyme, pancreatic dornase, which was approved for human use by inhalation in 1958 (Shak et al., 1990) but is no longer available. rhDNase reduces the viscosity of infected respiratory secretions when given by aerosol, by breaking down the DNA material in enzymatic fashion. This is illustrated in Figure 8–10. When mixed with purulent sputum from subjects with cystic fibrosis, rhDNase lowered the viscosity of the sputum (Shak et al., 1990). The nonflowing viscous gel of the sputum was changed to a flowing liquid by adding rhDNase. This was associated with a decrease in the size of the DNA in the sputum. The change in sputum viscosity with the addition of rhDNase is dose dependent, with greater reduction occurring at higher concentrations of the drug. In the study by Shak and colleagues, rhDNase had no effect on uninfected sputum.

Pancreatic dornase, termed *Dornavac* by the manufacturer, the product previously removed from the market, was a bovine pancreatic DNase. This product could cause serious bronchospasm when inhaled (Raskin, 1968). In addition, there was concern that the foreign protein might generate anti-DNase antibodies and cause allergic reactions. Differences between the human and bovine pancreatic DNase I molecules in an immunogenic region imply that some of the adverse reactions to pancreatic dornase could have been caused by an immune response. Serum antibodies to DNase were found in some patients who were given multiple doses of bovine pancreatic DNase (Shak et al., 1990). Adverse effects with bovine DNase may also have been caused by the presence of contaminating proteinases, trypsin and chymotrypsin, in the drug (Shak et al., 1990).

rhDNase is purified to produce a nonallergic DNase. Safety studies revealed no allergic bronchospastic response or serum anti-DNase antibodies with inhaled rhDNase in healthy subjects and those with cystic fibrosis (Aitken et al., 1992).

Reduction in Viscosity: (Pourability)			
	0 min.	15 min.	30 min.
Saline	0	+1	+1
rhDNase, 50 mcg/ml	0	+3	+4
Bovine DNase, 50 mcg/ml	0	+2	+4

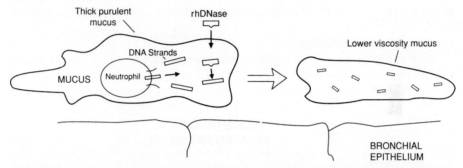

FIG 8–10. Illustration of the mode of action of rhDNase in reducing the viscosity of infected sputum. The table indicates viscosity reduction based on a qualitative assay of sputum pourability. *0*, no movement; *+1*, movement of <10% of sputum; *+2*, movement of 10% to 20%; *+3*, movement of 20% to 50%; *+4*, movement of all sputum freely. (Based on Shak S, Capon DJ, Hellmin R, Marsters SA, and Baker CL: Recombinant human DNase I reduces the viscosity of cystic fibrosis sputum, Pro Natl Acad Sci USA 87:9188, 1990.)

Aerosol Delivery of rhDNase

In the study by Aitken et al. (1992), the rhDNase was aerosolized with an Acorn II jet nebulizer using an expiratory filter. The dose in the nebulizer was 2.5 ml of rhDNase, with a concentration of 4 mg/ml. Since the nebulizer output is specified at 0.25 ml/min, the dose delivered is time dependent at a nominal rate of 1 mg/min. Dosages were varied in the study and delivered 3 times daily.

Inhaled Amiloride

Identification

Amiloride is a diuretic that acts in the kidneys to block sodium reabsorption. Loss of sodium prevents the reabsorption of water, increasing urinary water loss.

Clinical Use

Amiloride has been investigated by inhalation in cystic fibrosis as a means to reverse the ion exchange defect that is thought to cause viscous, dehydrated mucus.

Mode of Action

As previously described with rhDNase, the gene responsible for chloride transport out of airway epithelial cells is abnormal. Sodium is absorbed into the epithelium, along with an osmotic equivalent of water, leaving thick, dehydrated mucus. Amiloride, as a sodium channel blocker, inhibits the sodium absorption from secretions in the airway lumen. This is shown in Figure 8–11.

Aerosol Administration

In a study by App et al. (1990), amiloride was delivered by Pari Standard and Pari Boy nebulizers (Germany) powered at 6 L/min. A dose of 3 ml of a 10^{-3} mol/L solution of amiloride was used and was estimated to deliver 0.07

MODE OF ACTION
INHALED AMILORIDE

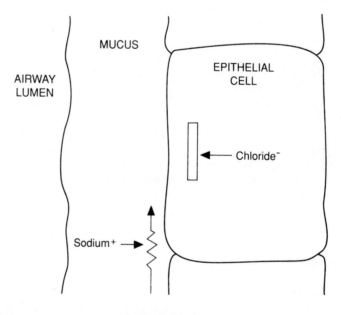

Amiloride Blocks

FIG 8–11. The mode of action of inhaled amiloride is based on its inhibition of sodium absorption from mucus.

mg of drug in a 10-minute treatment. Frequency of treatment was twice a day during the study. Both mucociliary clearance and cough clearance of secretions substantially improved. The effect of amiloride on mucociliary clearance lasted about 40 minutes.

Other Mucolytic Agents

Sodium bicarbonate is a weak base that has been used occasionally as a 2% solution for aerosol or direct tracheal irrigation, in amounts ranging from 2 to 5 ml. As a base, the bicarbonate solution acts to increase local bronchial pH, which weakens bonding among the saccharide side chains of the mucous molecule. As a result, mucous viscosity and elasticity are lowered. Systemic pH is unaffected in the amounts used, although local bronchial irritation may occur with topical pH above 8.0 in the lung.

Propylene glycol can reduce gel structure by releasing hydrogen bonding (Barton and Lourenco, 1973) of water in the gel. Propylene glycol is also used with aerosols for its hygroscopic properties to stabilize particle size by preventing evaporation. However, it can inhibit the growth of *Mycobacterium tuberculosis,* a fact that is relevant when obtaining sputum specimens to check for tuberculosis organisms.

Potassium iodide has been shown to decrease mucus elasticity (Martin et al., 1980), but it is generally considered as a stimulant expectorant (see Chapter 14, Cold and Cough Agents). A proteolytic effect was reported by Lieberman and Kurnick (1964). Martin et al. (1980) stated that the concentrations of potassium iodide required for a dispersant effect on mucus are harmful to cilia.

Glyceryl guaiacolate is usually considered an expectorant rather than a mucolytic. It does improve mucociliary clearance in chronic bronchitis (Wanner, 1977).

S-carboxymethylcysteine (Mucodyne) is a mucolytic agent investigated in Great Britain. It decreases sputum viscosity in vitro but is not considered effective (Thomson et al., 1975) for mucolysis when administered orally. The drug is a derivative of the amino acid cysteine, which has a sulfhydril group (—SH) intended to split the disulfide bonds of the glycoprotein chains of mucus, reducing its viscosity. However, S-carboxymethylcysteine has the —SH group blocked by a carboxylic acid residue and cannot liberate the —SH group for mucolysis.

Sodium 2-mercaptoethane sulfonate (Mistabron) is a compound containing a sulfhydril group. It acts in a fashion similar to acetylcysteine in reducing mucous viscosity. A 3-ml dose of a 20% solution has been inhaled by aerosol twice daily with pulmonary function improvement in cystic fibrosis (Weller et al., 1980). The drug is more active in vitro than acetylcysteine; in vivo efficacy is more difficult to compare. This drug is not currently available in the United States but is used in Great Britain.

Effect of Bland Aerosols on Mucus

Bland aerosols include distilled water, physiological saline (0.9%), and hyper- and hypotonic saline. Historically, aerosols of water and saline have been used for humidity in intermittent positive pressure breathing, for sputum induction, and also for liquefying secretions. There is no evidence that bland aerosols reduce mucus to a less viscous state by topical hydration or mixing. Evidence is that the mucus gel layer serves to protect and insulate the airway surface and is resistant to the addition or removal of water (Dulfano et al., 1973). A short-term aerosol treatment with 3 to 5 ml of water or saline adds considerably less than 1 ml of liquid to the lung (Asmundsson et al., 1970). Continuous aerosol treatment of small subjects with high-output devices *can* add substantial amounts of water to the lung and cause runny, watery secretions, as documented in infants.

Although short-term, bland aerosols do not directly liquefy mucus, they have been found to increase lung clearance and sputum production and cause productive coughing (Pavia et al., 1978). This effect is probably a vagally mediated reflex production of cough and mucous secretion due to the irritant nature of the bland aerosol and is the same mechanism as that of sputum induction. The greater the difference in tonicity, such as with hyper- or hypotonic solution, the more irritant the effect. Therefore bland aerosols are essentially expectorants. Since they act by irritating the airway, they may not be as suitable as oral expectorants, which are discussed with cough and cold agents in Chapter 14.

Future Mucus-Controlling Agents

To improve mucus transport, both elasticity and viscosity must be considered. Mucolytics have been targeted only at lowering the viscosity of mucus. Under the normal physiology of ciliary movement, logic dictates that thicker and denser strands of mucus would be moved more efficiently by ciliary contact and elastic recovery than would thin, low-viscosity solutions. The conceptual analogy is that of raking water—little transport will occur. This assumes mucus clearance is being optimized *physiologically*. Endotracheal aspiration of secretions using suction would be easier with low-viscosity mucus. Results of a study by Dulfano and Adler (1975) and that of another by Gelman and Meyer (1979) support the view that elasticity is extremely important for mucus transport. The former study found that high elastic recoil and low viscosity represent the best rheologic combination for maximal velocity by the mucociliary type of system. Other studies have appeared to reach conflicting conclusions (Giordano et al., 1978; Martin et al., 1980). Two factors may account for the variability of research studies: the non-Newtonian viscosity of mucus, and the initial rheologic state of secretions.

It has been suggested that the treatment of bronchial hypersecretion would be better aimed at *normalizing* the rheological properties of mucus to optimize transport, rather than at simply lysing or liquifying bronchial secretions as traditionally done. It is suggested that the term *mucolytic* be replaced by *mucus-controlling* to connote such an approach to secretion clearance. In this view of mucous control, there is a normal range of elasticity and viscosity, as illustrated in Figure 8–12 using arbitrary units. Puchelle (1980) has distinguished three possible states that would determine the treatment approach to be used:

1. Strongly cross-linked mucus has high elasticity *and* viscosity, and traditional mucolytic agents such as sulfhydril compounds (acetylcysteine) or proteolytic enzymes would restore normal transport properties by lowering both viscosity and elasticity.

2. With low viscoelasticity, restructuring or cross-linking agents would increase both viscosity and elasticity to improve transport. Such agents have been termed *mucospissic* and may be seen in future developments (Davis and Deverell, 1977; King, 1983).

3. With highly viscous but normally elastic mucus, a drug that selectively lowers viscosity but not elasticity, as promised by research with letosteine, is indicated. Such a condition may occur with bronchial inflammation states.

Currently there are no drugs available as mucus-controlling agents in the United States that will selectively modify viscosity or elasticity. The traditional

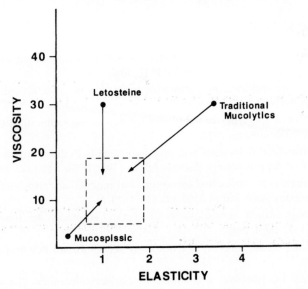

FIG 8–12. Conceptual representation of an optimal range of viscosity and elasticity of mucus for mucociliary transport.

mucolytic agents contain the sulfhydril group that substitutes for the disulfide bond in mucus. Examples are N-acetylcysteine, dithiothreitol, glutathione, and cysteamine (Davis and Deverell, 1977). Previous proteolytic enzymes such as pancreatic dornase (Dornavac), chymin, or trypsin are also effective mucolytics but are hazardous due to their possible antigenic effect or lack of specificity. The new agent, rhDNase, avoids this side effect but is still mucolytic in its effect. Letosteine, which is being investigated in Europe, is a thiazolidine derivative of mercaptoethylacetate; it has been studied in vitro with a 5-mg/ml concentration and was found to have most of its activity in lowering viscosity rather than changing elasticity (Puchelle, 1980).

A group of agents with mucospissic activity, to cause improved gelation, is also being investigated and includes sodium tetraborate, Congo red, and tetracycline (Davis and Deverell, 1977). These agents can cause a 50% change in mucus consistency in 2 to 12 minutes. The thickening effect of tetracycline can occur with oral and aerosol administration, although more so with direct aerosol. It may be that tetracycline binds to mucus proteins to increase viscosity and elasticity, although exact binding sites remain unclear.

Further investigation may produce clinically useful agents tailored to specific secretion problems, as illustrated in Figure 8–12. The first step has been to recognize the complex rheologic nature of mucous gel and the necessity of cross-linking to provide adequate elasticity for efficient ciliary transport. A second step has been an increased understanding of the structure of mucus and regulation of its production.

BIBLIOGRAPHY

Aitken ML et al: Recombinant human DNase inhalation in normal subjects and patients with cystic fibrosis, JAMA 267(14):1947, 1992.

App EM et al: Acute and long-term amiloride inhalation in cystic fibrosis lung disease, Am Rev Respir Dis 141; 605, 1990.

Asmundsson T et al: Efficiency of nebulizers for depositing saline in human lung, Am Rev Respir Dis 108:506, 1973.

Barton AD: Aerosolized detergents and mucolytic agents in the treatment of stable chronic obstructive pulmonary disease, Am Rev Respir Dis 110:104S, 1974.

Barton AD, Lourenco RV: Bronchial secretions and mucociliary clearance: biochemical characteristics, Arch Intern Med 131:140, 1973.

Basbaum CB: Supplement: airway mucin. Chairman's summary. Am Rev Respir Dis 144(suppl):S2, S3, Sept 1991.

Basbaum C et al: Cellular mechanisms of airway secretion, Am Rev Respir Dis 137:479, 1988.

Davis SS, Deverell LC: Rheological factors in mucociliary clearance. The assessment of mucotropic agents using an *in vitro* model, Mod Probl Paediatr 19:207, 1977.

Denton R et al: Viscoelasticity of mucus. Its role in ciliary transport of pulmonary secretions, Am Rev Respir Dis 98:380, 1968.

Dulfano JJ, Adler KB: Physical properties of sputum. VII. Rheologic properties and mucociliary transport, Am Rev Respir Dis 112:341, 1975.

Dulfano JJ, Adler KB, Wooten O: Physical properties of sputum. IV. Effects of 100 percent humidity and water mist, Am Rev Respir Dis 107:130, 1973.

Gelman RA, Meyer FA: Mucociliary transference rate and mucus viscoelasticity: dependence on dynamic storage and loss modulus, Am Rev Respir Dis 120:553, 1979.

Giordano AM, Holsclaw D, Litt M: Mucus rheology and mucociliary clearance: normal physiologic state. Am Rev Respir Dis 118:245, 1978.

Hirsch SR: Airway mucus and the mucociliary system. In Middleton E Jr, Reed CE, Ellis EF, eds: Allergy: principles and practice, ed 2, St Louis, 1983, CV Mosby.

Hodgkin JE, ed: Chronic obstructive pulmonary disease. Current concepts in diagnosis and comprehensive care, Park Ridge, Ill, 1979, American College of Chest Physicians.

Iravani J, Melville GN: Mucociliary activity in the respiratory tract as influenced by prostaglandin E_1. Respiration 32:305, 1975.

Kaliner M et al: Human respiratory mucus, J Allergy Clin Immunol 73:318, 1984.

Kilburn K: A hypothesis for pulmonary clearance and its implications, Am Rev Respir Dis 98:449, 1968.

King M: Mucus and mucociliary clearance, Respir Care 28:335, 1983.

King M et al: On the transport of mucus and its rheologic simulants in ciliated systems, Am Rev Respir Dis 110:740, 1974.

Lieberman J: Dornase aerosol effect on sputum viscosity in cases of cystic fibrosis, JAMA 205:114, 1968.

Lieberman J, Kurnick NB: The induction of proteolysis in purulent sputum by iodide, J Clin Invest 43:1892, 1964.

Lopez-Vidriero MT: Airway mucus: production and composition, Chest 80(suppl):799, Dec 1981.

Lourenco GV: Bronchial mucous secretions: introduction, Chest 63(suppl):55S, 1973.

Lundgren JD, Shelhamer JH: Pathogensis of airway mucus hypersecretion, J Allergy Clin Immunol 85:399, 1990.

Macy AM: Preventing hepatotoxicity in acetaminophen overdose, Am J Nurs 79:301, 1979.

Marin MG: Pharmacology of airway secretion, Pharmacol Rev 38:273, 1986.

Martin R, Litt M, Marriott C: The effect of mucolytic agents on the rheologic and transport properties of canine tracheal mucus, Am Rev Respir Dis 121:495, 1980.

Matthews LW et al: Studies in pulmonary secretions. I. The overall composition of pulmonary secretions from patients with cystic fibrosis, bronchiectasis and laryngectomy, Am Rev Respir Dis 88:199, 1963.

Nowell JA, Tyler WS: Scanning electron microscopy of the surface morphology of mammalian lungs, Am Rev Respir Dis 103; 313, 1971.

Pavia D, Thomson ML, Clarke SW: Enhanced clearance of secretions from the human lung after the administration of hypertonic saline aerosol, Am Rev Respir Dis 117:199, 1978.

Pinnock CB et al: Relationship between milk intake and mucus production in adult volunteers challenged with rhinovirus-2, Am Rev Respir Dis 141:352, 1990.

Puchelle E et al: Drug effects on viscoelasticity of mucus, Eur J Respir Dis 61(suppl 110):195, 1980.

Raskin P: Bronchospasm after inhalation of pancreatic dornase, Am Rev Respir Dis 98:597, 1968.

Reid L: Measurement of the bronchial mucous gland layer, Thorax 15:132, 1960.

Reid L, Clamp JR: Biochemical and histochemical nomenclature of mucus, Br Med Bull 34:5, 1978.

Sackner MA: Effect of respiratory drugs on mucociliary clearance, Chest 73(suppl):958S, 1978.

Shak S et al: Recombinant human DNase I reduces the viscosity of cystic fibrosis sputum, Proc Natl Acad Sci USA 87:9188, 1990.

Sheffner AL et al: The *in vitro* reduction in viscosity of human tracheo-bronchial secretions by acetylcysteine, Am Rev Respir Dis 90:721, 1964.

Shimura S et al: Bronchorrhea sputum in bronchial asthma, Am Rev Respir Dis 137:A14, 1988, (abstract).

Spier R, Witebsky E, Paine JR: Aerosolized pancreatic dornase and antibiotics in pulmonary infections: use in patients with post-operative and non-operative infections, JAMA 178:878, 1961.

Sturgen J, Reid L: An organ culture study of the effects of drugs on secretory activity of human bronchial submucosal gland, Clin Sci 43:533, 1972.

Thomson ML et al: No demonstrable effect of S-carboxymethylcysteine on clearance of secretions from the human lung, Thorax 30:669, 1975.

Turner-Warwick M, Openshaw P: Sputum in asthma, Postgrad Med J 63(suppl 1):79, 1987.

Unger L, Unger AH: Trypsin inhalation in respiratory conditions associated with thick sputum: its use in bronchiectasis, acute atelectasis, infectious bronchitis, bronchial asthma, emphysema, and tracheostomized patients with poliomyelitis, JAMA 152:1109, 1953.

Wanner A: Clinical aspects of mucociliary transport, Am Rev Respir Dis 116:73, 1977.

Wanner A, Rao A: Clinical indications for and effects of bland, mucolytic, and antimicrobial aerosols, Am Rev Respir Dis 122:79, 1980.

Weller PH et al: Controlled trial of intermittent aerosol therapy with sodium 2-mercaptoethane sulphonate in cystic fibrosis, Thorax 35:42, 1980.

9

Surfactant Agents

Chapter 9 presents surfactant agents, specifically exogenous surfactant products, and concepts useful in understanding these products. There are two agents currently available: colfosceril palmitate (Exosurf) and beractant (Survanta). These are used to treat and prevent respiratory distress syndrome (RDS) of the newborn. The following outlines the topics discussed.

- Physical principles of surface-active agents
- Previous surfactant agents used in respiratory care
- Exogenous surfactants
- Clinical application of exogenous surfactants

PHYSICAL PRINCIPLES OF SURFACTANT AGENTS

The use of surfactant, or surface-active, agents in respiratory care predates the release of the exogenous surfactants currently applied in RDS of newborns. Surface-active agents have been used in an attempt to reduce the adhesiveness of mucus (Alevaire, Tergemist), to reduce the froth of pulmonary edema (ethyl alcohol), and most recently to replace missing pulmonary surfactant in RDS (exogenous surfactants).

The following terms and concepts form the basis for an understanding of the application of surfactant preparations and their effects in the airway.

Surfactant: Surface-active agent that lowers surface tension. Examples include soap and various forms of detergent. Surfactants, or surface-active agents, have also been termed *detergents* for this reason.

Surface Tension: Force caused by attraction between like molecules that occurs at liquid-gas interfaces and that holds the liquid surface intact. The unit of measure for surface tension is usually dynes per centimeter, which indicates the force required to cause a 1-cm rupture in the surface film. Because a liquid's molecules are more attracted to each other than to the surrounding gas, a droplet or spherical shape usually results (Fig 9–1, *A*).

Laplace's Law: Physical principle that describes and quantifies the relation between the internal pressure of a drop or bubble, the amount of surface tension, and the radius of the drop or bubble (Fig 9–1, *B*).

A. SURFACE TENSION

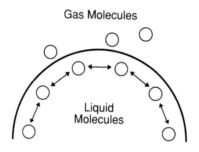

B. LAPLACE'S LAW

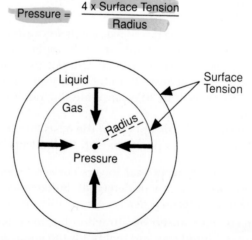

FIG 9–1. A, Illustration of the concept of like liquid molecules producing the attractive force resulting in surface tension. **B,** Illustration of Laplace's Law.

For a bubble (i.e., a liquid film with gas inside and out), Laplace's Law is:

$$\text{Pressure} = (4 \times \text{surface tension})/\text{radius}$$

Application to the Lung

Since an alveolus has a liquid lining, surface-tension forces apply. The higher the surface tension of the liquid, the greater the compressing force inside the alveolus, which can cause collapse or difficulty in opening the alveolus. In foamy, bubbly pulmonary edema, the surface tension of the liquid preserves the bubble. In both cases, lowering the surface tension will ease alveolar opening or cause the foam bubbles to collapse and liquefy.

PREVIOUS SURFACTANT AGENTS IN RESPIRATORY CARE

Ethyl Alcohol

Alcohol has been applied in acute fulminating pulmonary edema, in which the airway is obstructed with serous exudate. The exudate has sufficient surface tension to form a mass of bubbles or foamy froth that blocks gas exchange, precipitating acute hypoxemia. Ethyl alcohol has been given by nebulization, or more commonly by direct tracheal instillation in a dilute strength of 30% to 50%, to lower the surface tension of the foam and to reduce the froth to a liquid state, which can be cleared by tracheobronchial aspiration (suctioning). This concept is illustrated in Figure 9–2.

EFFECT OF SURFACE-ACTIVE AGENT
PULMONARY EDEMA

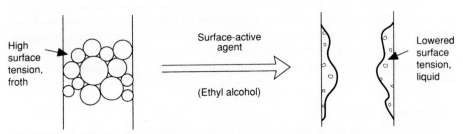

FIG 9–2. Illustration of the effect of alcohol on high–surface-tension foam to reduce the frothy bubbles to a liquid state.

Mode of Action

Alcohol has the following surface tension at the concentrations given:

100% Strength: 22 dynes/cm

50% Strength: 28 dynes/cm

30% Strength: 32 dynes/cm

Frothy sputum is estimated to have a surface tension of approximately 60 dynes/cm. The addition of alcohol was thought to lower the surface tension of the foamy exudate, reducing it to a liquid, clearable state. Since alcohol can dissolve in water through hydrogen bonding, theoretically physical mixing can occur between the alcohol and the aqueous exudate.

Disadvantages

There is lack of an approved clinical use of alcohol in this application. Efficacy is not well established by controlled studies, which would be difficult to perform. Ethyl alcohol is toxic to membranes and has been shown by Greiff et al. (1991) to cause a bidirectional increase in permeability across the airway mucous membrane. Exudation of plasma tracer substances onto the mucosal surface of the airway was substantial. This is a process seen in airway inflammation, indicating that alcohol causes inflammatory provocation of the airway. More sophisticated hemodynamic monitoring and the availability of improved diuretics and cardiotonics must make this therapy obsolete, unless a clear advantage can be shown in the future.

Mucus-Wetting Agents (Detergents)

Two agents in this category (Alevaire and Tergemist), which have been removed from the market, were intended to alter the surface tension of mucus. The agents were prescribed to improve water penetration and facilitate transport and expulsion of adhesive mucus (Miller et al., 1954). Both agents were actually compounds with the following ingredients:

Alevaire: tyloxapol (Superinone, 0.125%), bicarbonate (2.0%), glycerin (5.0%).

Tergemist: sodium ethasulfate (0.125%), potassium iodide (0.1%).

The compounds were prescribed on a maintenance basis for chronic bronchitis. Interestingly, alcohol in the form of vodka was also used by some physicians as a maintenance drug given by nebulization to reduce adhesiveness of mucus by its effect on surface tension. Perhaps the side effect of slight intoxication contributed to patient approval and compliance with this therapy.

Mode of Action

In mucus, the attraction between water molecules is greater than the attraction between lipophilic groups of the macromolecule and water. Lipophilic groups tend to be pushed together to reduce the interfacial area of contact between lipophilic and water molecules. The resulting contacts of water and lipophilic groups are termed *hydrophobic bonds* and provide junction points in the mucus gel (Marriott and Richards, 1974). It was thought that detergents may interact with mucus to produce emulsification, just as they do with grease and water. The lipophilic group on the detergent associates with that in the mucus, since the polar groups of the detergent orient to project into the aqueous phase and associate with the water molecules (Fig 9–3). Consequently the mucus gel will be "dissolved," or better, dispersed into smaller particles. Sears and Stanitski (1983), in discussing solutions, give a good illustration of this basic action of detergents. The proposed mechanism of emulsification was described by Tainter et al. (1955).

Efficacy

Whether detergents actually have this emulsifying effect on mucus in vivo is questionable. The consensus ultimately was that clinical efficacy of surface-active agents with mucous (as opposed to frothy edema) secretions could not be demonstrated, and that some of the clinical effects seen could be due to the added ingredients (bicarbonate, glycerin, and potassium iodide), all of which have some mucolytic properties (Paez and Miller, 1971; Palmer, 1957). Surface tension is probably not the important property of mucus, as much as the viscosity/elasticity ratio of mucus previously discussed in Chapter 8. Tylox-

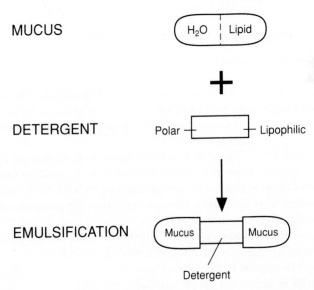

FIG 9–3. Illustration of the theoretical effect of detergents, or "wetting agents," in emulsifying mucus to lower airway adhesion. Such agents have been withdrawn for lack of efficacy.

apol *can* reduce surface tension and is an ingredient in a synthetic surfactant mixture discussed next.

EXOGENOUS SURFACTANTS

Resp. Distress Syndrome

Introductory Overview

The term *exogenous* refers to the fact that these are surfactant preparations from outside the patient's body. These preparations may be obtained from other humans, from animals, or by laboratory synthesis. The clinical use of exogenous surfactants has been to replace the missing pulmonary surfactant of the premature, or immature, lung in RDS of the newborn. These agents have also been investigated for use in adult respiratory distress syndrome (ARDS) and may prove to be beneficial, although results have not been entirely consistent (Holm and Matalon, 1989; Morton, 1990).

There are currently two exogenous surfactant preparations approved for general clinical use: Exosurf (Burroughs Wellcome Co.) and Survanta (Ross Laboratories). A brief historical perspective of the development of successful exogenous surfactants is given, and the composition of natural pulmonary surfactant is described. The four categories of surfactant preparations are listed, with each described briefly, followed by a more detailed description of the two products currently available.

History and Development of Exogenous Surfactants

1929—Von Meergaard shows that lungs are more difficult to inflate with air than with liquid.

1956—Clements measures the surface tension of lung fluid extracts.

1958—Dipalmitoylphosphatidylcholine (DPPC) is identified by Clements and associates as the main surface-active component of pulmonary surfactant.

1959—Avery and Mead show that surface tension is higher in the lungs of infants with hyaline membrane disease than in healthy infants.

1964—Aerosols of synthetic DPPC are attempted in RDS, with little success.

1972—Enhorning and Robertson demonstrate the effectiveness of surfactant replacement in premature animals.

1980—Fujiwara and associates report success in artificial surfactant therapy in infants by using a lyophilized artificial surfactant.

1990—Exosurf is approved for general use.

1991—Survanta is approved for general use.

The discovery of DPPC in 1958, combined with an understanding that surface tension is abnormally high in RDS, led to the development of the exogenous surfactant products Exosurf and Survanta. Their application in RDS is to normalize lung compliance. Although DPPC is the primary surface-active ingredient of natural surfactant, the use of DPPC alone was not successful in maintaining surface tension in immature lungs. Other components of pulmonary surfactant, described in the next section, were needed to reproduce the surface properties of natural surfactant.

Composition of Pulmonary Surfactant

Pulmonary surfactant is a mixture of phospholipids, neutral lipids, and proteins specific to the mixture. Surfactant is produced by alveolar type II cells, and its primary, although not necessarily only, function is to regulate the surface-tension forces of the liquid alveolar lining. Surfactant lowers surface tension as it is compressed during expiration, thus reducing the amount of pressure and inspiratory effort necessary to reexpand the alveoli during a succeeding inspiration.

Components of Surfactant

Figure 9–4 illustrates the source, composition, and basic function of pulmonary surfactant in the alveolus. Each of the major components is described.

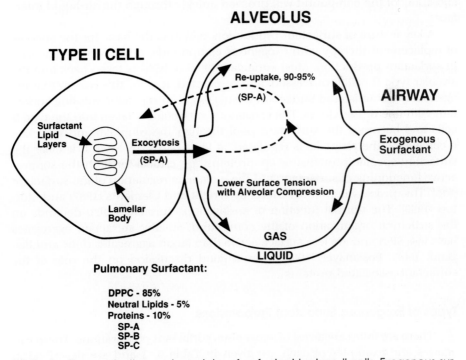

Pulmonary Surfactant:

DPPC - 85%
Neutral Lipids - 5%
Proteins - 10%
   SP-A
   SP-B
   SP-C

FIG 9–4. The production and reuptake of surfactant by type II cells. Exogenous surfactant is also taken up, to become part of the surfactant pool for alveoli.

DPPC, also known as lecithin, is the main surface-active component of surfactant. This substance is a phospholipid and constitutes approximately 85% of the mixture.

Surfactant protein A (SP-A) is a high-molecular-weight glycoprotein probably synthesized and secreted by the type II alveolar cell. This protein is specific to surfactant and has also been denoted by SP-35 and apoprotein A or SAP-35 (Jobe and Ikegami, 1987). SP-A seems to regulate both secretion and exocytosis of surfactant from the type II cell, as well as the reuptake of surfactant for recycling and reuse.

Surfactant proteins B and C (SP-B, SP-C) are low-molecular-weight, hydrophobic proteins that improve the adsorption and spreading of the phospholipid throughout the air-liquid interface in the alveolus.

Production and Regulation of Surfactant Secretion

The surfactant lipids are synthesized in the type II alveolar cells and stored in vesicles termed *lamellar bodies* (Fig 9–4). The surfactant in the lamellar bodies is then secreted by exocytosis out of the type II cell and into the alveolus. SP-A and SP-B facilitate the formation of an intermediate form of surfactant called *tubular myelin,* before it reaches the air-liquid interface. SP-C also helps to "break" the lipid layers of surfactant, so that adsorption and spreading of the compound will proceed quickly through the air-liquid interface.

A key feature of surfactant production, which is the basis for the success of replacement therapy with exogenous compounds, is the recycling activity in surfactant production. Most surfactant (90% to 95%) is taken back into the alveolar type II cell, reprocessed, and resecreted. It is for this reason that exogenously administered surfactant is successful in replacing missing surfactant with one or two doses. The exogenous surfactant is taken into the type II cells and becomes the surfactant pool through the reuptake and recycling mechanism. The reuptake is regulated, at least partly, by SP-A. It is clear the surfactant-specific proteins, or apoproteins, are critical for both the surface-active functioning of surfactant and the metabolic regulation of the surfactant pool. This process is well described by Wright and Clements (1987) and Morton (1990). The normal function of endogenous surfactant also depends on the structural organization of the compound. Smaller surfactant aggregates have less SP-A and are less surface active than larger aggregates (Jobe and Ikegami, 1987). Possmayer (1990) gives a good discussion on the role of the surfactant-associated proteins.

Types of Exogenous Surfactant Preparations

There are four categories of exogenous surfactant preparations. These categories and examples of each are given in Table 9–1 and are described in

TABLE 9–1.

Types of Surfactant Preparations and Examples

Category	Description	Examples
Natural	Surfactant removed from human or animal by alveolar lavage or amniotic fluid harvesting	Human surfactant
Modified natural	Surfactant from natural sources (human or animal) with addition or removal of substances	Survanta, Surfactant TA, Curosurf, Infasurf
Artificial	Surfactant that is prepared by mixing in vitro synthesized substances that may or may not be in natural surfactant	Exosurf
Synthetic natural	Surfactant prepared in vitro with genetic engineering	None at present

this section. A more complete technical description is found in Jobe and Ikegami (1987).

Natural Surfactant

Natural surfactant is an apt descriptive term for the category of surfactants that are obtained from animals or humans by means of alveolar wash or from amniotic fluid. The large surface-active aggregates of natural surfactant are recovered from the fluid by centrifugation or simple filtration. Since this is a natural surfactant, the ingredients necessary for effective function to regulate surface tension are present. Specifically these include the surface proteins needed for adsorption and spreading. Depending on the source, natural surfactants can be expensive and time consuming to obtain and prepare. In addition, there is concern over contamination with infective agents or allergic reaction to foreign proteins.

Modified Natural Surfactant

There are surfactant preparations obtained from natural sources, such as human or animal lungs, and modified by the addition or removal of certain components. Examples of modified natural surfactants are given in Table 9–1 and include Survanta. **Survanta,** as an example, is obtained as an extract of minced cow lung, supplemented with other ingredients such as DPPC, palmitic acid, and tripalmitin. Usually, the modifications to the natural surfactant material are designed to improve their functioning in the lung, to reduce protein contamination and for sterility. Although Survanta contains the hydrophobic proteins SP-B and SP-C, the protein SP-A is missing, and this may shorten the duration of effect.

Other examples of a modified natural surfactant include **Surfactant TA,** prepared by the Tokyo-Akita Co. in Japan, and used by Fujiwara and associates in their 1980 work. Surfactant TA is a reconstituted chloroform-methanol extract from minced bovine lungs, with DPPC and other lipids added. **Curosurf** is another modified natural surfactant obtained as a porcine lung extract. **Infasurf** is a chloroform-methanol extract of fluid lavaged from calf lung, and like Survanta, contains only the surfactant proteins SP-B and SP-C, but not SP-A (Notter et al., 1985).

Artificial Surfactant

Artificial surfactants are mixtures of synthetic components. An example is provided by **Exosurf,** which is composed of DPPC, cetyl alcohol, and tyloxapol. The phospholipid, DPPC, can be synthesized in the laboratory. The characteristic feature of artificial surfactants is that none of the ingredients is obtained from natural sources, such as human or cow lung. A major advantage of this class of surfactant is its freedom from contaminating infectious agents and additional foreign proteins that may be antigenic to the recipient. A possible disadvantage is the lack of equivalent performance between the organic chemicals substituted for the naturally occurring surfactant proteins, such as SP-A, SP-B, or SP-C.

Synthetic Natural Surfactant

An ideal solution to the problems that are of concern in both natural and artificial surfactants would be genetically engineered surfactant. In such a preparation the phospholipid, lipid, and protein ingredients of the natural surfactant aggregate would be produced by cloning of the gene or genes responsible for human surfactant, with in vitro synthesis. There are no products available for general use at this time, but work progresses in their development. The gene encoding SP-A has been identified, sequenced, and translated (Floros et al., 1985). The genes for human surfactant proteins B and C have also been cloned (Avery and Merritt, 1991). It is anticipated that a genetically engineered surfactant will be available within the next 10 years.

CLINICAL APPLICATION OF EXOGENOUS SURFACTANTS

Clinical Indications

Exogenous surfactants are clinically indicated for the following applications:

1. Prevention of RDS in very low birth weight infants.
2. Prevention of RDS in other infants with evidence of immature lungs.
3. Retroactive or "rescue" treatment of infants with RDS.

The basic problem in RDS is lack of pulmonary surfactant due to lung immaturity. This results in high surface tensions in the liquid-lined, gas-filled alveoli. Increased ventilating pressure is required to expand the alveoli during
inspiration, which will lead to ventilatory and respiratory failure in the infant
without ventilatory support. This concept and the effect of exogenous surfactant are shown in Figure 9–5.

Exogenous surfactants are also being investigated for efficacy in the treatment of ARDS, although this is not an approved clinical application at this
time.

Available Surfactant Preparations

Exosurf

Description.   Exosurf is a protein-free, artificial surfactant preparation
consisting of the following components in a 10-ml vial:

Colfosceril palmitate (108 mg)
Cetyl alcohol (12 mg)
Tyloxapol (9 mg)

Colfosceril palmitate is another name used for DPPC. Exosurf is stored as
a powder that also contains sodium chloride to adjust osmolality, and the pH

RDS

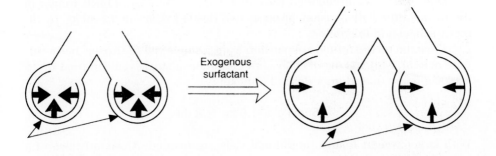

- High surface tension
- Low compliance
- Increased work of breathing

- Lowered surface tension
- Increased compliance
- Decreased work of breathing

FIG 9–5.   Illustration of the pathogenesis of RDS and the effect of exogenous surfactants to improve lung compliance.

of the powder is adjusted with sodium hydroxide (base) or hydrochloric acid. The powder form is reconstituted with 8 ml of preservative-free sterile water. The reconstituted suspension is milky white, has a pH in the range of 5 to 7, and each milliliter of solution contains the following:

> Colfosceril palmitate (13.5 mg)
> Cetyl alcohol (1.5 mg)
> Tyloxapol (1.0 mg)

As a synthetic, or artificial mixture prepared in the laboratory, Exosurf does not contain any of the surfactant-associated proteins (SP-A, SP-B, or SP-C). Cetyl alcohol is a 16-carbon form of alcohol (hexadecanol) that acts as a spreading agent for DPPC at the liquid-air alveolar interface, since the proteins SP-B and SP-C are not contained in the artificial mixture. The tyloxapol additive (a polymeric long-chain alcohol) also acts to help disperse the DPPC and cetyl alcohol. A summary of prescribing information with complete details on the Exosurf product is given in the manufacturer's literature.

Indications for Use.   The general indication for use of Exosurf is the presence or risk of RDS of the newborn, previously described. Specific guidelines for its use are the following:

1. Prophylactic therapy of infants less than 1350-g birth weight.
2. Prophylactic therapy of infants with birth weights greater than 1350 g with evidence of pulmonary immaturity and at risk for RDS.
3. Rescue treatment of infants who have developed RDS.

Dose.   The recommended dose of Exosurf is 5 ml/kg of birth weight of the reconstituted suspension, given as two divided doses of 2.5 ml/kg, by direct tracheal administration.

Since the reconstituted suspension from a single vial of Exosurf has a volume of 8 ml, with 108 mg of colfosceril palmitate, a single vial can treat up to a 1600-g infant, based on a dose of 5 ml/kg:

$$5 \text{ ml/kg} \times 1.6 \text{ kg} = 8 \text{ ml}$$

With larger weight infants, additional vials are needed. A second dose of 5 ml/kg is administered 12 hours after the first, with a third dose, if needed, administered 12 hours after the second.

Administration.   Exosurf is instilled directly into the endotracheal tube through a side-port adapter that fits on the endotracheal tube and has a Luer-Lok. The first half of the dose is administered in bursts, timed to coincide with inspiration. The dose is given with the infant in midline position. The infant is then rotated to the right for half a minute and ventilated. The second half of the dose is then given, again in midline position, and the infant is rotated to the left.

Complete details of preparing the suspension, dosage, and administration are in the manufacturer's literature, which should be thoroughly read before using the drug.

Survanta (Beractant)

Description. Survanta (beractant) is considered a modified natural surfactant. It is a mixture with natural bovine lung extract, to which is added colfosceril palmitate (DPPC), palmitic acid, and tripalmitin. These last three ingredients are used to standardize the composition of the drug preparation, as well as to reproduce the surface-tension–lowering properties of natural surfactant. The colfosceril, or DPPC, is the same phospholipid contained in Exosurf. The ingredients are suspended in 0.9% saline. The composition of Survanta, given in the product literature, is as follows:

Phospholipids (25 mg/ml)
Triglycerides (0.5 to 1.75 mg/ml)
Free fatty acids (1.4 to 3.5 mg/ml)
Protein (<1.0 mg/ml)

The extract from minced bovine lung contains natural phospholipids; neutral lipids; fatty acids; and the low-molecular-weight, hydrophobic surfactant proteins SP-B and SP-C. The hydrophilic, large-molecular-weight protein SP-A is not contained in Survanta. SP-A helps regulate surfactant reuptake and secretion by the type II cell. However, the addition of SP-A to Survanta by Yamada et al. (1990) did not improve the biophysical (spreading, absorption) *or* physiological (lung compliance charge) activities of the mixture.

Survanta is available from Ross Laboratories as a vial containing 8 ml of suspension, with a concentration of 25 mg/ml, in a 0.9% sodium chloride solution. This gives a maximal total dose of 200 mg of phospholipids in a single vial of 8 ml of suspension.

Indications for Use. The general indications for Survanta are the same as those of all exogenous surfactants—the prevention (prophylaxis) and treatment (or rescue) of RDS in the newborn:

1. Prophylactic therapy of premature infants of less than 1250 g birth weight or with evidence of surfactant deficiency and risk of RDS.
2. Rescue treatment of infants with evidence of RDS.

Dose. The recommended dose of beractant is 100 mg/kg of birth weight. Since there are 25 mg/ml in the beractant suspension, this is equivalent to a dose of 4 ml/kg of birth weight.

As an example, a 2000-g (2-kg) infant would require 8 ml, or the entire vial of suspension.

Unlike Exosurf, Survanta does not require reconstitution since it is marketed as a suspension.

Administration. Beractant suspension is off-white to light brown. If settling has occurred in the suspension, the vial can be swirled gently but should not be shaken.

The calculated dose is given in quarters, one fourth at a time. The dose is given from a syringe and instilled into the trachea through a 5-French catheter placed into the endotracheal tube. The catheter is removed, and the infant is manually ventilated or returned to the ventilator for 30 seconds or until stable. The remaining doses are given in similar fashion.

Repeat doses of beractant are given no sooner than 6 hours later if there is evidence of continuing respiratory distress. The manufacturer's literature recommends that manual hand-bag ventilation *not* be used for the repeat dose in place of mechanical ventilation. Ventilator adjustment may be necessary, however.

The preceding general description of beractant (Survanta) is intended to be instructional. Complete prescribing information from the manufacturer should be reviewed when using this product.

Hazards and Complications of Surfactant Therapy

Some of the complications in exogenous surfactant therapy are due to the dosage procedure, and others can be caused by the therapeutic effect of the drug itself. In the dosage procedure, relatively large volumes of suspension are instilled in neonatal-sized airways, and this can block gas exchange, causing desaturation and bradycardia.

The effect of the drug in improving pulmonary compliance can lead to overventilation, excessive volume delivery from pressure-limited ventilation, and overoxygenation with dangerously high Pao_2 levels. As a result, the following complications or hazards can occur with surfactant therapy.

Airway Occlusion, Desaturation, and Bradycardia. Since the current method of administration is by direct tracheal instillation, a large volume of surfactant suspension may cause an acute obstruction of infant airways, with subsequent hypoxemia and bradycardia (Jobe, 1991). Repetitive small additions of the dose and a transient increase in ventilating pressure may help distribute the surfactant to the periphery. Administration methods are summarized briefly with the product, and details are in the manufacturer's literature.

High Arterial Oxygen (Pao$_2$) Values.   A good response to exogenous surfactant will result in better (higher) lung compliance, increased functional residual capacity, and concomitant improvement in oxygenation. Fractional inspired oxygen (Fio$_2$) settings must be lowered if Pao$_2$ improves to prevent overoxygenation and the possibility of retrolental fibroplasia.

Overventilation and Hypocarbia.   As lung compliance improves, peak ventilating pressure, expiratory baseline pressures, and ventilatory rate must be adjusted, or overventilation and pneumothorax may occur.

Apnea.   Apnea has been noted to occur with the intratracheal administration of surfactant.

Pulmonary Hemorrhage.   In a study of infants weighing less than 700 g at birth, the incidence of pulmonary hemorrhage was 10% with Exosurf compared with 2% in the control group. This increase was not seen in infants greater than 700 g at birth. Pulmonary hemorrhage was more frequent in infants who were younger, smaller, male, and with a patent ductus arteriosus (manufacturer's insert, Burroughs Wellcome Co.).

In general, complications of prematurity may affect the response to exogenous surfactant.

Selection and Administration

Now that exogenous surfactant products are available for general clinical use in the United States, new questions on their use are beginning to be addressed.

1. Which surfactant does the clinician choose? This question is really one of degree of efficacy and risk of adverse reaction, which can only be addressed by comparative data on individual products such as Survanta and Exosurf, under similar circumstances of use.

2. Which diseases will benefit from exogenous surfactant therapy? In addition to RDS of the newborn, meconium aspiration syndrome, pneumonia, and ARDS are potential target diseases for surfactant therapy. Data are becoming available on efficacy with these applications.

3. When should surfactant be given for therapy in RDS? The advantage of rescue treatment is that there is no need to predict or anticipate the onset of RDS. The need for the treatment is clearly evident in the presence of RDS.

With prophylactic therapy, there is the possibility of needless treatment, with possible adverse effects and unnecessary expense. The prophylactic approach administers surfactant as soon as possible after birth. There is discussion on waiting several hours after birth before giving surfactant, or even to withhold surfactant until and unless there is mild, or even moderate, RDS present.

   4. Are there other methods of administering surfactant preparations? An alternative to direct tracheal instillation is nebulization, and this is being investigated (Lewis et al., 1991). Other questions concern the use of high-frequency ventilation, extracorporeal membrane oxygenation, and even liquid ventilation for the administration of a surfactant.

BIBLIOGRAPHY

Avery ME, Merritt TA: Surfactant-replacement therapy, N Engl J Med 324:910, 1991.

Floros J, Phelps DS, Taeusch HW: Biosynthesis and in vitro translation of the major surfactant-associated protein from human lung, J Biol Chem 260:495, 1985.

Fujiwara T et al: Artificial surfactant therapy in hyaline membrane disease, Lancet 1:55, 1980.

Greiff L et al: Effects of histamine, ethanol, and a detergent on exudation and absorption across guinea pig airway mucosa in vivo, Thorax 46:700, 1991.

Holm BA, Matalon S: Role of pulmonary surfactant in the development and treatment of adult respiratory distress syndrome, Anesth Analg 69:805, 1989.

Jobe AH: The role of surfactant therapy in neonatal respiratory distress, Respir Care 36:695, 1991.

Jobe A, Ikegami M: Surfactant for the treatment of respiratory distress syndrome, Am Rev Respir Dis 136:1256, 1987.

Lewis J et al: Nebulized vs. instilled exogenous surfactant in an adult lung injury model, J Appl Physiol 71:1270, 1991.

Marriott C, Richards JH: The effects of storage and of potassium iodide, urea, N-acetyl-cysteine and triton X - 100 on the viscosity of bronchial mucus, Br J Dis Chest 68:171, 1974.

Merritt TA et al: Prophylactic treatment of very premature infants with human surfactant, N Engl J Med 315:785, 1986.

Miller JB et al: Alevaire inhalation for eliminating secretions in asthmatic sinusitis, bronchiectasis and bronchitis of adults, Ann Allergy 12:611, 1954.

Morton NS: Exogenous surfactant treatment for the adult respiratory distress syndrome? A historical perspective, Thorax 45:825, 1990 (editorial).

Notter RH et al: Lung surfactant replacement in premature lambs with extracted lipids from bovine lung lavage: effects of dose, dispersion techniques, and gestational age, Pediatr Rev 19:569, 1985.

Paez PN, Miller WF: Surface active agents in sputum evacuation: a blind comparison with normal saline solution and distilled water, Chest 60:312, 1971.

Palmer KNV: Effect of an aerosol detergent in chronic bronchitis, Lancet 1:611, 1957.

Possmayer F: The role of surfactant-associated proteins, Am Rev Respir Dis 142:749, 1990 (editorial).

Sears CT Jr, Stanitski CL: Chemistry for the health-related sciences: concepts and correlations, ed 2, Englewood Cliffs, NJ, 1983, Prentice-Hall.

Tainter ML et al: Alevaire as a mucolytic agent. N Engl J Med 253:764, 1955.

Wright JR, Clements JA: Metabolism and turnover of lung surfactant, Am Rev Respir Dis 135:427, 1987.

Yamada T et al: Effects of surfactant protein-A on surfactant function in preterm ventilated rabbits, Am Rev Respir Dis 142:754, 1990.

10

Corticosteroids in Respiratory Care

There are currently four corticosteroids available in the United States for inhalation as an aerosol:

Dexamethasone (Decadron Respihaler)
Beclomethasone dipropionate (Beclovent, Vanceril)
Triamcinolone acetonide (Azmacort)
Flunisolide (AeroBid)

Their primary purpose is to treat asthma through their anti-inflammatory effect. The following topics are discussed to understand the use and mechanisms of action with corticosteroids:

- Physiological characteristics of corticosteroids
- Nature of an inflammatory response
- Pharmacological properties of corticosteroids
- Aerosolized corticosteroids
- Hazards and side effects of corticosteroids
- Clinical application of aerosol corticosteroids
- Androgenic (Anabolic) corticosteroids

INTRODUCTION

Corticosteroids are a complex group of drugs. These agents act within the endocrine system rather than the nervous system.

PHYSIOLOGICAL CHARACTERISTICS OF CORTICOSTEROIDS

Identification and Source

Corticosteroids are a group of chemicals secreted by the adrenal cortex and are referred to as *adrenal cortical hormones.* The adrenal, or suprarenal, gland is composed of two portions (Fig 10–1). The inner zone is the adrenal medulla and produces epinephrine. The outer zone is the cortex, the source of corticosteroids. There are actually three types of hormones produced by the adrenal cortex: glucocorticords (e.g., cortisol), mineralocorticoids (e.g., aldosterone), and sex hormones such as androgens and estrogens. The mineralocorticoid aldosterone regulates body water by increasing the amount of sodium reabsorption in the renal tubules. Androgenic corticosteroids such as testosterone, the male sex hormone, cause secondary sex characteristics to appear and will be discussed briefly in the section on androgenic corticosteroids. The corticosteroids used in pulmonary disease are all analogues of cortisol, or *hydrocortisone* as it is also termed.

Following is a list of the major developments in the introduction of corticosteroids, specifically the glucocorticoids, for treatment of asthma.

1949—Hench and others report the anti-inflammatory activity of compound E (cortisone) in rheumatoid arthritis.

1950—Cortisone is reported to be effective in asthma.

1951—Cortisone is given by aerosol.

1956—Treatment of asthma with aerosolized hydrocortisone is reported.

1957–1958—Use of aerosolized prednisolone in asthma is reported.

1962—Aerosolized form of dexamethasone is reported.

1972—Topically active aerosolized steroids become available to treat asthma in the United Kingdom.

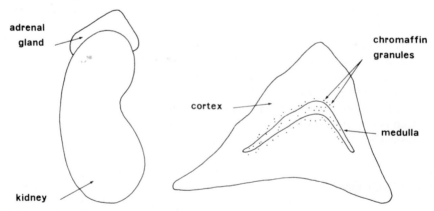

FIG 10–1. Location and cross section of the adrenal, or suprarenal, gland.

1976—Topically active aerosol beclomethasone dipropionate is available in the United States.

1984—Triamcinolone acetonide and flunisolide are approved for use in the United States.

Cortisone was isolated in 1935 by Kendall as compound E and synthesized in 1948. Its anti-inflammatory action was reported in rheumatoid arthritis by Hench and coworkers in 1949. It was found to be effective in asthma in the early 1950s, and since the 1970s there has been increasing development and introduction of aerosolized glucocorticoids for maintenance therapy of asthma.

Hypothalamic-Pituitary-Adrenal Axis

The side effects of corticosteroids and the rationale for aerosol or alternate-day therapy can be understood if the production and control of endogenous (the body's own) corticosteroids is grasped. The pathway for release and control of corticosteroids is the hypothalamic-pituitary-adrenal (HPA) axis (Fig 10–2).

Stimulation of the hypothalamus causes impulses to be sent to the area known as the median eminence, where corticotropin releasing factor (CRF) is released. CRF circulates through the portal vessel to the anterior pituitary gland, which then releases adrenocorticotropic hormone (ACTH) into the bloodstream. ACTH in turn stimulates the adrenal cortex to secrete glucocorticoids such as cortisol. Cortisol and glucocorticoids in general regulate the metabolism of carbohydrates, fats, and proteins, generally to increase levels of glucose for body energy. This is the reason cortisol and its analogues are called *glucocorticoids*. They can also cause lipolysis, redistribution of fat stores and breakdown of tissue protein stores. These actions are the basis for many of the side effects seen with glucocorticoid drugs. The breakdown of proteins for use of the amino acids (gluconeogenesis) is responsible for muscle wasting, and the effects on glucose metabolism can increase plasma glucose levels. The latter is sometimes referred to as *steroid diabetes.*

HPA Suppression With Steroid Use

One of the most notable side effects of treatment with glucocorticoid drugs (exogenous corticosteroids) is adrenal suppression, or more generally, HPA suppression. When the body produces *endogenous* glucocorticoids, there is a normal feedback mechanism within the HPA axis to limit production. As glucocorticoid levels rise, release of CRF and ACTH is inhibited, and further adrenal production of glucocorticoids is stopped. This feedback inhibition of the hypothalamus and the pituitary gland can be seen in Figure 10–2 and is analogous to the servomechanism by which a thermostat regulates furnace production of heat by monitoring temperature levels. Unfortunately, the body can-

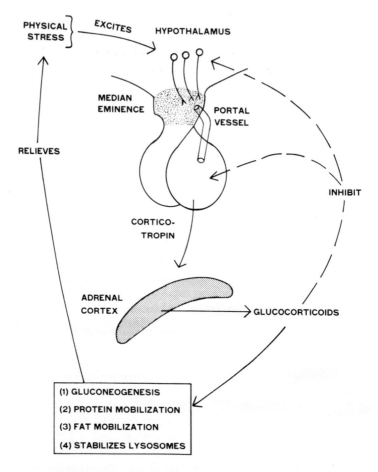

MECHANISM FOR REGULATION OF GLUCOCORTICOID SECRETION

FIG 10–2.   HPA axis regulation of corticosteroid secretion.

not distinguish between its own *endogenous* glucocorticoids and *exogenous* glucocorticoid drugs. Administration of glucocorticoid drugs raises the body's level of these hormones, and this inhibits the hypothalamus and pituitary gland, which in turn decreases adrenal production. This is referred to as *HPA suppression,* or specifically *adrenal suppression.* It is seen with systemic administration of corticosteroids, begins after a single day, and is substantial after a week of oral therapy at usual doses. One of the primary reasons for using aerosolized glucocorticoids is to minimize adrenal, or HPA, suppression both by minimizing the dosage and localizing the site of treatment.

If a patient has received oral corticosteroids and adrenal suppression has occurred, then weaning from the exogenous corticosteroids through use of tapered-dose therapy allows time for recovery of the body's own adrenal secretion. It should be noted that aerosolized corticosteroids do not deposit sufficient amounts of drug to replace the missing output of a suppressed adrenal gland. Therefore a patient with adrenal suppression cannot be abruptly withdrawn from oral corticosteroids and placed on an aerosol dosage. The aerosol should be started and the oral agent tapered off slowly at the same time.

Diurnal Steroid Cycle

The production of the body's own glucocorticoids also follows a rhythmic cycle, termed a *diurnal* or *circadian rhythm.* This daily rise and fall of glucocorticoid levels in the body is shown in Figure 10–3. On a daily schedule of daytime work and nighttime sleep, cortisol levels are highest in the morning around 8 AM. These high plasma levels inhibit further production and release of glucocorticoids and ACTH by the HPA axis, because of the feedback mechanism previously presented. The high levels mobilize the body's energy resources in response to the anticipated stress and challenge of earning a living! During the day, plasma levels of both ACTH *(dotted line)* and cortisol *(solid line)* gradually fall. As the glucocorticoid level falls, the anterior pituitary is reactivated to begin releasing ACTH, which in turn stimulates production of cortisol by the adrenal cortex. This lag between the increased ACTH and cortisol levels is seen in Figure 10–3. One of the reasons for jet lag and the delay in adjusting to night shift from day shift is that this diurnal and regular rhythm of corticosteroid levels becomes out of synchronization with the time zone and the work time. Although the worker needs to sleep at 8 o'clock after working all night, the body is wide awake with energy stores being released.

Alternate-Day Steroid Therapy

Alternate-day therapy mimics the natural diurnal rhythm by giving a steroid drug early in the morning, when normal tissue levels are high. Thus, suppression of the hypothalamic-pituitary system occurs at the same time it normally would with the body's own steroid, and on the alternate day the regular diurnal secretion in the HPA system can resume. Tissue side effects are minimized since the drug is administered at the time when tissues are nor-

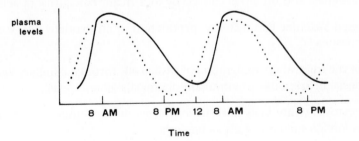

FIG 10–3. Diurnal variations in ACTH *(dotted line)* and cortisol *(solid line).*

mally exposed to high corticosteroid levels by the body's rhythm. Use of an intermediate-acting corticosteroid drug, with a duration of 12 to 36 hours, allows drug therapy to be restricted to alternate days.

NATURE OF THE INFLAMMATORY RESPONSE

One of the major therapeutic effects seen with analogues of the natural (endogenous) adrenal cortical hormone hydrocortisone is an anti-inflammatory action. Glucocorticoid analogues of natural (endogenous) hydrocortisone are used for this effect in treating asthma, which is an inflammatory process in the lungs. To understand the anti-inflammatory activity of the glucocorticoid drugs used in asthma, the nature of inflammation in general and airway inflammation in particular will be reviewed briefly.

Inflammation

A general definition of inflammation is the response of vascularized tissue to injury. An excellent and still-applicable description of inflammation was given in the first century A.D. by Celsus: "rubor et tumor cum calore et dolore." This is translated as redness and swelling, with heat and pain. This is the most general description of an inflammatory reaction to injury, such as a cut, wound infection, a splinter, burn, scrape, or bee sting.

An update of the description by Celsus occurred in the 1920s with Lewis Thomas's characterization known as the *triple response:*

Redness: local dilatation of blood vessels, occurring in seconds.

Flare: reddish color several centimeters from the site, occurring 15 to 30 seconds after injury.

Wheal: local swelling, occurring in minutes.

The process of inflammation producing the visible results described by Celsus, Thomas, and others is caused by four major categories of activity:

Increased Vascular Permeability: production of an exudate into surrounding tissues.

Leukocytic Infiltration: emigration of white cells through capillary walls (diapedesis) in response to attractant chemicals (chemotaxis).

Phagocytosis: white cells and macrophages (in the lungs) ingest and process foreign material such as bacteria.

Mediator Cascade: histamine and chemoattractant factors are released at the site of injury, and various inflammatory mediators such as complement and arachidonic acid products are generated.

Inflammation in the Airway

Inflammation can occur in the lungs in response to a variety of causes. These include direct trauma (gunshot wound, stabbing), indirect trauma (blunt chest injury), inhalation of noxious or toxic substances (chlorine gas, smoke), respiratory infections and systemic infections producing septicemia and septic shock with a respiratory distress syndrome. The two most common inflammatory diseases seen in respiratory care are chronic bronchitis, usually caused by tobacco smoking, and asthma, which can be caused by a range of triggers and involves a complex pathophysiology.

Since glucocorticoids are a mainstay for treating asthma, and asthma is a disease characterized by inflammation in the lungs, the following summary of airway inflammation is based on the sequence seen in asthma.

The inflammatory process in the lung begins with a triggering stimuli that causes the release of the following **chemical mediators:**

1. Histamine.
2. Heparin.
3. Eosinophil chemotactic factor of anaphylaxis (ECF-A).
4. Neutrophil chemotactic factor of anaphylaxis (NCF-A).
5. Bradykinin.
6. Lymphokines.
7. Arachidonic acid metabolites:
   a. Cyclooxygenase pathway:
      (1) thromboxane A_2 (TXA$_2$).
      (2) prostaglandins D_2, E_2, F_{2a} (PGD$_2$, PGE$_2$, PGF$_{2a}$).
      (3) prostacycline (PGI$_2$).
   b. Lipoxygenase pathway:
      (1) Leukotriene B_4 (LTB$_4$).
      (2) Slow-reacting substance of anaphylaxis (SRS-A).
         a. Leukotriene C_4 (LTC$_4$).
         b. Leukotriene D_4 (LTD$_4$).
         c Leukotriene E_4 (LTE$_4$).
      (3) Platelet-activating factor.

This "chemical cascade" comes from mast cells in lung tissue, from phospholipids in the cell membrane, from lymphocytes or other leukocytes, and from serum precursors. A conceptual representation of the overall process is given in Figure 10–4. After an insult to the asthmatic airway by an allergen, cold air, viral infection, or noxious gas, mast cells begin to release mediators including histamine. These mediators of inflammation act in the surrounding tissues and/or blood vessels to attract eosinophils (ECF-A), neutrophils (NCF), and lymphocytes. As previously described, blood vessels increase their permeability, leaking exudate into tissues of the airway and releasing neutrophils and monocytes. Macrophages are drawn to the airway.

Phospholipids in the cell membrane of mast cells and other cells are converted by phospholipase A_2 to arachidonic acid and then to a variety of bronchoactive and vasoactive substances by the two metabolic paths shown. The term *eicosanoid* is used to refer to the chemical mediators listed previously, which are the products of the two pathways.

The immediate response of the airway to chemicals such as histamine is bronchospasm. This produces the early-phase decrease in expiratory flow rates illustrated in Figure 10–4. Although the early bronchoconstriction of smooth muscle may self-limit or respond to the beta agonists described in Chapter 5, the progression of cellular events can continue. The migration of white cells, lymphocytes, and further development of inflammation-producing chemicals such as the arachidonic acid metabolites all contribute to build an inflammatory response in the lung (Kay, 1987). In addition to smooth muscle

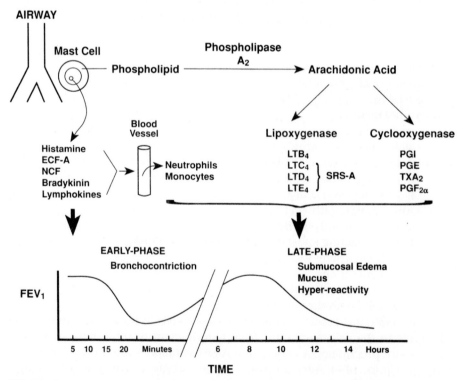

FIG 10–4. Development of inflammation in the airway, producing a biphasic deterioration in expiratory flow rates.

spasm, there is mucous secretion and mucosal swelling due to increased vascular permeability. There is increase in eosinophils and neutrophils that migrate to the airway, shedding of airway cells (desquamation), and hyperplasia of goblet cells. The result is mucus plugging of the airway, complicated by the cellular debris in the bronchial lumen. In fact the pathologic condition of bronchial asthma has been described as "chronic desquamating eosinophilic bronchitis" (Reed, 1990). These airway changes lead to further bronchial hyperreactivity seen in asthma. There are many detailed reviews of chemical mediators of lung inflammation.*

These events that follow the initial bronchospasm can occur hours later and produce what is termed the *late-phase reaction* (Fig 10–4), unless the inflammatory progression is stopped with treatment.

PHARMACOLOGICAL PROPERTIES OF CORTICOSTEROIDS

The inflammatory process can be reduced or blocked by the anti-inflammatory effects of glucocorticoids. The beneficial effect of glucocorticoids in asthma, as well as in other diseases of inflammation, is due to their ability to inhibit the number and activity of inflammatory cells.

Mode of Action

Nuclear Model

The mode of action of corticosteroids in causing their effects has been well reviewed in several sources: Kaliner, 1985; Morris, 1985a and 1985b; Sertl, 1990; Szefler, 1991; Townley and Suliaman, 1987. The February 1990 supplement of the *American Review of Respiratory Disease* is entirely devoted to a comprehensive review of the pharmacological properties and clinical application of corticosteroids.

Although the mechanism by which these agents exert their effects is not completely understood, a nuclear model for corticosteroid action is usually given (Munck et al., 1990). In addition to this nuclear mechanism (Fig 10–5), there may be other actions caused by direct stimulation of tissue receptor sites by corticosteroids. In the nuclear model, a steroid molecule diffuses into a cell, binds to a specific receptor, and forms a complex. The steroid-receptor complex enters the cell nucleus and influences the synthesis of messenger ribonucleic acid *(MRNA)*; this causes production of new proteins by the cell.

The particular result produced by the steroid depends on the type of cell involved, such as a lymphocyte or a neutrophil. The effect of the steroid in the body is caused by the changes produced in the cell. These include the production of protein such as lipocortin and changes in cell proliferation rates

*Barnes (1987), Drazen and Austen (1987), Friedman and Kaliner (1987), Gundel et al. (1986), Henderson (1987), O'Byrne (1986), Schulman (1986), and Schwartz (1987).

GLUCOCORTICOID: MODE OF ACTION

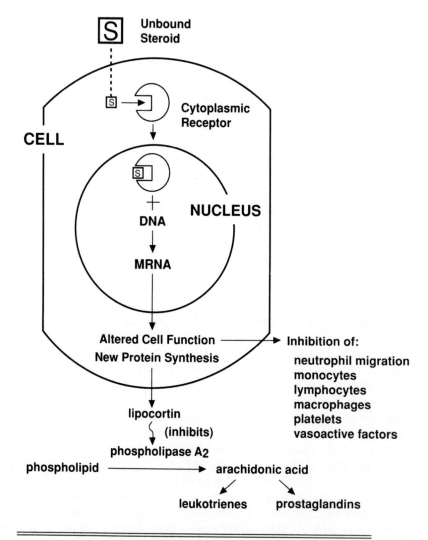

RESULT: SUPPRESSION OF INFLAMMATION

FIG 10–5. Conceptualization of the nuclear model for corticosteroid action.

or in cell surface receptors. Ultimately, as seen in Figure 10–5, the cells and mediators responsible for generating an inflammatory response are modified to inhibit the process, as described next. Because the effects are mediated by such a nuclear pathway, there is a time lag between 2 and 24 hours for various steroid effects to become evident.

Effect on the Inflammatory Response

Some of the specific effects of glucocorticoids in reducing inflammation are as follows:

1. Blockade of arachidonic acid metabolites in inhibition of phospholipase A_2, including prevention of SRS-A (LTC_4, LTD_4, LTE_4) synthesis and prevention of prostaglandin (PGE, PGF, TXA) synthesis.
2. Decrease of monocytes, eosinophils, and basophils.
3. Decrease of lymphocytes and suppression of type IV delayed hypersensitivity reaction.
4. Inhibition of late-phase inflammatory response.
5. Increase in beta-receptor density on cell surfaces.
6. Redistribution of neutrophils (demargination).

There is controversy over whether glucocorticoids prevent IgE-mediated mast cell release of mediators in humans. Their effect may be on subsequent steps of the process caused by mast cell mediators. The situation is complicated by the recent recognition of different types of mast cells in humans.

Two of the better known effects of glucocorticoids are their blockade of arachidonic acid products and their effect on leukocytes. The inhibition of arachidonic acid metabolites by glucocorticoids is shown in Figure 10–5. Glucocorticoids cause synthesis of a protein, lipocortin, which inhibits the phospholipase A_2 enzyme from converting phospholipid to arachidonic acid. This prevents generation of eicosanoids, the cyclooxygenase and lipoxygenase products of arachidonic acid. Thus, glucocorticoids inhibit prostaglandin synthesis and in general all of the inflammatory mediators derived from arachidonic acid.

Leukocytes such as monocytes, macrophages, neutrophils, and basophils are also essential to the inflammatory response and are attracted to an area of injury by the chemotactic factors identified among the chemical mediators of inflammation listed previously. Neutrophils usually adhere ("marginate") to the capillary endothelium of storage sites in the lung. Glucocorticoids cause depletion of these stores and reduce their accumulation at inflammatory sites and in exudates. This is often termed *demargination* and can increase the number of neutrophils in circulation as the cells leave their storage sites. An overall increase in the white cell count can then be seen in patients on glucocorticoids. Glucocorticoids affect other leukocytes by inhibiting the number of monocytes, basophils, and eosinophils. This can also be seen in the differential count of these cells. An allergic asthmatic patient who would otherwise have a higher than normal eosinophil count, will show a low count after initiation of drug therapy. Finally, glucocorticoids constrict the microvasculature to reduce leakage of the above cells and fluids into inflammatory sites.

Effect on Beta Receptors

Beta-adrenergic agents are among the most potent inhibitors of mast cell release, yet the asthmatic patient in an acute episode may be unresponsive to these drugs. A very beneficial effect of glucocorticoids is their ability to restore responsiveness to beta-adrenergic stimulation (Svedmyr, 1990). This effect is seen within 1 to 4 hours after intravenous administration of glucocorticoids and is the rationale for administering a bolus of steroid in status asthmaticus when managing an acute episode. Even though steroid action is slow, the sooner glucocorticoids are given, the sooner the asthmatic patient will begin to respond to beta-adrenergic drugs, and supported ventilation may be avoided. Glucocorticoids enhance beta-receptor stimulation by increasing the number and availability of beta receptors on the cell surfaces, and by increasing affinity of the receptor for beta agonists. There is also evidence that glucocorticoids prolong endogenous, circulatory catecholamine action by inhibiting the uptake-2 mechanism (extraneuronal uptake) discussed in Chapter 4.

AEROSOLIZED CORTICOSTEROIDS

Pharmacological Properties of Topical Steroids

There are a number of corticosteroid preparations such as hydrocortisone, cortisone, prednisone, prednisolone, and methylprednisolone, all of which have anti-inflammatory activity. However, they produce undesirable systemic side effects when used to treat asthma, an inflammation of the lung.

Early Trials of Aerosol Steroids

The attempt to introduce aerosolized corticosteroids directly into the lung to avoid systemic side effects began in 1951, shortly after the identification of steroids. The development of this effort, which resulted in the currently available aerosolized steroid agents, was highlighted previously in this chapter.

Glucocorticoid receptors are similar throughout the body, and therefore it has not been feasible to develop a steroid that would control bronchial inflammation without causing systemic side effects when given orally or intravenously. These side effects include adrenal suppression and cushingoid symptoms such as moon face, edema, central fat deposition (humpback). The alternative is to target the lung locally with an aerosol formulation.

Cortisone, hydrocortisone, prednisone, and finally dexamethasone were all tried by aerosol between 1951 and 1963; although all produced the desired therapeutic effect of reduced airway inflammation, each unfortunately caused hypercortical effects and adrenal suppression. In each agent, the therapeutic dose was large enough to lead to systemic absorption, with the resulting side effects. Because of this, the aerosol route was not especially beneficial compared with the oral route for long-term administration. Until 1976, dexamethasone, in its metered-spray formulation, remained the aerosolizable steroid of choice despite this fact. However, the introduction of the newer synthetic analogues of hydrocortisone, which have a high topical anti-inflammatory activity, paved the way for effective use of aerosolized steroids with little systemic side effects. These agents include beclomethasone, triamcinolone, flunisolide, and the investigational agent budesonide.

Topical/Systemic Activity Ratios

Specifically these agents have a high ratio of topical to systemic activity. Check and Kaliner (1990) reviewed the chemical principles involved in the development of these steroid analogues, to achieve local effect in the lungs with less potential for systemic absorption and side effects. The high topical/systemic activity ratios of aerosolized corticosteroids are facilitated by the following combination of factors:

1. Direct introduction into the airway by aerosol.
2. Nonpolar, water-insoluble preparations with less potential for systemic absorption.
3. Rapid inactivation of drug absorbed into the plasma.
4. Intrinsic topical anti-inflammatory effect (measured by skin blanching, which reflects vasoconstriction).

The topical potency of the aerosolized agents in relation to cortisol is as follows (Check and Kaliner, 1990; Harris, 1975):

Cortisol:	0.1
Dexamethasone:	0.8
Triamcinolone-16,17-acetonide:	100.0
Beclomethasone-17,21-dipropionate	500.0

Of the compounds listed, beclomethasone dipropionate has the highest topical potency in humans. It also has the lowest systemic potency, as measured in animals (Check and Kaliner, 1990), when compared with triamcinolone or flunisolide.

Aerosolized Corticosteroid Agents

There are currently four aerosolized steroid agents, all of which are glucocorticoids, available for inhalational use in the United States at the time of this edition. They are the following:

Dexamethasone sodium phosphate (Decadron Respihaler)
Beclomethasone dipropionate (Beclovent, Vanceril)
Triamcinolone acetonide (Azmacort)
Flunisolide (AeroBid)

These agents, along with their strengths and recommended dosages, are listed in Table 10–1. All of the agents are synthetic analogues of hydrocortisone and are marketed in metered-dose inhalers. There is not currently a nebulizer solution marketed in the United States for inhalational use, although nasal spray solutions (e.g., flunisolide) are available. With the exception of dexamethasone, these agents possess the high topical/systemic potency ratio described, to make them suitable for control of asthma with minimal systemic side effects.

The basic steroid structure and the chemical structures of the four aerosol agents are shown in Figure 10–6. A brief description of each of the aerosol agents is given below. A more detailed review of the structure-activity relations of these agents can be found in Check and Kaliner (1990).

Dexamethasone Sodium Phosphate (Decadron Respihaler)

Dexamethasone is the oldest of the four aerosolized agents for inhalation and has an anti-inflammatory activity 30 times that of hydrocortisone, with 0.6 mg equivalent to a 20-mg dose of hydrocortisone. This is one of the first successfully aerosolized agents and has a long biologic and plasma half-life. Plasma half-life refers to the presence of the drug in the blood, whereas biologic half-life refers to its effect on tissue.

TABLE 10–1.

Corticosteroids Available by Aerosol for Inhalation Administration

Drug	Strength (μg/puff)	Dosage
Dexamethasone sodium phosphate (Decadron Respihaler)	84	Adults, 3 puffs tid, qid; Children, 2 puffs tid, qid
Beclomethasone dipropionate (Beclovent, Vanceril)	42	Adults, 2 puffs tid, tid; Children, 1–2 puffs tid, qid
Triamcinolone acetonide (Azmacort)	100	Adults, 2 puffs tid, qid; Children, 1–2 puffs tid, qid
Flunisolide (Aerobid)	250	Adults, 2 puffs bid; Children, 2 puffs bid

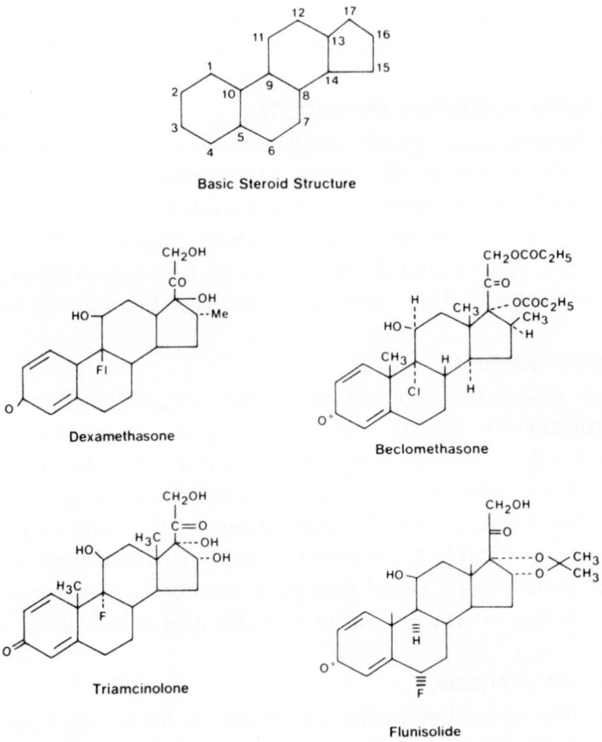

Basic Steroid Structure

Dexamethasone

Beclomethasone

Triamcinolone

Flunisolide

FIG 10–6. Basic steroid structure and structures of four aerosolized corticosteroids.

Beclomethasone Dipropionate (Vanceril, Beclovent)

Beclomethasone was the second aerosolized corticosteroid available in the United States. This is an effective anti-inflammatory aerosol for use in controlling asthma that requires steroid therapy. In severe asthma, a dosage of 12 to 16 inhalations per day may be initiated and then adjusted downward. The drug's success as an aerosol in reducing or replacing the use of systemic steroids is due to its high topical/systemic activity ratio previously discussed.

An aerosol dose of 400 µg is approximately equivalent to 5 to 10 mg of oral prednisone. It has a topical/systemic potency ratio approximately 500 times that of dexamethasone. The low systemic effect of beclomethasone is due to the following factors:

1. Swallowed drug is slowly absorbed from the gastrointestinal tract.
2. Most of what is absorbed is quickly (half-life in the liver = 10 minutes) broken down in its first passage through the liver, preventing high plasma levels.
3. Beclomethasone has a high intrinsic topical activity.

4. There is good absorption of the drug across the pulmonary epithelium, but rapid first-pass inactivation prevents systemic accumulation.

Triamcinolone Acetonide (Azmacort)

Triamcinolone is also topically active and was available as Aristocort and Kenalog before its release as an aerosol. Triamcinolone acetonide is nonpolar and water insoluble, resulting in a lower potential for systemic absorption. This drug is slightly less topically active than beclomethasone dipropionate (Check and Kaliner, 1990). High initial dosages of 12 to 16 inhalations per day may be needed in severe asthma. This agent is marketed with a built-in spacer device.

Flunisolide (AeroBid)

Flunisolide is another topically active aerosol preparation, similar in potency to triamcinolone, and is said to be longer acting. The name AeroBid indicates the dosage schedule, which is twice daily. Flunisolide shows a peak plasma level after inhalation between 2 and 60 minutes, indicating good absorption from the lungs, as with beclomethasone. The half-life in plasma with inhalation is approximately 1.8 hours and similar to that with oral or intravenous dosages, indicating a rapid first-pass metabolism. The pharmacokinetics of flunisolide has been studied by Chaplin and co-workers (1980).

Other Aerosol Steroids

Other steroids are either under investigation for aerosol use or are used in countries outside the United States. These include betamethasone valerate (Bextasol), budesonide (Pulmicort), and clobetasol.

Intranasal Steroids

Several of the aerosolized steroids are available in nasal insufflators and are used for seasonal rhinitis, nasal polyps, and allergic or inflammatory nasal conditions. They are the following:

Dexamethasone (Decadron Turbinaire): two sprays (168 μg) into each nostril 2 to 3 times daily.

Flunisolide (Nasalide): two sprays (50 μg) in each nostril 2 times daily.

Beclomethasone (Beconase, Vancenase): one spray (42 μg) in each nostril 2 to 4 times daily.

Triamcinolone (Nasacort): two sprays (110 μg) in each nostril once a day.

HAZARDS AND SIDE EFFECTS OF STEROIDS

Systemic Administration of Steroids

The complicating side effects of systemic steroid treatment are well known and provide the motivation to transfer to aerosolized, inhaled steroids when possible. These complications arise from the physiological effects of steroids on the body. These physiological effects are often exaggerated with systemic drug therapy, because potency and plasma levels are higher than with the body's own steroids. Complications of systemic therapy are reviewed by Truhan and Ahmed (1989). These complications are summarized as follows:

1. Suppression of the HPA axis by exogenous steroids may occur, causing inhibition of ACTH release and cortisol secretion from the adrenal gland. The length of time to recover from this suppression varies with patient, dose, and duration of treatment.
2. With sufficient dose and duration, immunosuppression can be caused by systemic use of steroids. This can lead to increased susceptibility to infection by bacterial, viral, or fungal agents.
3. There can be psychiatric reactions, ranging from insomnia and mood changes, to manic-depressive or schizophrenic psychoses.
4. Cataract formation has been noted, and rarely intraocular pressure may increase with systemic steroid therapy.
5. Myopathy of striated skeletal muscle can occur.
6. Steroid-induced osteoporosis is debated but is thought to be a limitation of extended steroid therapy. Aseptic necrosis of the bone is also caused by steroid therapy.
7. Peptic ulcer is thought to be a complication of steroid therapy, but evidence for this is debated. Patients may often be receiving other ulcerogenic medications such as aspirin or nonsteroid anti-inflammatory drugs.
8. Fluid retention can occur due to the sodium-sparing effects of glucocorticoids, giving a puffy appearance.
9. Hypertension may accompany the fluid retention or be aggravated by it.
10. Corticosteroids given systemically can increase the white blood cell count, with an increase in neutrophils and a decrease in lymphocytes and eosinophils.
11. There are a number of dermatogical changes with steroid therapy, including a redistribution of subcutaneous fat causing the cushingoid appearance of central obesity, and moon face.
12. Growth of children can be slowed by prolonged systemic therapy, since corticosteroids retard bone growth and epiphyseal maturation.
13. Corticosteroids lead to gluconeogenesis and antagonize glucose uptake, causing hyperglycemia. This can lead to a reversible steroid-induced diabetes.

Inhalation of Aerosolized Steroids

The rationale for the introduction of inhaled aerosolized steroids was to eliminate or reduce the side effects seen with systemic therapy. However, even aerosolized steroids can cause side effects. These are divided into systemic side effects caused by the inhaled aerosol and topical side effects from the aerosolized drug.

Systemic Side Effects from Aerosol

Each of the following can complicate the use of aerosolized steroids, especially when transferring from oral therapy to the inhaled route.

1. Adrenal insufficiency may occur after transfer from systemic to inhaled aerosolized steroids. Weaning from systemic steroids to allow recovery of adrenal cortex and HPA function and careful monitoring of pulmonary function can help to control this problem.

2. There may be a recurrence of allergic inflammation in other organs, such as nasal polyps or atopic dermatitis, following cessation of systemic steroids.

3. Acute severe episodes of asthma may occur following withdrawal from oral steroids and transfer to inhaled forms. Aerosolized steroids may not be adequate to control asthma, especially during periods of stress, and short courses of oral drug may be necessary ("burst" therapy).

4. Suppression of HPA function is nonexistent or small at low doses of inhaled aerosolized steroids and increases with higher doses. Clinically relevant suppression is rare at inhaled doses below 800 μg per day (Geddes, 1992).

5. There are questions about the effect of inhaled steroids on growth when used with prepubertal children. A study by Wolthers and Pedersen (1992) found a reduction in rate of lower leg growth with inhaled budesonide compared with placebo. Murphy and Kelly (1992) caution that knowledge of the complete safety profile with inhaled steroids in children is incomplete.

Topical Side Effects from Aerosol

Two of the most common side effects that are caused by the topical application of inhaled steroids in the respiratory tract are oropharyngeal candidiasis (oral thrush) and dysphonia. Several other complications and precautions with the inhaled route are listed below:

1. Orophyaryngeal fungal infections with *Candida albicans* or *Aspergillus niger* may occur in the mouth, pharynx, or larynx with aerosolized steroid treatment. Some form of this may be seen in up to one third of patients on the aerosol formulations, but such an infection responds to topical antifungal agents and seems to diminish with continued aerosol steroid use (Reed, 1990). Occurrence and severity are dose related and more likely in patients who are also taking oral steroids. The use of a spacer device and gargling after treatment can reduce orophyarnygeal deposition of the steroid and the incidence or severity of such infections.

2. Dysponia, hoarseness and changes in voice quality, also may occur with inhaled steroids in one third of patients. This can be minimized with use of a spacer and by gargling. The effect is primarily caused by adductor vocal cord paresis, which is thought to be a local steroid-induced myopathy (Williams et al, 1983).

3. Cough and bronchoconstriction occasionally may occur after inhalation of an aerosolized steroid (Reed, 1990).

4. Use of aerosolized corticosteroids during an acute severe asthmatic episode represents a risk, since the aerosol route is not recommended in such cases, and steroids are not themselves bronchodilators.

5. Incorrect use of the metered-dose inhaler also represents a possible risk factor, since inadequate amounts of the topical inhaled steroid will be delivered.

CLINICAL APPLICATION OF AEROSOLIZED STEROIDS

Indications for Use

Systemic corticosteroids are used for a wide variety of conditions, usually with the therapeutic goal of reducing inflammation. These applications range from contact dermatitis to rheumatoid arthritis and systemic lupus erythematosus.

Aerosolized steroids are indicated for the following uses:

1. Control of asthma.
2. Treatment of related corticosteroid-responsive bronchospastic states not controlled with other therapy.

Intranasal aerosolized steroid preparations are used for treatment of allergic or inflammatory nasal conditions, including seasonal or perennial rhinitis.

Use in Asthma

Corticosteroids have traditionally been used in asthma, both by oral and intravenous routes, as well as by aerosol. However, the increased emphasis on asthma as a disease of inflammation leading to bronchial hyperresponsiveness has shifted the use of inhaled aerosolized steroids from second- or third-line therapy to first-line, primary therapy. Current considerations in the clinical application of steroids in asthma are presented in the *Guidelines for the Diagnosis and Management of Asthma*, prepared by the National Asthma Education Program (NAEP) Expert Panel and published by the Department of Health and Human Services (August 1991). A recent discussion of the scientific basis of steroid treatment in asthma is also available in the February supplement, Corticosteroids: Their biologic mechanisms and application to the treatment of asthma, *American Review of Respiratory Disease* (February, 1990).

The following summarizes the principles of steroid use in asthma, based on these findings and guidelines:

- Bronchial hyperresponsiveness is characteristic of asthma and is related to the degree of airway inflammation (Barnes, 1990).
- The basic pathologic condition of asthma, previously emphasizing bronchospasm, is now described as "chronic desquamating eosinophilic bronchitis" (Reed, 1990).
- The use of inhaled corticosteroids should be considered as primary therapy in managing moderate and severe asthma. Several points are related to the use of inhaled steroids:

1. Inhaled steroids should be attempted in an effort to replace chronic therapy with oral steroids (Guidelines, Chapter 4).
2. Successful aerosol treatment may require an initial clearing of the airways by use of oral steroids (Morrow-Brown et al, 1972; Reed, 1990).
3. If asthma is not controlled by inhaled steroids and other types of drug therapy, a short burst of oral steroids may be required to prevent or lessen acute exacerbations (Guidelines, Chapter 7).
4. The use of inhaled anti-inflammatory agents such as corticosteroids may benefit all asthmatic patients other than those with only mild, episodic symptoms (Guidelines, Chapter 7).
5. There is evidence that the addition of an inhaled corticosteroid to first-line beta-agonist maintenance treatment of asthma reduces morbidity and airway hyperresponsiveness (Kerstjens et al., 1992).
6. Although inhaled corticosteroids are excellent anti-inflammatory agents and acceptable for primary therapy of moderate asthma in children, the NAEP recommends a trial of cromolyn sodium (see Chapter 11) before using the inhaled steroid (Guidelines, Chapter 7).

The efficacy, as well as side effects, of aerosol steroids are dose dependent. This has two implications.

First, high-dose inhaled steroids can be tried in cases of severe, persistent asthma to replace or reduce oral corticosteroid dependence. High doses of inhaled steroids are 2 to 4 times the usual recommended dose. Oral steroid therapy can be reduced slowly while monitoring the patient's pulmonary function (Guidelines, Chapter 4).

Second, although more control may be achieved with high doses of inhaled steroids, side effects (including systemic ones) are also likely to increase with inhaled dosages above 1 mg/d. However, if oral steroids can be replaced or even reduced, this can be an overall improvement in the risk/benefit ratio (Geddes, 1992).

Aerosolized steroids are not considered to be indicated in the emergency management of acute, severe asthmatic episodes (Reed, 1990). Systemic administration is indicated in this situation (Guidelines, Chapter 8).

Aerosol treatment is more effective when administered in several dosages throughout the day (Reed, 1990).

All aerosolized corticosteroids should be administered for oral inhalation using an auxiliary, reservoir (spacer), device to reduce the risk of oropharyngeal candidiasis or other fungal infections.

Use in COPD

The use of steroids in chronic obstructive pulmonary disease (COPD) is debated. Corticosteroids can be beneficial in improving flow rates in patients with chronic bronchitis or acute respiratory failure. With stable COPD, especially severe disease, corticosteroids may be helpful in improving lung function. However, a study by Eliasson and others (1986) estimated that the proportion of stable COPD patients showing improvement with corticosteroids is small. Therefore, pulmonary function results, symptoms, and change in response to beta agonists should be evaluated when determining whether corticosteroids will benefit a COPD patient. Because of the serious side effects with these agents, they should be discontinued if improvement cannot be shown. The availability of the anticholinergic agent ipratropium also now offers an alternative to both beta agonists and corticosteroids for use in COPD.

ANDROGENIC (ANABOLIC) CORTICOSTEROIDS

Testosterone is a hormone, generally referred to as the male sex hormone, which is the third type of steroid secreted by the adrenal cortex. This hormone is androgenic, is responsible for secondary male sex characteristics, and is present in both men and women, although to a lesser degree in women. The hormone also causes anabolic effects such as an increase in muscle and lean body mass (the prefix *ana-* means building up). Derivatives of testosterone have been developed in an effort to minimize the androgenic or masculinizing effects and still maintain the anabolic effects. Medical uses of these derivatives, which are termed *anabolic steroids*, include stimulation of red blood cells in certain forms of anemia and stimulation of sexual development in hypogonadal male patients.

The structure of testosterone, cortisol, and anabolic steroid derivatives are pictured in Figure 10–7. The common steroid nucleus is clearly seen in all of these agents. Testosterone can also be converted by the body to estradiol (Fig 10–7), which is an estrogenic or feminizing hormone. One of the side effects of anabolic steroids is gynecomastia, which implies that these testosterone derivatives can also be converted to estrogens. Generally, testosterone and its derivatives bind with an androgen receptor in the cytoplasm of skeletal muscles, prostate gland, and other organs. The steroid-receptor complex then causes the cell nucleus to increase ribonucleic acid synthesis and in turn protein synthesis in cell ribosomes. There is no question that the anabolic steroids increase nitrogen retention and body mass, as well as enhance muscle growth in castrated male animals and in normal female animals. Anabolic steroid therapy is effective in stimulating muscular development in castrated men or those otherwise deficient in natural androgens. Following is a partial list of therapeutic androgenic steroids:

Ethylestrenol (Maxibolin)
Methandrostenolone

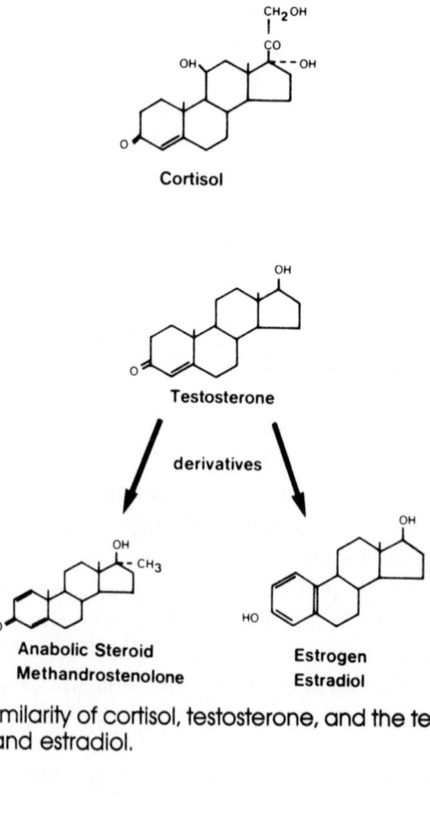

FIG 10–7. Structural similarity of cortisol, testosterone, and the testosterone derivatives methandrostenolone and estradiol.

Nandrolone (Deca-Durabolin)
Oxandrolone (Anavar)
Oxymetholone (Anadrol-50)
Stanozolol (Winstrol)

Use in Sports

Since the 1950s, anabolic steroids have been increasingly used by athletes for their effect in increasing body weight and muscle mass. The increased muscle mass is perceived to be associated with improved performance, endurance, and strength. Controversy over the use of such agents centers on whether performance is really improved and on the potential for hazardous side effects. There is little question that the drugs do produce marked side effects in both men and women as listed below:

Side Effects in the Men

Acne
Increased aggressiveness and sexual appetite
Kidney dysfunction
Reduced testicular size
Reduced sperm count
Breast enlargement
Premature baldness
Prostate gland enlargement

Side Effects in the Women

Masculinization
Interference with menstrual cycle
Excessive facial and body hair
Clitoral enlargement
Deepening of the voice

In men, the side effects are generally due to interference with the hypothalamic-pituitary-gonadal regulation and to conversion of anabolic agents to estrogens. In women, masculinizing side effects predominate due to the androgenic nature of the steroids, which is the basis for the humorous though seldom accurate stereotype of the female athlete. Two review articles are cited in the Bibliography on the subject of anabolic steroids (Haupt, 1984; Lamb, 1984) as is an editorial report in the *Journal of the American Medical Association* (1987).

BIBLIOGRAPHY

Barnes PJ: Inflammatory mediator receptors and asthma, Am Rev Respir Dis 135(suppl):S26, 1987.

Brockbank W, Brebner H, Pengelly CDR: Chronic asthma treated with aerosol hydrocortisone, Lancet ii:807, 1956.

Carryer HM et al: The effect of cortisone on bronchial asthma and hay fever occurring in subjects sensitive to ragweed pollen, J Allergy 21:282, 1950.

Chaplin MD et al: Flunisolide metabolism and dynamics of a metabolite, Clin Pharmacol Ther 27:402, 1980.

Check WA, Kaliner MA: Pharmacology and pharmacokinetics of topical corticosteroid derivatives used for asthma therapy, Am Rev Respir Dis 141(suppl):S44, Feb 1990.

Drazen JM, Austen KF: Leukotrienes and airway responses, Am Rev Respir Dis 136:985, 1987.

Eliasson O et al: Corticosteroids in COPD: a clinical trial and reassessment of the literature, Chest 89:484, 1986.

Fisch BR, Grater WC: Dexamethasone aerosol in respiratory tract disease, J New Drugs 2:298, 1962.

Friedman MM, Kaliner MA: Human mast cells and asthma, Am Rev Respir Dis 135:1157, 1987.

Geddes DM: Inhaled corticosteroids: benefits and risks, Thorax 47:404, 1992 (editorial).

Gelfand ML: Administration of cortisone by the aerosol method in the treatment of bronchial asthma, N Engl J Med 245:203, 1951.

Gundel RH et al: The leukotrienes: pharmacologic and clinical implications for respiratory care, Respir Care 31:137, 1986.

Harris DM: Some properties of beclomethasone dipropionate and related steroids in man, Postgrad Med J 57(suppl 4):20, 1975.

Haupt HA, Rovere GD: Anabolic steroids: a review of the literature, Am J Sports Med 12:469, 1984.

Hench PS et al: The effect of a hormone of the adrenal cortex (17-hydroxy-11-dehydrocorticosterone, compound E) and of pituitary adrenocorticotropic hormone on rheumatoid arthritis, Mayo Clin Proc 24:181, 1949.

Henderson WR Jr: Lipid-derived and other chemical mediators of inflammation in the lung, J Allergy Clin Immunol 79:543, 1987.

Kaliner M: Mechanisms of glucocorticosteroid action in bronchial asthma, J Allergy Clin Immunol 76:321, 1985.

Kay AB: Mediators and inflammatory cells in allergic disease, Ann Allergy 59:35, 1987.

Kerstjens HAM et al: A comparison of bronchodilator therapy with or without inhaled corticosteroid therapy for obstructive airways disease, N Engl J Med 327:1413, 1992.

Lamb DR: Anabolic steroids in athletics: how well do they work and how dangerous are they? Am J Sports Med 12:31, 1984.

Morris HG: Mechanisms of glucocorticoid action in pulmonary disease, Chest 88(suppl):133S, Aug 1985a.

Morris HG: Mechanisms of action and therapeutic role of corticosteroids in asthma, J Allergy Clin Immunol 75:1, 1985b.

Morrow-Brown H, Storey G, George WHS: Beclomethasone dipropionate: a new steroid aerosol for the treatment of allergic asthma, Br Med J 1:585, 1972.

Munck A et al: Glucocorticoid receptors and actions, Am Rev Respir Dis 141(suppl):S2, Feb 1990.

Murphy S, Kelly HW: Evaluation of therapy for childhood asthma, Am Rev Respir Dis 146:544, 1992 (editorial).

National Asthma Education Program: Guidelines for the diagnosis and management of asthma. Bethesda, Md, 1991, U.S. Department of Health and Human Services, National Institutes of Health.

O'Byrne PM: Airway inflammation and airway hyperresponsiveness, Chest 90:575, 1986.

Peters GA, Henderson LL: Prednisolone aerosol in asthmatic bronchitis: a preliminary report. Proc Staff Meet Mayo Clinic 33:57, 1958.

Reed CE: Aerosol glucocorticoid treatment of asthma: adults. Am Rev Respir Dis 141(suppl):S82, Feb 1990.

Schulman GS: The role of mast cell derived mediators in airway hyperresponsiveness, Chest 90:578, 1986.

Schwartz LB: Mediators of human mast cells and human mast cell subsets. Ann Allergy 58:226, 1987.

Steroids in sports. After four decades, time to return these genies to bottle? (Medical News & Perspectives) JAMA 257:421, 1987 (editorial).

Svedmyr N: Action of corticosteroids on beta-adrenergic receptors, clinical aspects, Am Rev Respir Dis 141(suppl):S31, Feb 1990.

Szefler SJ: Glucocorticoid therapy for asthma: clinical pharmacology, J Allergy Clin Immunol 88:147, 1991.

Townley RG, Suliaman F: The mechanism of corticosteroids in treating asthma, Ann Allergy 58:1, 1987.

Truhan AP, Ahmed AR: Corticosteroids: a review with emphasis on complications of prolonged systemic therapy, Ann Allergy 62:375, 1989.

Williams AJ et al: Dysphonia caused by inhaled steroids: recognition of a characteristic laryngeal abnormality, Thorax 38:813, 1983.

Wolthers OD, Pedersen S: Controlled study of linear growth in asthmatic children during treatment with inhaled glucocorticoids, Pediatrics 89:839, 1992.

11

Antiasthmatic Aerosol Agents

Chapter 11 discusses the antiasthmatic drugs cromolyn sodium and nedocromil sodium. Both drugs are for prevention of asthmatic episodes. The major topics presented are:

- History and identification of cromolyn sodium
- Pathophysiological characteristics of asthma
- Mode of action of cromolyn sodium
- Formulations of cromolyn sodium
- Side effects of the drug
- Clinical use of cromolyn sodium
- Nedocromil sodium

HISTORY AND IDENTIFICATION

In January 1965 a bischromone, later known as cromolyn sodium, was synthesized in the laboratory of the Fisons Corporation (Bedford, Mass.). Dr. Roger Altounyan, an investigator of the drug who himself has asthma, found that prior inhalation of cromolyn sodium inhibited and reduced his symptoms (Altounyan, 1967). This drug, a synthetic derivative of khellin, the active ingredient found in the Mediterranean plant *Ammi visnaga*, was first introduced for clinical use in 1967 and became available for use in the United States in 1973.

Cromolyn sodium, or *disodium cromoglycate* as it is also termed, is used as a prophylactic agent to prevent asthmatic reactions. It is a unique agent, different in structure and activity from the drug groups considered in previous chapters. The structure of cromolyn sodium is shown in Figure 11–1. The basic catecholamine, xanthine, and steroid structures are given for compari-

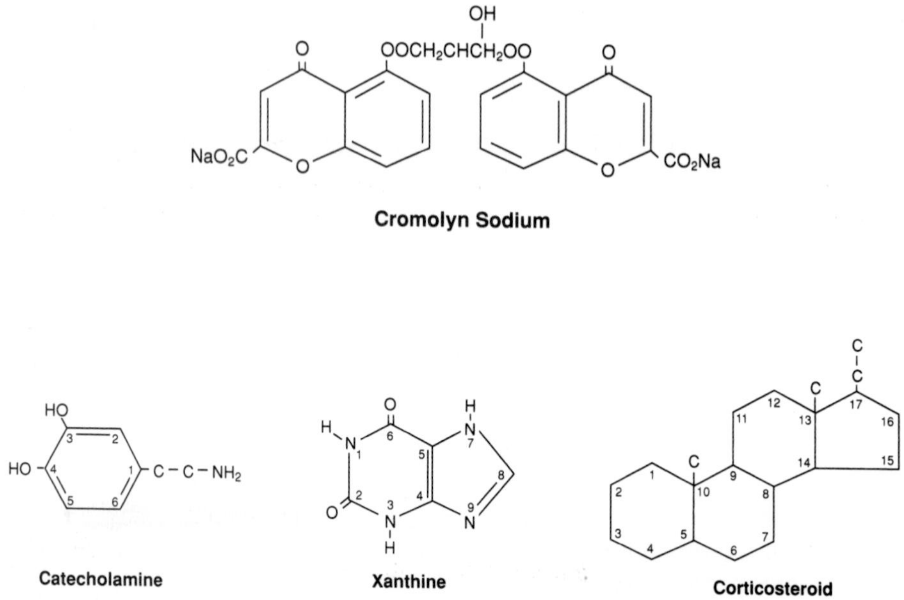

FIG 11-1. Chemical structure of cromolyn sodium, or disodium cromoglycate, in comparison with the basic catecholamine, xanthine, and corticosteroid structures.

son. Cromolyn is not related to beta agonists, xanthines, theophylline, or antiinflammatory glucocorticoids. Its mode of action also differs from these drug groups. Cromolyn does not block cholinergic, muscarinic receptors and has no intrinsic bronchodilating capability.

Cromolyn is usually described as a mast cell stabilizer. Since its release in the United States, cromolyn has been considered as a second-line drug in the management of asthma. Clinical studies have repeatedly shown that it is effective as a first-line maintenance drug for asthma and should be considered instead of corticosteroids and theophylline in controlling asthmatic reactions because of its safety and effectiveness (Bernstein, 1985b). Contrary to popular myth, cromolyn is also effective in adult asthmatic patients and for allergic and nonallergic asthma (Petty et al., 1989). A review of the effect of cromolyn on nonspecific bronchial hyperresponsiveness can be found in Hoag and McFadden (1991).

A brief overview of the pathophysiological characteristics of asthma, and of the hypersensitivity reaction of allergic asthma in particular, will be presented as a basis for understanding the mode of action of cromolyn.

PATHOPHYSIOLOGICAL CHARACTERISTICS OF ASTHMA

The nature of lung inflammation, as well as the major chemical mediators and the blood cells involved (such as the various leukocytes), was reviewed in the preceding chapter when discussing the use of corticosteroids in asthma. Cromolyn sodium acts in a very different way to block the sequence of events that result in an asthmatic reaction. Figure 11–2 illustrates in a simplified outline the pathogenesis of asthma. McFadden (1984) provides an excellent review of the nature and causes of asthma. Bronchial asthma is defined as an intermittent, reversible narrowing of the airways accompanied by increased secretions, mucosal edema, and damage to bronchial epithelium. In a report by the National Asthma Education Program (1991), a panel of experts stresses airway inflammation and increased airway responsiveness to a variety of stimuli in its definition of asthma. Wheezing, cough, dyspnea, and hypoxemia result from this process.

Causes of Asthmatic Episodes

Asthma has been differentiated as allergic, or extrinsic, and nonallergic, or intrinsic. The different causes of the asthmatic response are seen in Figure 11–2. Immunological (allergic) and nonimmunological (nonallergic) stimuli can trigger the asthmatic response. Immunological stimuli are allergens, such as dander, grass clippings, pets, ragweed, dusts, or molds, and involve an antigen-

PRODUCTION OF ASTHMATIC RESPONSE

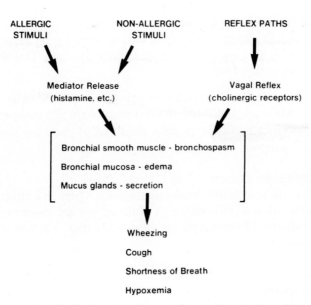

FIG 11–2. Conceptual illustration of various paths resulting in the asthmatic response.

antibody reaction. They are termed *immunological* because the immune system, with its antibodies, is involved. Nonimmunological stimuli include exercise, cold air, or stress and do not involve an antibody (i.e., immune response). There are also reflex mechanisms that lead to bronchial reactivity and that can be triggered by irritant gases (sulfur dioxide) or aerosols. The cholinergic reflex path was presented in Chapter 6. It is likely that nonimmunological stimuli cause both mediator release *and* reflex stimulation of bronchioles through cholinergic pathways. Since allergic asthma triggered by antigen-antibody reaction involving mast cell release of mediators is the most researched and best understood pathway, a brief review of this sequence is given.

Allergic Asthmatic Response

The allergic response in asthma is essentially an immune response, and a *mistaken* response at that, somewhat akin to a military guard firing at a stray cow in a war zone instead of at the real enemy.

There are basically two branches of the immune response:

Sensitized lymphocytes (cellular immunity)
Circulating antibodies (humoral immunity)

Cellular Immunity.   Cellular immunity is responsible for tissue rejection in transplants and for the purified protein derivative reaction in the skin test for tuberculosis exposure. This is termed a *type IV*, or *delayed*, type of hypersensitivity.

Humoral Immunity.   Humoral immunity is mediated by the antibodies that are involved in allergic asthma, as well as the routine protection of the body against mumps, measles, polio, and other diseases. The terms *antigen* and *antibody* are defined below:

Antigen: Substance that is capable of provoking antibodies and/or cellular immunity when administered to an immunologically competent animal.

Antibody: Serum globulin or protein modified to combine and react with its specific antigen.

Immunoglobulin Groups

Antibodies are also called immunoglobulins. There are approximately 30 serum proteins, such as albumin, and of these, five are immunoglobulins, or substances capable of becoming specific antibodies. Immunoglobulins are grouped as follows:

1. Major class.
   a. Immunoglobulin G (IgG), 80%.
   b. Immunoglobulin A (IgA), 10%.
   c. Immunoglobulin M (IgM), 5% to 10%.

2. Minor class.
   a. Immunoglobulin D (IgD), trace.
   b. Immunoglobulin E (IgE), trace.

Antibodies offer defense against invading organisms by being specific to the organism. The basic sequence is exposure to an organism (virus, etc.), with a specific antibody developing against that organism, and then upon reexposure, the antibody will react specifically with the organism. This antigen-antibody reaction *inactivates* or kills the organism, preventing any disease resulting from exposure to the organism.

Immunoglobulin G. IgG is the antibody most responsible for protection against the common diseases usually encountered in growing up, which is why the clinical condition of agammaglobulinemia (lack of gammaglobulin, IgG) is life threatening.

Immunoglobulin A. IgA exists as serum IgA and secretory IgA, probably playing an important role in protecting the respiratory tract from infectious viruses or bacteria. IgA is found in salivary and bronchial secretions, tears, milk, and the gastrointestinal tract. Secretory IgA is characterized by the presence of a "secretory piece," which is thought to provide resistance to degradation by proteolytic enzymes. Secretory IgA guards against respiratory tract infections such as influenza, poliovirus, or rhinovirus. Patients who lack respiratory tract IgA experience recurrent pulmonary infections. Since the lung is essentially open to a contaminated environment, IgA provides a first line of defense.

Immunoglobulin E. IgE is the antibody of interest for allergic asthma ever since this substance was discovered and studied by Ishizaka and coworkers in 1966. IgE is also known as *reagin*, or reaginic antibody. The sequence of IgE antibody formation and mast cell release of mediators is shown in Figure 11–3. IgE is a circulating, or humoral, immunoglobulin, but once it is *sensitized*, or made specific to a certain antigen or allergen, it will attach to cells known as *mast cells*. The term *cytophilic antibody* describes this affinity of IgE for cell surfaces. The mast cell contains granules that are storehouses of the chemical mediators of lung inflammation, discussed in Chapter 10. After attachment of the allergen-specific IgE, the mast cell is sensitized. Upon reexposure to the allergen, the allergen couples ("bridges") with the IgE, and this causes release of the granules containing the mediators of inflammation. This process is termed *mast cell degranulation.*

Mast Cell

Mast cells are specialized cells whose function in the healthy individual is not completely understood. These cells are found in organs rich in con-

MAST CELL RELEASE OF MEDIATORS

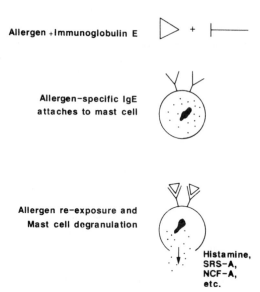

Allergen +Immunoglobulin E

Allergen−specific IgE
attaches to mast cell

Allergen re−exposure and
Mast cell degranulation

Histamine,
SRS−A,
NCF−A,
etc.

FIG 11–3. Antigen-induced mast cell release of chemical mediators of inflammation.

nective tissue, occurring primarily in the skin, and in intestinal and respiratory tract submucosa. In the lung, the mast cell is located near peribronchial nerve and vascular areas. The basophil, found in the bloodstream, is analogous to the tissue mast cell. The mast cell has 100,000 to 500,000 surface receptor sites for the constant, or Fc portion, of IgE. A single mast cell has approximately 1000 secretory granules that contain chemical mediators of inflammation: histamine, heparin, slow-reacting substance of anaphylaxis, platelet activating factor, and esoinophilic chemotactic factor of anaphylaxis.

When an individual with sensitized mast cells (i.e., cells with IgE specific to an antigen [allergen]), is exposed to the antigen, the mast cell *degranulates* and releases potent chemical inflammatory agents into the surrounding sites. In general, these chemicals increase vascular permeability, cause contraction of smooth muscle, increase mucus secretion, and cause vasodilatation with edema. In the *lung*, this reaction produces the potentially lethal airway obstruction of asthma, characterized by bronchospasm, mucus plugging, and mucosal edema. Kay (1987), Friedman and Kaliner (1987), Schulman (1986), and Kaliner (1985) all provide well-referenced reviews of the role of mast cell mediators in asthma.

Site of Mast Cells. The site where the mast cell is located determines the clinical condition. If mast cell degranulation occurs in the *nasal mucosa*, then one has rhinitis and sinusitis. In the *skin*, urticaria with itching and angioedema occur. *Intestinal* mast cells are implicated in food allergies. Mastocytosis is a disorder that involves the proliferation of mast cells in tissues. Since there are large numbers of mast cells in tissues exposed to the environment (skin and respiratory and intestinal tracts), it is suggested that they constitute one of the first lines of immunologic defense, possibly against parasitic diseases (Kaliner, 1979). There is a great deal of research currently elucidating the nature of human mast cells and showing that there are actually subspecies of human mast cell types. Such findings indicate the possibility of heterogeneous roles for mast cell subtypes (Schwartz, 1987).

Control of Mast Cell Degranulation.   Degranulation of mast cells in the lung is regulated by autonomic nerve paths. Beta-sympathomimetic agents, discussed in Chapter 5, are potent inhibitors of mast cell mediator release. Likewise, parasympatholytic agents, discussed in Chapter 6, can block cholinergic reflex stimulation and reduce mediator release.

CROMOLYN SODIUM: MODE OF ACTION

Pretreatment with inhaled cromolyn sodium results in inhibition of mast cell degranulation, thereby blocking release of the chemical mediators of inflammation. This is illustrated in Figure 11–4. By its action, cromolyn is effective in blocking the late-phase reaction in asthma, as corticosteroids can. The late-phase reaction in asthma was discussed previously in Chapter 10, when reviewing corticosteroids.

Cromolyn prevents the extrusion of the granules containing the mediators of inflammation to the cell exterior. For this reason, cromolyn is often classified as a "mast cell stabilizer." The exact mechanism by which this inhibition is accomplished is not completely understood, but the following details of cromolyn activity and mast cell function are known:

1. The mode of action of cromolyn sodium is *prophylactic;* pretreatment is necessary for inhibition of mast cell degranulation.
2. Cromolyn sodium may inhibit mediator release by preventing calcium influx necessary for microfilament contraction and extrusion of mast cell granules (Orr, 1973; Orr et al., 1972).
3. Cromolyn sodium does not have an antagonistic effect on any of the chemical mediators themselves.
4. Cromolyn sodium does not operate through the cyclic AMP system and does not affect alpha or beta receptors.
5. Antibody formation, attachment of antibody (IgE) to the mast cell,

CROMOLYN SODIUM (INTAL)

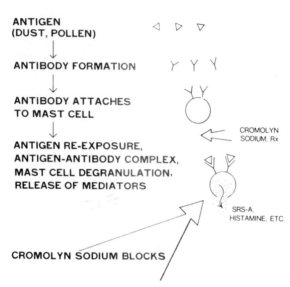

ANTIGEN
(DUST, POLLEN)
↓
ANTIBODY FORMATION
↓
ANTIBODY ATTACHES
TO MAST CELL
↓
ANTIGEN RE-EXPOSURE,
ANTIGEN-ANTIBODY COMPLEX,
MAST CELL DEGRANULATION,
RELEASE OF MEDIATORS

CROMOLYN
SODIUM, Rx

SRS-A,
HISTAMINE, ETC.

CROMOLYN SODIUM BLOCKS

FIG 11–4. Mode of action of cromolyn sodium in preventing mast cell degranulation.

 and antigen-antibody union are *not* prevented by cromolyn, only release of mediators.
6. Cromolyn sodium can prevent or attenuate the late-phase response in an asthmatic episode, which can otherwise cause more severe airway obstruction 4 to 6 hours after initial bronchoconstriction (McFadden, 1987; O'Byrne et al., 1987).

The protective effect of cromolyn in inhibiting mast cell degranulation has been captured by using the scanning electron microscope and is shown in the sequence in Figure 11–5. Initial understanding of cromolyn's activity focused on allergy-triggered mast cell release of mediators, and therefore the drug came to be considered useful primarily in allergic asthma. There is evidence that the activity of cromolyn is not limited to preventing allergen-stimulated asthma. Cromolyn inhibits mast cell mediator release caused by nonallergic stimuli and may even reduce reflex-induced asthma (Fig 11–6). The latter requires about twice the usual dose of cromolyn. Understanding of the broader protection given by cromolyn has supported its successful use in allergic and nonallergic asthma and specifically with exercise-induced asthma. This view of the broader pharmacological activity of cromolyn is discussed by Bernstein (1985a and 1985b).

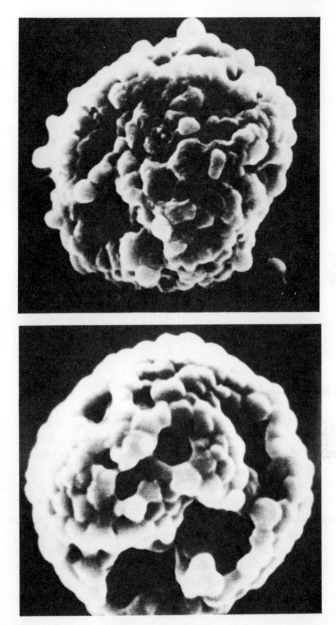

FIG 11–5. Degranulation of a mast cell. **A,** Mast cell undergoing gross degranulation shows free granules. **B,** The pores now occupy a large area of the cytoplasm.

(Continued.)

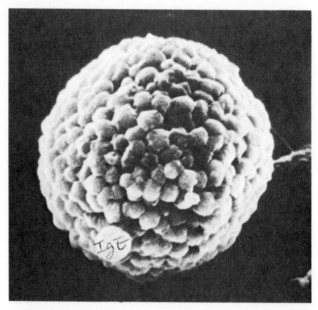

FIG 11–5.   (cont.).   C, A sensitized mast cell fails to degranulate after challenge when pretreated with cromolyn sodium. (Courtesy Fisons Corp, Bedford, Mass.)

FORMULATIONS OF CROMOLYN SODIUM

Cromolyn sodium is marketed for inhalation as Intal and Aarane. Table 11–1 lists the currently available forms of the drug and recommended dosages. With any dosage form for inhalation, about 8% to 10% of the drug is absorbed from the lung, giving a peak plasma level 5 to 30 minutes after inhalation, with a duration of action of 4 to 6 hours. All three forms used for lung application (Spinhaler, Ampule, metered-dose inhaler [MDI]) require proper breathing patterns for the particular mode of delivery. Package inserts should be reviewed by practitioners to properly instruct patients. Advantages and disadvantages of each delivery method should be considered to tailor the best form of the drug to the patient's abilities and needs. The three delivery forms for inhalation of the drug are equivalent in the protection afforded in reducing symptom severity and wheezing. Cromolyn is also available in solutions for nasal and ophthalmic application.

Spinhaler (Dry-Powder Inhaler)

The original formulation of the drug was 20 mg of dry powder contained in a gelatin capsule. The capsule was placed in a specially designed inhaler

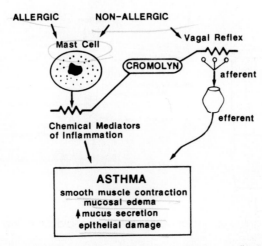

STIMULI

FIG 11–6. Illustration of the protection given by cromolyn sodium with allergic- and nonallergic-induced mediator release, and with reflex asthmatic responses.

apparatus, the Spinhaler. This device has a movable sleeve that pierces the capsule to release the powder. When the patient inhales from the Spinhaler, a small propeller ("turbo") spins to disperse the powder into a fine, uniform cloud. High inspiratory flow rates are needed (40 to 100 L/min) to obtain suitably small particles. The device is seen in Figure 11–7. The patient should be instructed to inhale as rapidly and deeply as possible, with a breath hold of up to 10 seconds if possible. Discussion of dry-powder inhalers as a method of aerosol administration was presented in Chapter 2. Because the dry pow-

TABLE 11–1.

Delivery Methods and Dosages for Pulmonary, Ophthalmic, Nasal, and Oral Application of Cromolyn Sodium

Delivery Method	Strength	Usual Dosage
Capsule with dry powder	20 mg/caps.	1 capsule, inhaled qid
Ampules with liquid	20 mg/amp.	1 ampule, inhaled qid
MDI	0.8 mg/puff	2 puffs, qid
Eye drop solution (Opticrom)	4% (40 mg/ml)	1–2 drops each eye, 4–6 times daily
Nasal solution (Nasalcrom)	4% (40 mg/ml)	1 spray each nostril, 3–6 times daily
Oral solution (Gastrocrom)	100 mg/caps.	2 capsules, orally, qid (contents dissolved in water)

THE SPINHALER TURBO-INHALER

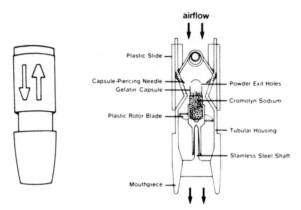

FIG 11–7. Sketch of the Spinhaler device used for inhalation of the dry-powder form of cromolyn sodium.

der can be irritating on inhalation, causing coughing or bronchoconstriction, and requires flow rates as well as coordination difficult for young children below age 5 years, the liquid solution may be preferred.

Finally, it should be emphasized to patients who use the capsules and inhaler device that the capsules *are not to be swallowed.* The drug is ineffective for asthma prophylaxis when taken orally, and the capsules are intended for inhalational use.

Ampule for Nebulization

The ampule contains the same dose as the dry powder, 20 mg in 2 ml of aqueous solution (a 1% strength). This solution can be nebulized in any small reservoir device powered by compressed air, which will produce suitably small particles of 3 to 5 μm. Additional diluent will be needed for most nebulizers to function well. Slow tidal breathing reduces the need for inspiratory maneuvers seen with the turbo inhaler or the MDI, although longer administration times and lack of portability become a disadvantage.

Metered-Dose Inhaler

The MDI is the most easily carried device and employs lower doses than the turbo inhaler or nebulized solution—only 2 mg per dose rather than 20 mg per dose. This is typical of the dose ratio of MDIs vs. nebulizers.

Ophthalmic Solution (Opticrom)

A 4% solution of cromolyn is available as Opticrom for use in treating ocular symptoms of allergic conjunctivitis. The drug is effective within 7 days and is poorly absorbed from the eye into the body, giving a localized effect. After initiation of the eye solution at regular intervals as prescribed, there is a decrease in the allergic symptoms of itching, tearing, redness, or discharge.

Nasal Solution (Nasalcrom)

Cromolyn is available as a 4% solution for treatment of seasonal and perennial allergic rhinitis. As with the inhaled solution, protection requires prior administration, although the drug does not need to be taken outside of seasonal exposure to allergens. The solution is delivered by using a metered pump spray device.

Oral Solution (Gastrocrom)

A 100-mg capsule of cromolyn sodium has been released for oral use and is indicated for the management of systemic mastocytosis.

Mastocytosis: Condition involving the formation of clumps of mast cells in the skin. These may appear as brown areas that itch. Other organs may be involved. Symptoms include diarrhea, vomiting, and abdominal pain, as well as itching of the skin (urticaria).

In this use of cromolyn, the powder contents of the capsule are dissolved in one-half glass of hot water, to which cold water is added. Usual starting dosage is 200 mg q.i.d., one-half hour before meals and at bedtime.

SIDE EFFECTS

Cromolyn sodium is a safe drug. It has an effectiveness similar to theophylline in controlling asthma, with a better therapeutic margin than theophylline (McFadden, 1987). In studies comparing the two agents, subjects using theophylline reported more side effects, including nervousness, nausea, school behavioral problems, and more office visits. The overall incidence of adverse effects with cromolyn has been reported at 2% (Settipane et al., 1979). With the dry-powder form, the most common reactions are throat irritation, hoarseness, dry mouth, cough, a feeling of chest tightness, or bronchospasm. Prior inhalation of a β_2 agent may prevent this, or the nebulized solution and the MDI form may be tried. Nasal congestion may be seen after beginning cromolyn sodium use. Dermatitis, myositis (muscle tissue inflammation), and gastroenteritis occurred in a very few patients.

CLINICAL USE OF CROMOLYN SODIUM

Three points should be emphasized concerning the clinical application of cromolyn sodium with asthma and hyperreactive airway states.

First, the drug is only prophylactic and should not be used during acute bronchospasm. This is based on its mode of action, since the drug must be already present to prevent mast cell degranulation. *It has no bronchodilating action* and in fact may cause further bronchial irritation as an aerosol.

Second, abrupt withdrawal of oral corticosteroids and substitution of cromolyn sodium in asthmatic patients can result in inadequate adrenal function. Cromolyn has no effect on the adrenal system, and tapered withdrawal of corticosteroids is necessary while beginning cromolyn use with patients.

Third, it may take from 2 to 4 weeks for improvement in the patient's symptoms, enabling a decrease in concomitant therapy such as bronchodilator or steroid use.

Dosage Regulation

The protective effect of cromolyn in allergic, nonallergic, or reflex-induced asthma is dose dependent. The following observations on dosage regulation are based on Bernstein (1985a and 1985b).

The usual dosage of 20 mg 4 times daily (80 mg/d) with the turbo-inhaler or nebulized solution in some cases can be reduced to a maintenance dosage of 40 to 60 mg/d after the patient is stabilized for 1 or 2 months. Likewise, if stimuli for asthma increase in severity (e.g., heavy exercise in cold weather [skiing] as opposed to walking in warm weather), higher dosages or addition of a beta agonist may be required. For seasonal allergy, cromolyn should be started at least *1 week* before allergen exposure. The drug will protect if given *30 minutes* before a specific allergen exposure (e.g., cat fur), and a *single dose 15 minutes* prior to exercise on an occasional instead of continuous basis is effective. As stated previously, the degree of exercise and the conditions must be considered in estimating the protection required. *Long-term* continual maintenance with cromolyn may be needed for patients with reflex-induced asthma or for those with late-phase reactions or with severe bronchial reactivity and lability.

Other Clinical Uses of Cromolyn

Cromolyn has been used effectively to inhibit a variety of inflammatory disorders besides asthma, thus further supporting a theory of broader-based pharmacological activity. Some of those uses reported in the literature include the following.

Control of Food Allergies. Cromolyn has been given orally, in ranges of 25 to 100 mg t.i.d., dissolved in water, for prevention of allergy reactions to food (Gerrard, 1979; Nizami et al., 1977).

Systemic Mastocytosis. Cromolyn has been used for the treatment of diarrhea in systemic mastocytosis, the accumulation of mast cells in the tissues (Nizami et al., 1977). The formation of cromolyn as Gastrocrom for this use was previously listed.

Oral Ulcers. Cromolyn has been used for treating ulcers on the oral mucosa by using a toothpaste with 2½% concentration of cromolyn (Frost, 1973).

Inflammatory Bowel Disease. There are reports of using cromolyn for treating nonspecific inflammatory bowel disease, such as Crohn's disease, colitis, and proctitis (Heatley et al., 1975; Mani et al., 1976).

In all clinical uses of cromolyn, it is critical that subjects use the drug properly in each of its formulations. This is especially true with inhalational use where lower plasma levels, and presumably decreased protection, occur with poor inhalational techniques (Bernstein, 1985b).

NEDOCROMIL SODIUM (TILADE)

Nedocromil sodium is an agent that was approved for general clinical use by the Food and Drug Administration on December 30, 1992, and therefore is one of the newest aerosol agents in respiratory care. The drug is an inhaled, prophylactic antiasthmatic agent and is extensively reviewed by Gonzalez and Brogden (1987). Nedocromil is marketed by Fisons Corporation as Tilade in an MDI.

Nedocromil is considered a second-generation antiasthmatic agent and is a cromolyn-like drug in its action and clinical use. The structures of cromolyn and nedocromil are given for comparison in Figure 11–8. The drug is a disodium salt of a pyranoquinolone dicarboxylic acid. The following summary describes the essential features of the new agent.

Mode of Action

Nedocromil sodium, like cromolyn, inhibits mediator release (histamine) from mast cells and the formation of the inflammatory mediators leukotriene C4 and prostaglandin D2. Nedocromil also inhibits mediator release from other cells, such as neutrophils, eosinophils, macrophages, monocytes, and platelets.

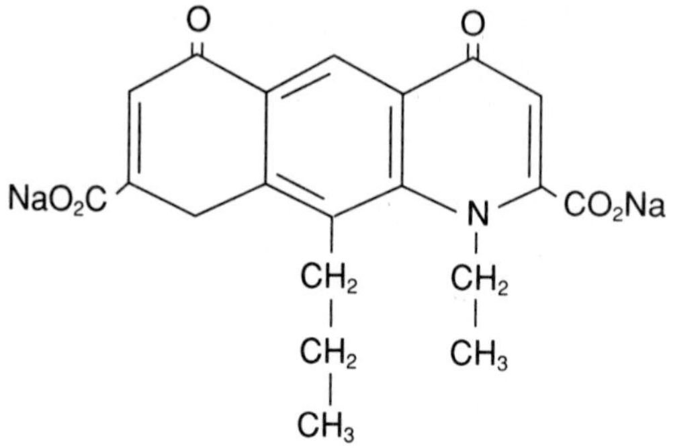

Nedocromil Sodium

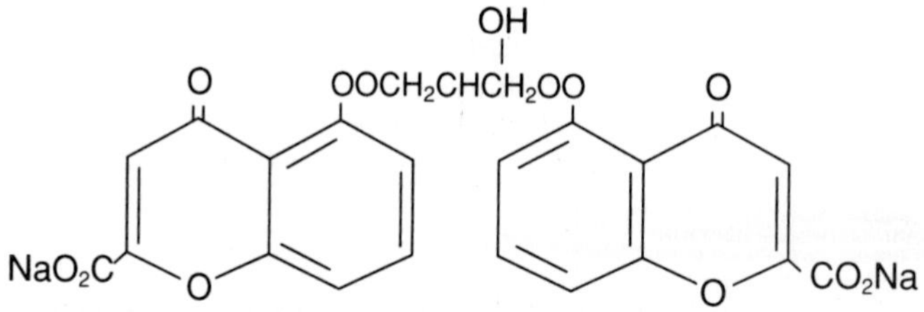

Cromolyn Sodium

FIG 11–8. Chemical structures of nedocromil sodium and cromolyn sodium.

Because of its action, nedocromil should be used prophylactically (as with cromolyn), and it is effective in preventing the late-phase reaction in asthma.

Side Effects

Nedocromil was well tolerated in both healthy volunteers and asthmatic subjects. The most commonly reported side effects are listed below (Gonzalez and Brogden, 1987):

Unpleasant taste (13.6%)
Headache (4.8%)
Nausea (4.0%)
Vomiting (1.8%)
Dizziness (1% to 2%)

Clinical Use

Nedocromil has been shown to be effective by inhalation in treating asthma in adults and children over 12 years. It may also be effective for allergic rhinitis (intranasally as a 1% spray) and allergic conjunctivitis (ophthalmic drops 2% solution).

Dosage and Administration

Nedocromil is available as an MDI, with 1.75 mg per actuation, with approximately 112 metered inhalations per canister.

The recommended dosage by MDI for maintenance therapy in asthma is two inhalations 4 times a day. It is not intended for use in acute asthmatic episodes.

BIBLIOGRAPHY

Altounyan REC: Inhibition of experimental asthma by a new compound—disodium cromoglycate (Intal), Allergy 22:487, 1967.

Bernstein IL: Cromolyn sodium, Chest 87(suppl):68S, Jan 1985a.

Bernstein IL: Cromolyn sodium in the treatment of asthma: coming of age in the United States, J Allergy Clin Immunol 76:381, 1985b.

Friedman MM, Kaliner MA: Human mast cells and asthma, Am Rev Respir Dis 135:1157, 1987.

Frost M: Cromoglycate in aphthous stomatitis, Lancet 389; 2, 1973.

Gerrard JW: Oral cromoglycate: its value in the treatment of adverse reactions to food, Ann Allergy 42:135, 1979.

Gonzalez JP, Brogden RN: Nedocromil sodium: a preliminary review of its pharmcodynamic and pharmacokinetic properties, and therapeutic efficacy in the treatment of reversible obstructive airways disease, Drugs 34:560, 1987.

Heatley RV et al: Disodium cromoglycate in the treatment of chronic proctitis, Gut 16(7):559, 1975.

Hoag JE, McFadden ER Jr: Long-term effect of cromolyn sodium on nonspecific bronchial hyperresponsiveness: a review, Ann Allergy 66:53, 1991.

Ishizaka K, Ishizaka T, Hornbrook MM: Physicochemical properties of human reaginic antibody. IV. Presence of a unique immunoglobulin as a carrier of reaginic activity, J Immunol 97:75, 1966.

Kaliner M: Mast cell mediators and asthma, Chest 87(suppl):2S, Jan 1985.

Kaliner MA: The mast cell—a fascinating riddle, N Engl J Med 301:498, 1979 (editorial).

Kay AB: Provoked asthma and mast cells, Am Rev Respir Dis 135:1200, 1987.

Mani V et al: Treatment of ulcerative colitis with oral disodium cromoglycate: a double-blind controlled trial, *Lancet* I:439, 1976.

McFadden ER Jr: Cromolyn: first-line therapy for chronic asthma? J Respir Dis 8:39, 1987.

McFadden ER Jr: Pathogenesis of asthma, J Allergy Clin Immunol 73:413, 1984.

National Asthma Education Program: Guidelines for the diagnosis and management of asthma. Bethesda, Md, 1991, U.S. Department of Health and Human Services, National Institutes of Health.

Nizami RM, Levin PK, Baboo MT: Oral cromolyn sodium therapy in patients with food allergy: a preliminary report, Ann Allergy 39:102, 1977.

O'Byrne PM, Dolovich J, Hargeave FE: Late asthmatic responses, Am Rev Respir Dis 136:740, 1987.

Orr TSC: Mast cells and allergic asthma, Br J Dis Chest 67:87, 1973.

Orr TSC, Hall DE, Allison AC: Role of contractile microfilaments in the release of histamine from mast cells, Nature 236:350, 1972.

Petty TL et al: Cromolyn sodium is effective in adult chronic asthmatics, Am Rev Respir Dis 139:694, 1989.

Schulman ES: The role of mast cell derived mediators in airway hyperresponsiveness, Chest 90:578, 1986.

Schwartz LB: Mediators of human mast cells and human mast cell subsets, Ann Allergy 58:226, 1987.

Settipane GA, Klein DE, Boyd GK: Adverse reactions to cromolyn, JAMA 241:811, 1979.

12

Aerosolized Anti-Infective Agents

There are two anti-infective agents currently approved for administration as inhaled aerosols: pentamidine isethionate (NebuPent) and ribavirin (Virazole). Pentamidine is used to prevent or treat *Pneumocystis carinii* pneumonia (PCP) in patients with the acquired immunodeficiency syndrome (AIDS), while ribavirin is used for treating respiratory syncytial virus (RSV) infection. A third use of aerosolized anti-infective agents is the treatment of respiratory infections in cystic fibrosis. Topical application of antibiotics has also been used to prevent respiratory infections in patients on ventilators. The following topics are presented in this chapter:

- Aerosolized pentamidine
- Ribavirin
- Aerosolized antibiotics
- Topical antibiotics in patients on ventilators

AEROSOLIZED PENTAMIDINE

Description of Drug

Pentamidine isethionate is an antiprotozoal agent that is active against *P. carinii*, the causative organism for PCP. Chemically it is an aromatic diamidine, whose structure is seen in Figure 12–1. Pentamidine has been used for years to treat protozoal infections. Waskin (1991) gives a clear review of the drug's uses, pharmacokinetics, and effects, with source references. The following summarizes the drug's activity in the body.

The drug was first synthesized in 1937 and has been used since the 1940s to treat African sleeping sickness, or trypanosomiasis. Pentamidine is also ef-

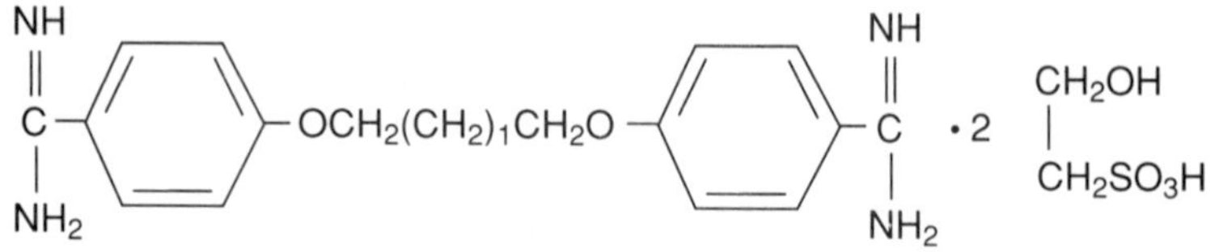

Pentamidine Isethionate

FIG 12–1. Chemical structure of pentamidine isethionate (NebuPent).

fective against other protozoal infections, including leishmaniasis, pneumocystosis, and babesiosis (a disease caused by an erythrocytic protozoal parasite).

Pentamidine can be given parenterally or as an inhaled aerosol but is not absorbed with oral administration. When given parenterally, either intravenously or intramuscularly, the drug distributes quickly to the major organs (liver, kidneys, lungs, pancreas). There it binds to tissues and is stored for months. After a single intramuscular dose, the drug can be detected in the urine 270 days later.

When given by inhaled aerosol, pentamidine reaches substantially higher concentrations in the lung than when given intravenously (Montgomery et al, 1988). The inhaled drug first binds to lung tissue. Although plasma levels are much less than with parenteral administration, the drug is slowly absorbed into the circulation and distributed to body tissues, as with parenteral administration. As a result, prolonged aerosol administration can result in systemic accumulation.

Approximately 75% of the drug is excreted in the urine and 25% in feces over the months following administration.

Indication for Use

Both systemic and aerosol administration of pentamidine are used for the treatment of PCP, which occurs as a common opportunistic respiratory infection in AIDS subjects.

Inhaled pentamidine (NebuPent) is specifically approved by the Food and Drug Administration (FDA) for the prevention of PCP in patients infected with the human immunodeficiency virus (HIV). The criteria given with the product are the following:

1. History of one or more episodes of PCP.
2. Peripheral CD4+ lymphocyte count of 200 cells/mm^3 or less.

General recommendations for prophylaxis of PCP have been published by the Centers for Disease Control (CDC, now the Centers for Disease Control and Prevention) in *Morbidity and Mortality Weekly Report* for HIV-positive adults (CDC, 1992) and for children (CDC, 1991).

In addition to the prophylactic use of aerosolized pentamidine, the aerosolized form has also been used for treatment of acute episodes. The first report by Montgomery and associates in 1987 was for therapy of acute episodes of PCP.

Rationale for Aerosol Administration

The rationale for aerosol administration of pentamidine to treat or prevent PCP is based on at least three reasons:

1. PCP is located in the alveolar region of the lung, and inhaled aerosol administration targets drug delivery to the lung.
2. Parenteral administration of pentamidine is associated with numerous and serious systemic side effects, to be reviewed subsequently.
3. Aerosolized pentamidine produces substantially higher lung concentrations than intravenous administration, as previously noted.

The San Francisco prophylaxis trial, published in 1990, showed that 300 mg of aerosolized pentamidine every 4 weeks was effective in preventing PCP in patients with HIV infection (Leoung et al., 1990).

Description of PCP

P. carinii is a protozoal parasite. Protozoa are simple, unicellular members of the animal kingdom. Exact taxonomy is yet to be established. An excellent review of *P. carinii* and PCP is in Levine and White (1988). The following is a brief summary of key points.

The organism was first noted in the lungs of guinea pigs by Chagas in 1909 and by Carinii in 1910. In 1912, Delanoe and Delanoe named this new organism *P. carinii* to describe the cystic form in the lungs and its earlier discoverer. Mammals are commonly infected with the organism at an early age, probably through an airborne vector. Disease occurs when there is suppression of the immune system. Prior to the AIDS pandemic, PCP was reported in malnourished infants in the 1940s and 1950s and in premature infants able to survive in the 1970s.

The life cycle of *P. carinii* is illustrated in Figure 12–2. The organism seems to attach to epithelial lung cells and is termed a *trophozoite*. The trophozoite form gradually evolves into a cystic form, with internal sporozoites. The sporozoites are released from the cyst, beginning a new cycle of reproduction. When

LIFE CYCLE, P. CARINII

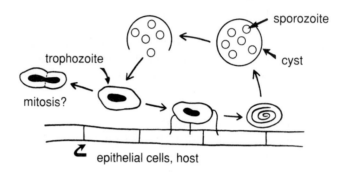

trophozoite

sporozoite

cyst

mitosis?

epithelial cells, host

P. CARINII PNEUMONIA (PCP)
Pathology

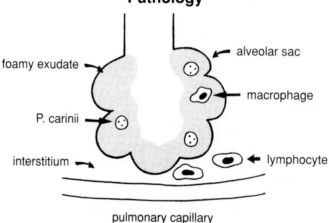

foamy exudate

alveolar sac

macrophage

P. carinii

interstitium

lymphocyte

pulmonary capillary

- foamy intra-alveolar exudate
- mild/moderate interstitial lymphocytes
- mild infiltration of alveolar macrophages

FIG 12–2. Pathogenesis of PCP.

not contained by a competent immune system, *P. carinii* causes the pneumonia termed PCP, also seen in Figure 12–2. This produces a foamy intraalveolar exudate that contains cysts of *P. carinii*. There is mild-to-moderate interstitial infiltration of lymphocytes, and macrophages are present in the alveoli. The common radiographic appearance of diffuse bilateral interstitial or alveolar infiltrates results. Pentamidine and trimethoprim-sulfamethoxazole (TMP-SMX) are effective against PCP and are usually given parenterally to manage an acute episode.

Mode of Action of Pentamidine

The exact mode of action of pentamidine is not known. The drug's toxic effect on *P. carinii* may be due to multiple actions. Pentamidine blocks synthesis of ribonucleic acid (RNA) and deoxyribonucleic acid (DNA), inhibits oxidative phosphorylation, and interferes with folate transformation (Levine and White, 1988; Mathewson, 1989; Waskin, 1991). Resistance to pentamidine by *P. carinii* has not been shown, and this may be due to the multiple effects of the drug on the organism's metabolism (Waskin, 1991).

Side Effects

It was the side effects seen with systemic therapy of PCP by using either pentamidine or TMP-SMX that provided part of the rationale for aerosol administration of pentamidine. Although both of these drugs are effective in a majority of patients with PCP when given systemically, over 50% of patients experience adverse effects.

Side Effects With Parenteral Pentamidine

Side effects with parenteral administration of pentamidine are reviewed by Corkery and associates (1988a) and by Waskin (1991). Numerous references can be found in these citations for the effects listed. The following effects have been reported with parenteral use of pentamidine:

- Pain, swelling, and abscess formation at the site of injection with intramuscular administration.
- Thrombophlebitis and urticarial eruptions with intravenous administration.
- Hypoglycemia (up to 62% of patients), with a cumulative cytotoxic effect on pancreatic beta cells.
- Impaired renal function and azotemia.
- Hypotension.
- Leukopenia.
- Hepatic dysfunction.

Side Effects With Aerosol Administration

Side effects with aerosol administration can be differentiated into local airway effects and systemic effects. Although the aerosol route of administration targets the lung locally, adverse systemic effects have been reported.

Local airway effects with aerosol administration have included the following:

- Cough and bronchial irritation (36% in Leoung et al, 1990).
- Shortness of breath.
- Bad taste (bitter or burning) of the aerosol impacting in the oropharynx.
- Bronchospasm and wheezing (11% in Leoung et al, 1990).
- Spontaneous pneumothoraces (Martinez et al, 1988).

In addition, the following adverse systemic reactions have occurred with aerosolized pentamidine:

- Conjunctivitis.
- Rash.
- Neutropenia.
- Pancreatitis (Hart, 1989).
- Renal insufficiency.
- Dysglycemia (hypoglycemia and diabetes).
- Digital necrosis in both feet (Davey et al., 1989).
- Appearance of extrapulmonary *P. carinii* infection.

Because of the pharmacokinetics of pentamidine, reviewed qualitatively above when describing the drug, chronic treatment with the aerosol can lead to tissue accumulation in the body, causing some of the same side effects as with parenteral administration.

Preventing Airway Effects

Use of a beta-adrenergic bronchodilator before inhaling aerosolized pentamidine can reduce or prevent local airway reaction, including reduction of coughing or wheezing. Ipratropium has also been shown to prevent bronchoconstriction (Quieffin et al., 1991). The airway reaction may be caused by the sulfite moiety in isethionate, which is known to cause airway irritation (Fine et al, 1987), or by the drug itself (Corkery et al., 1990). This effect can be reduced by use of a nebulizing system that produces very small particles, which will lessen airway deposition and increase alveolar targeting (Corkery et al., 1988a).

Administration of Aerosolized Pentamidine

Details of dosage and administration of NebuPent, the aerosolized brand of pentamidine, can be found in the manufacturer's literature. The following summary is not intended to replace the more detailed instructions that accompany the drug.

Dosage

The approved dosage of aerosolized pentamidine for prophylaxis of PCP in AIDS subjects is 300 mg given by inhalation once every 4 weeks. This dosage may be altered by physicians, in treating individual patients.

NebuPent, the brand of pentamidine approved for inhalation as an aerosol, is supplied as a dry powder, with 300 mg in a single vial. This must be reconstituted with 6 ml of sterile water for injection (not saline, which can cause precipitation) added to the vial. The entire 6 ml of reconstituted solution is placed into the nebulizer.

Administration

Approval of aerosolized pentamidine by the FDA was for administration with the Respirgard II nebulizer. This is a small-volume nebulizer system, powered by compressed gas and fitted with a series of one-way valves and an expiratory filter (Fig 12-3). This nebulizer system has been described by Montgomery and associates (1988). The Respirgard II should be powered with a flow rate of 5 to 7 L/min from a 50-psi source, or alternatively, by controlling the flow with a 22- to 25-psi pressure source connected to the small-bore tubing of the nebulizer. Pressures below 20 psi are not sufficient to produce the

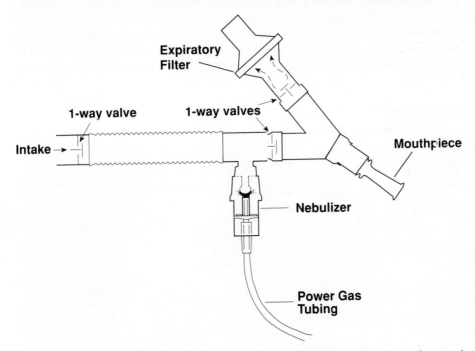

FIG 12-3. Diagram of the Respirgard II nebulizer system shows one-way valves and expiratory filter to scavenge exhaust aerosol.

desired particle size necessary for peripheral delivery of the drug. These requirements with the Respirgard II are found in the manufacturer's literature and further discussed in Corkery (1988a).

Nebulizer Performance

Although nebulized pentamidine was approved for general clinical use with the Respirgard II nebulizer system, other nebulizers are used to administer the drug. Table 12–1 summarizes various reports in the literature on the particle sizes produced by different nebulizers with pentamidine.

The general requirement for effective nebulization of pentamidine is a particle size or distribution of sizes with a mass median diameter (MMD) of 1 to 2 μm (Corkery, 1988a). This is needed for two reasons:

1. To achieve peripheral intraalveolar deposition targeted at the location of the microorganism.
2. To reduce or prevent airway irritation seen with larger particles, which will deposit more in larger airways (Corkery et al., 1988a).

Of particular interest is the study by Vinciguerra and Smaldone (1990), which compared treatment time and patient tolerance of aerosolized pentamidine with the Respirgard II and the AeroTech II. They found that treatment times are substantially shorter with the AeroTech II than with the Respirgard II. Patient cough occurs more with the AeroTech II, although this is said to have no impact on patient tolerance. Furthermore, 150 mg with the AeroTech

TABLE 12–1.

Particle Size Produced by Nebulizing Systems Used to Deliver Aerosolized Pentamidine for Inhalation

Nebulizer	MMD (μm)	Reference
AeroTech II	1.0 (at 10 L/min)	Smaldone et al, 1988
	2.0 (at 7 L/min)	Corkery et al, 1988b
Respirgard II	0.76 (at 6 L/min)	Smaldone et al, 1988
	0.93 (at 7 L/min)	Corkery et al, 1988b
	1.24 (at 6 Lpm)	Dolovich et al, 1990
Fisoneb USN	2.5 (on minimum)	Smaldone et al, 1988
	5.0 (at 7 L/min)*	Corkery et al, 1988b
	2.6 (on minimum)	Dolovich et al, 1990
Pulmosonic USN	4.2 (at 7 L/min)	Corkery et al, 1988b
Porta-sonic USN	1.6 (at 7 L/min)	Corkery et al, 1988b
	1.95 (at 6 L/min)	Dolovich et al, 1990
Fan Jet	4.3 (at 7 L/min)	Corkery et al, 1988b

*Auxiliary gas flow was used to drive aerosol from chamber.

II has been shown to be an equivalent monthly dosage to 300 mg with the Respirgard II (Vinciguerra and Smaldone, 1990; Smaldone, et al., 1988)

Smaldone and co-workers (1988) also examined the efficiency of three nebulizers used to deliver pentamidine: the AeroTech II, the Respirgard II, and the ultrasonic nebulizer Fisoneb. Efficiency was defined as follows: drug inspired as a percentage of the dose in the nebulizer. Their results are listed below:

AeroTech II: 21% efficiency.
Respirgard II: 4.6% efficiency.
Fisoneb: 16% efficiency.

Their testing conditions used a tidal volume of 750 ml and a respiratory rate of 20 per minute. Details can be found in the referenced study.

Environmental Exposure

There are two concerns regarding environmental exposure of health care workers or others when pentamidine is nebulized. The first is exposure to the drug itself from the exhaust aerosol. The second is risk of infection with tuberculosis, a disease associated with AIDS.

Drug Exposure

Pentamidine is not known to be teratogenic, based on its use in pregnant women with African sleeping sickness (trypanosomiasis), although detailed clinical data were not kept. The drug is not mutagenic, and its carcinogenic potential is considered minimal (Waskin, 1991).

An abstract by Montgomery and co-workers (1989) reported the results of a study on the amount of secondhand exposure to aerosolized pentamidine. They conclude that the health care worker receives one-millionth of the patient's dose, even in an unventilated 36-m^3 treatment room (Montgomery et al., 1989). However, Smaldone and others (1991) report low levels of pentamidine in the urine of five of 14 practitioners with chronic exposure to the drug. A follow-up study also shows intermittent pentamidine in the urine of four of five health care workers (O'Riordan and Smaldone, 1992). The investigators conclude that exposure probably occurs during treatment interruptions usually caused by coughing episodes.

Health care workers have complained of conjunctivitis and bronchospasm when aerosolizing the drug (Waskin, 1991). On the basis of these reports, and the long tissue half-life of pentamidine, contact with the drug should be held to a minimum or prevented if possible. The precautions given in the following section to reduce the risk of tuberculosis transmission will also reduce drug exposure with the aerosol. In addition, the following suggestions are given for administering the drug.

1. Use a nebulizer system with one-way valves and expiratory filter.
2. Stop nebulization if the patient takes the mouthpiece out of the mouth (a thumb control on the power gas tubing gives more control).

Risk of Tuberculosis

The risk of tuberculosis when treating AIDS patients with nebulized pentamidine is due to the following factors:

1. There is an association of tuberculosis with AIDS.
2. Tuberculosis has an airborne mode of transmission.
3. Pentamidine aerosol can cause coughing and expulsion of droplet nuclei containing tuberculosis bacilli.

The precautions given in the next section could reduce the risk of both drug exposure and tuberculosis infection, when using aerosolized pentamidine.

Environmental Precautions

The following suggestions for control of environmental contamination from aerosolized drug or infectious organisms are summarized from Fallat and Kandal (1991), from Chaisson and McAvinue (1991), from the guidelines from the Centers for Disease Control (CDC, 1990), and from the American Respiratory Care Foundation.

Since aerosolized pentamidine is considered to be useful and effective in preventing PCP in AIDS subjects, these precautions can help practitioners design safe programs for administration of pentamidine.

1. Use nebulizers producing an MMD of 1 to 2 μm to increase alveolar targeting and lessen large airway deposition and cough production.
2. Always use a suitable expiratory filter and one-way valves with the nebulizer.
3. Instruct patients to turn off the nebulizer when talking or when taking it out of the mouth.
4. Screen patients for cough history and pretreat with a beta agonist, with sufficient lead time for effect in reducing the bronchial reactivity.
5. Administer aerosol in a negative pressure room, with six air changes per hour, or consider using an isolation booth/hood assembly with an exhaust fan and air directed through a high-efficiency filter.
6. Use barrier protection (gloves, mask, eyewear) for health care workers.
7. Screen HIV subjects for tuberculosis and treat where evidence of infection exists.

8. Do not allow treatment subjects to mix with others until coughing subsides.
9. Health care workers should be periodically screened for tuberculosis.
10. Pregnant women and nursing mothers should avoid exposure to the drug, and all practitioners should limit their exposure to the extent possible.

Although measures exist to radically limit environmental contamination with aerosolized pentamidine, many of these are expensive, such as negative pressure rooms and improvement of ventilation exchange in older buildings. Others are difficult, such as the wearing of effective high-efficiency masks in a busy clinical setting for prolonged periods. The use of room disinfection with UV light was reviewed by Riley and Nardell (1989) but is debated (Chaisson and McAvinue, 1991).

Clinical Application

Fahy and coworkers (1992) examined the effect of prophylactic use of nebulized pentamidine on the severity of subsequent bouts of PCP, as well as the sensitivity of sputum diagnostic testing for PCP. They conclude that hospitalization is less common in those treated prophylactically, but the treatment does not lessen the clinical severity of PCP or lessen sensitivity of diagnostic testing for PCP in sputum.

Aerosol Therapy of Acute PCP

It is important to note the difference between the short-term use of aerosolized pentamidine and the prophylactic use. The use reported by Montgomery and associates in 1987 was a short-term use. In that report, aerosolized pentamidine was given to 15 AIDS patients experiencing a first episode of pneumonia caused by *P. carinii*. Patients received 600 mg of aerosolized pentamidine once a day for 21 days. Of the 15 patients, 13 responded to treatment.

Conte and coworkers (1990) compared aerosol pentamidine (600 mg) with intravenous pentamidine (3 mg/kg) in 45 patients with mild-to-moderate first episodes of PCP. Their conclusion was that the reduced-dose of intravenous pentamidine is more effective than aerosolized pentamidine for treating mild-to-moderate PCP. The study enrollment was in fact halted due to relapse, nonresponse, or early recurrence of symptoms in the aerosol group.

Aerosol Therapy for Prophylaxis

Some comparisons have also been made of aerosol prophylactic therapy and TMP-SMX (Bactrim). In a study by Martin and associates (1992), 133 HIV-infected patients received TMP-SMX 3 days a week, and 125 others received aerosolized pentamidine (NebuPent) 300 mg once a month. No patient on TMP-SMX developed PCP during the long-term study (2 years), while 17 patients on the aerosol regimen developed PCP. However, in the TMP-SMX group, 56% of subjects changed drug due to adverse reactions, while only 2% of the aerosol group did so. The authors conclude that TMP-SMX is the drug of choice to prevent PCP in these subjects, provided adverse effects are tolerated and clinically acceptable.

These results, together with reports of serious adverse effects with aerosolized pentamidine discussed previously, have caused a reevaluation of aerosol therapy with pentamidine for prophylaxis of PCP. Guidelines from the CDC published in 1989 recommended either oral TMP-SMX or aerosolized pentamidine for prophylaxis, but neither was preferred over the other. In the 1992 recommendations from the CDC, oral TMP-SMX was preferred over aerosol pentamidine for prophylaxis of PCP, provided adverse side effects from TMP-SMX were absent or acceptable.

With the potential for rapid changes in the treatment of AIDS victims and PCP, it will be essential for practitioners to monitor the literature for revisions to these recommendations.

RIBAVIRIN

Description of Drug

Ribavirin (Virazole) is classified as an antiviral drug that is active against several viruses: respiratory syncytial, influenza, and herpes simplex viruses. Chemically, it is a nucleoside analogue first synthesized in 1972 that resembles guanosine and inosine (Reines and Gross, 1988). It is virostatic, not virucidal, and inhibits both DNA and RNA (retrovirus) viruses. Ribavirin is one of a relatively finite group of antiviral agents. These agents are listed in Chapter 13 with general anti-infective agents.

When given by inhaled aerosol, ribavirin levels are much greater in respiratory secretions than in the bloodstream. Waskin (1991) gives a referenced summary of ribavirin kinetics. With 8 to 20 hours of aerosol treatment, peak plasma levels are 1 to 3 μg/ml, while respiratory secretion levels are greater than 1,000 μg/ml. The minimal inhibitory concentration for RSV is in the range of 4 to 16 μg/ml. The half-life of ribavirin is about 9 hours in plasma and about 1 to 2 hours in respiratory secretions, which is the rationale for the almost continuous administration by aerosol.

Ribavirin has been used throughout the world for a variety of viral infections, including RSV, influenza types A and B, and Lassa fever. Clinical trials of aerosolized ribavirin for severe RSV infection were conducted by Hall and associates (1983, 1985), and the results show substantial improvement with ribavirin treatment compared with placebo.

Indication for Use

Ribavirin has been approved as an inhaled aerosol for management of bronchiolitis and pneumonia caused by RSV. Specifically it is indicated for use in severe cases of RSV in infants and young children requiring hospitalization and/or supported ventilation, where underlying conditions of prematurity, immunosuppression, congenital heart disease, or other cardiopulmonary diseases increase the risk of morbidity or mortality from the RSV infection. Guidelines concerning use of ribavirin have been published by the American Academy of Pediatrics Committee on Infectious Diseases (1987).

Nature of Viral Infection

A short summary of viruses and viral infection is presented to establish key principles and concepts needed for understanding the difficulties in treating viral diseases, as well as the mode of action of ribavirin.

Virus: Obligate intracellular parasite, containing either DNA or RNA, that reproduces by synthesis of subunits within the host cell and that causes disease as a consequence of this replication.

Figure 12–4 illustrates the simple structure of a virus. These are primitive members of the animal kingdom, submicronic in size, that consist of a strand of DNA or RNA surrounded by a protein coat. A virus may or may not be surrounded by an envelope whose glycoprotein spikes are partially obtained from the host cell.

STRUCTURE OF A VIRUS

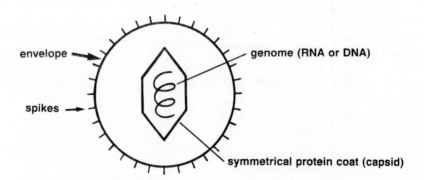

Virion: extracellular virus particle

FIG 12–4. Illustration of the structure of a virus shows the core of nucleic acid (DNA, RNA), protein coat, and an envelope.

The concept and sequence of a viral infection is shown in Figure 12−5. A virus enters the body through a variety of routes (oral, inhaled, mucous membranes), then invades a host cell. This is a multistep process consisting of phases in which the virus adsorbs to the cell, penetrates, uncoats, and goes through a process of recoding cell DNA (transcription, translation, synthesis), assembly, and shedding from the cell. The host cell may die in the process. Clinically, signs of a viral infection do not occur until after the initial latent

SEQUENCE OF VIRAL INFECTION

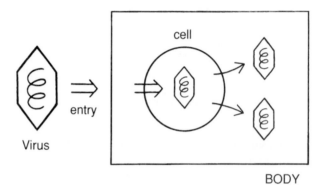

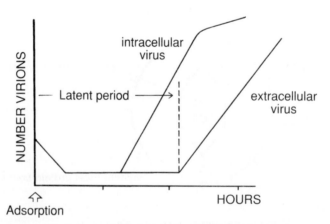

FIG 12−5. Illustration of the sequence of viral infection shows intracellular replication prior to dissemination in the body.

period when the virus leaves the cell (Fig 12–5). At this point infection is well-established. The diagnosis of viral illness is usually based on clinical signs, including symptoms, age of the patient, and time of year. Definitive diagnosis requires isolating the virus or demonstrating an antibody titer increase. Diseases produced by viruses include chickenpox, smallpox, fever blisters (herpes simplex virus), genital herpes, poliomyelitis, the common cold, AIDS, influenza, mumps, and measles.

Because of the nature of viral infection just outlined, antiviral drug therapy, whether for the common cold or for HIV, is difficult. In particular, there are three complications in managing viral diseases with drugs:

1. Attacking the intracellular virus may harm the host cell.
2. Viral replication is maximal before the appearance of symptoms.
3. Viruses have the property of antigenic mutability (i.e., they change their appearance to the immune system).

Respiratory Syncytial Virus Infection

General reviews of antiviral drug therapy can be found in Nicholson (1984), Mathewson (1986), and Bryson (1986).

RSV, which was isolated in 1956, can cause bronchiolitis and pneumonia. Almost all children are exposed to the virus by their second year of life, and in most the infection is mild and self-limiting. Outbreaks of RSV pneumonia are seasonal and peak during winter months (November through March), with some variation.

The name of the virus reflects its effects on cells, that is, to cause the formation of large, multinucleated cells called *syncytium*. The virus spreads easily by personal contact or hand contamination from surfaces. There is no effective vaccine to prevent RSV respiratory disease.

Mode of Action of Ribavirin

The mechanism of action by which ribavirin exerts its virostatic effect is not completely understood. Its viral inhibition is probably based on its structural resemblance to the nucleosides used to construct the DNA chain (Reines and Gross, 1988). Figure 12–6 shows the structures of the natural nucleoside guanosine, together with that of ribavirin, which as previously stated is a synthetic nucleoside analogue. During the formation and assembly of new viral protein within the cell, ribavirin is most likely taken up instead of the natural nucleoside to form the DNA chain. This prevents construction of viable viral particles and subsequent shedding of the virus into the bloodstream. A conceptual illustration of the process is shown in Figure 12–7. Ribavirin does not prevent the attachment or the penetration of RSV into the cell and does not induce interferon (Reines and Gross, 1988).

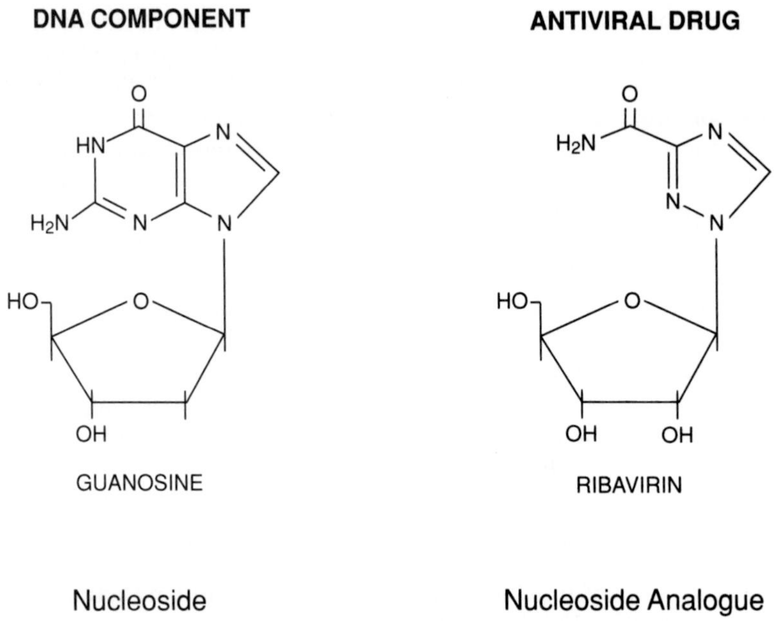

DNA COMPONENT

ANTIVIRAL DRUG

GUANOSINE

RIBAVIRIN

Nucleoside

Nucleoside Analogue

FIG 12–6. Similarity of the ribavirin molecule to the DNA precursor component, guanosine, may be the basis for the drug's virostatic effect.

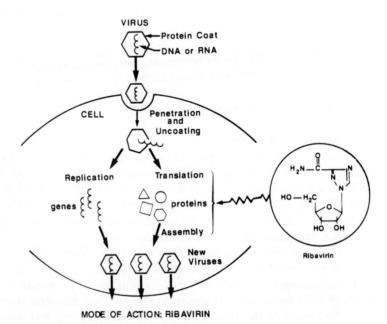

MODE OF ACTION: RIBAVIRIN

FIG 12–7. Illustration of the mode of action of ribavirin in blocking viral replication.

Side Effects

The side effects seen with aerosolized ribavirin are listed in the product literature and have been reviewed by Waskin (1991), who gives detailed references. The following summarizes the adverse effects reported and includes those seen with adults receiving the drug.

Pulmonary: deterioration of pulmonary function and worsening of asthma or chronic obstructive disease; pneumothorax, apnea, and bacterial pneumonia.

Cardiovascular: cardiovascular instability including hypotension, cardiac arrest, and digitalis toxicity.

Hematologic: effects on blood cells reported with oral or parenteral administration but not with aerosol use; reticulocytosis (excess of young erythrocytes in the circulation) reported with aerosol use.

Dermatologic/Topical: rash, eyelid erythema, and conjunctivitis.

Although the above effects have been reported, common effects clinically are pulmonary function deterioration and skin irritation from excess drug precipitation. Additional hazards with ventilator use include occlusion and impairment of expiratory valves and sensors, and endotracheal tube blockage from drug precipitate.

Dosage and Administration

The following is a descriptive summary of ribavirin dosage and administration. It is not intended to replace the detailed instructions contained in the manufacturer's literature, which should be reviewed prior to administering this drug. This includes the operating manual for the small-particle aerosol generator (SPAG) nebulizing system.

Dosage

Ribavirin is given in a 20-mg/ml solution that is administered by nebulizer (SPAG-2) for 12 to 18 hours per day, for a minimum of 3 days and not more than 7 days.

The drug is supplied as 6 g of powder in a 100-ml vial. The powder is reconstituted first in the vial with sterile USP water for injection or inhalation, transferred to the large-volume (500-ml) reservoir of the nebulizer, and further diluted to a total volume of 300 ml with sterile water. This gives a concentration of 6 g/300 ml, or 20 mg/ml, a 2% strength solution.

Administration

Clinical trials of ribavirin aerosol were carried out by using the SPAG, which is a large-volume nebulizing system. The drug was approved for general use with this aerosol generator. A diagram of the SPAG unit is shown in Figure 12–8. The SPAG is a large-volume, pneumatically powered nebulizer operating on a jet shearing principle, with baffling of aerosol particles, and with a drying chamber to further reduce particle size to a level of approximately 1.3-μm MMD. Solutions in the SPAG reservoir should be replaced after 24 hours. Residual solution in the reservoir should be discarded before adding newly reconstituted solution. The drug solution should always be visually inspected for particulate matter or discoloration before use.

The nebulizer is connected to a hood at the patient interface. The manufacturer (ICN Pharmaceuticals) specifically warns against administration of the drug with infants requiring mechanical ventilation, because of the risk of drug precipitation occluding expiratory valves and sensors or even the endotracheal tube. However, the sickest infants with RSV are likely to need ventilatory support, and there are reports of drug use with mechanical ventilation. Detailed information concerning precautions with ventilator use during administration of the drug can be found in Demers et al. (1986). A clinical study of aerosol administration with mechanical ventilation of infants with severe RSV infection was reported by Smith and coworkers (1991), who showed that treatment reduces duration of ventilation, oxygen support, and hospital stay.

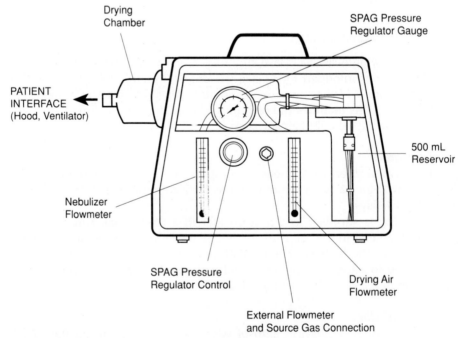

FIG 12–8. Diagram of the SPAG unit used for nebulizing ribavirin.

Although labor intensive, mechanical ventilatory administration of ribavirin actually simplifies environmental control.

Environmental Contamination

Health care workers are concerned about exposure to ribavirin. The drug has potential for mutagenic and carcinogenic effects, based on the results of in vitro and animal studies (Waskin, 1991). The effect on fertility is uncertain, but the drug has caused testicular lesions in rats. The effect during pregnancy is of particular concern because the drug is teratogenic or embryocidal in animal species.

Acute side effects reported by health care workers have included precipitation on contact lenses and conjunctivitis. A low concentration of drug in the blood of one clinical worker was reported in a California study when the drug was administered by oxygen tent (Harrison et al., 1988). However, Rodriguez and others (1987) report no toxic or adverse effects with ribavirin aerosol delivered by ventilator, oxygen tent, or hood in 19 nurses. No drug was detected in erythrocytes, plasma, or urine with this clinical exposure.

Minimal levels of ribavirin exposure are difficult to specify because of lack of dose-response data for humans (Harrison et al., 1988). Corkery and others (1989) state that the California Department of Health Services recommend an acceptable occupational airborne concentration for 8 hours of "limited" exposure to be 1/1000 of the lowest no-observed-effect level, which would be 2.5 $\mu g/m^3$.

Although to my knowledge there are no reports at this date of serious effects from drug exposure by aerosol, precautions to limit or avoid exposure to the drug are well-indicated, as advocated by Kacmarek (1990). Pregnant women, or those wishing to become pregnant, should avoid exposure to the drug if at all possible. In addition, environmental containment is superior to personnel barrier protection alone. ICN Pharmaceuticals makes available a containment system for use when the drug is aerosolized to an oxyhood, and several similar systems have been proposed in the literature (Cefaratt and Steinberg, 1992; Charney et al., 1990; Kacmarek and Kratohvil, 1992). All have common features of enclosure around the hood, with vacuum extraction and filtering of gas from the enclosure. Details needed for use can be found in the references given.

AEROSOLIZED ANTIBIOTICS

General Use of Aerosol Antibiotics

Aerosol delivery of antibiotics and direct endotracheal instillation were reported in the early 1970s and reviewed in both the 1974 and 1979 conferences on the scientific bases of respiratory care (Wanner and Rao, 1980; Williams, 1974). These trials were also reviewed in more detail, with reference to specific reports, in the second and third editions of this text. Readers are referred to those bibliographies.

Aerosol delivery of antibiotics has been tried for two general situations: gram-negative pulmonary infections and fungal pulmonary infections. In both cases, local targeting of the lung was intended to be adjunctive to systemic therapy and to reduce the toxicity seen with systemic therapy. The efficacy and benefit of this practice was not well established or generally practiced.

Aerosol Antibiotics in Cystic Fibrosis

One disease in which aerosolized antibiotics have been used more consistently for pulmonary infections is cystic fibrosis. Patients with cystic fibrosis are chronically infected with gram-negative organisms such as *Pseudomonas aeruginosa, Haemophilus influenzae, Pseudomonas cepacia,* and also with the gram-positive bacterium *Staphylococcus aureus.* In particular, chronic infection with *Pseudomonas* species leads to recurring acute respiratory infections. With the exception of the newer quinolone derivatives such as ciprofloxacin, antibiotics that are effective against *Pseudomonas* species do not give sufficient lung levels to inhibit bacteria when taken orally. This is referred to as *poor oral availability.* Antibiotics with poor oral availability for lung tissue include the aminoglycosides, penicillin derivatives, and cephalosporins. Consequently, either the intravenous or the inhaled aerosol route must be used. Aerosol administration is attractive because of reduced cost potential and ease of use at home. Furthermore, fluoroquinolones such as ciprofloxacin or norfloxacin are not as suitable for prolonged maintenance or preventive therapy as the agents given by inhalation, because of the risk of drug-resistant strains of bacteria (Neu, 1988).

A detailed review of the use of antibiotic therapy for respiratory infections in cystic fibrosis can be found in the August 1988 supplement to *Chest.* Consideration of antibiotic treatment by using aerosol therapy in this population of patients is provided by Hodson (1988).

Aerosol Administration

Aerosol administration of antibiotics is usually by nebulization (small-volume nebulizer). Several points should be noted when nebulizing such agents:

1. Antibiotic solutions such as gentamicin are more viscous than are bronchodilator solutions, and this may affect nebulizer performance. Compressors

must be suitably powerful, and high flow compressors are suggested. Flow rates of 10 to 12 L/min have also been suggested for suitably small particles (Newman et al., 1985, 1986).

2. Environmental contamination and practitioner exposure to aerosolized drug can be reduced by using expiratory filters with one-way valves and a thumb control, as with aerosolized pentamidine.

3. Antibiotic aerosols such as polymyxin or gentamicin may irritate the airway and cause bronchospasm, with decreased ventilatory flow rates (Dally et al., 1978; Dickie and de Groot, 1973; Wilson, 1981). Concomitant use of a beta agonist or pretreatment may be needed.

4. Physical incompatibility between some antibiotics has been noted (Hata and Fick, 1988). Aminoglycosides such as gentamicin are chemically inactivated by carbenicillin and piperacillin when mixed together. These drugs should be given in separate nebulizer treatments, which has the disadvantage of requiring twice the patient treatment time. Any antibiotic combination, or other drug combinations, should at least be inspected for visible changes, such as discoloration or precipitation, and not used if this is observed.

5. Specific written physician orders are needed to administer an antibiotic as an inhaled aerosol if the drug is not FDA-approved for this method of delivery.

A listing of selected reports of aerosolized antibiotics, both for cystic fibrosis and other respiratory diseases is given in Table 12–2.

TABLE 12–2.
Selected Reports of Aerosolized Antibiotics for Cystic Fibrosis and Other Diseases

Study	Drug	Dosage	Disease
Hodson et al, 1981	Gentamicin	80 mg bid	Cystic fibrosis
	Carbenicillin	1 g bid	
Wall et al, 1983	Tobramycin	80 mg bid	Cystic fibrosis
	Ticarcillin	1 g bid	
Kun et al, 1984	Gentamicin	20 mg bid	Cystic fibrosis
Littlewood et al, 1985	Colomycin	500,000 U bid	Cystic fibrosis
Stead et al, 1987	Ceftazidime	1 g bid	Cystic fibrosis
	Gentamicin	80 mg bid	
	Carbenicillin	1 g bid	
Steinkamp et al, 1989	Tobramycin	80 mg bid	Cystic fibrosis
Eisenberg and Oatway, 1971	Amphotericin B	10 mg qid	Coccidioidomycosis
Wright et al, 1979	Nystatin	100,000 U tid	Pulmonary aspergillosis
Stockley et al, 1985	Amoxicillin	500 mg bid	Bronchiectasis

TOPICAL ANTIBIOTICS FOR OROPHARYNGEAL DECONTAMINATION

Infection of the lower respiratory tract is a common complication of intubation and mechanical ventilation and increases with the duration of such support. The stomach and orophyarnyx are both sources of pathogens such as *S. aureus, Streptococcus pneumoniae,* and *H. influenzae* (Ruiz-Santana et al., 1987). Gram-negative colonization of the stomach may be facilitated by increases in gastric pH intended to reduce stress-induced peptic ulcer (Driks et al., 1987). These microorganisms spread to the tracheobronchial tree to cause respiratory infection, since normal clearing mechanisms (swallowing, coughing) are impaired.

There are reports of topical decontamination of the oropharynx and/or the stomach, with patients on ventilators, to reduce lower respiratory tract infection. The following antibiotics were used: norfloxacin, polymyxin E, amphotericin B (Aerdts et al., 1991); polymyxin B, neomycin, and vancomycin (Pugin et al., 1991); and polymyxin E, tobramycin, and amphotericin B (Stoutenbeek et al., 1987). The drugs are used in a paste or ointment form to coat the orophyarnyx or stomach. Levine and Niederman (1991) provide a good review of the risk of pneumonia with tracheal intubation and ventilatory support, as well as a review of topical antibiotic therapy to prevent respiratory infection.

BIBLIOGRAPHY

Aerdts SJA et al: Antibiotic prophylaxis of respiratory tract infection in mechanically ventilated patients: a prospective, blinded, randomized trial of the effect of a novel regimen, Chest 100:783, 1991.

American Academy of Pediatrics, Committee on Infectious Disease: Ribavirin therapy of respiratory syncytial virus, Pediatrics 79:475, 1987.

American Respiratory Care Foundation: Pentamidine aerosols and care giver safety, Dallas, Tex, 1992, AARC.

Bryson YJ: Antiviral agents, Clin Chest Med 7:453, 1986.

Cefaratt JL, Steinberg EA: An alternative method for delivery of ribavirin to nonventilated pediatric patients, Respir Care 37:877, 1992.

Charney W et al: Engineering and administrative controls to contain aerosolized ribavirin: results of simulation and application to one patient, Respir Care 35:1042, 1990.

Centers for Disease Control: Guidelines for prophylaxis against *Pneumocystis carinii* pneumonia for persons infected with human immunodeficiency virus. Morbid Mortal Weekly Rep 38(suppl 5):1, 1989.

Centers for Disease Control: Guidelines for preventing the transmission of tuberculosis in health-care settings, with special focus on HIV-related issues. Morbid Mortal Weekly Rep 39:1, 1990.

Centers for Disease Control: Guidelines for prophylaxis against *Pneumocystis carinii* pneumonia for children infected with human immunodeficiency virus. Morbid Mortal Weekly Rep 40:1, 1991.

Centers for Disease Control: Recommendations for prophylaxis against *Pneumocystis carinii* pneumonia for adults and adolescents infected with human immunodeficiency virus. Morbid Mortal Weekly Rep 41:1, 1992.

Chaisson RE, McAvinue S: Control of tuberculosis during aerosol therapy administration, Respir Care 36:1017, 1991.

Conte JE Jr et al: Intravenous or inhaled pentamidine for treating *Pneumocystis carinii* pneumonia in AIDS. A randomized trial, Ann Intern Med 113:203, 1990.

Corkery KJ, Luce JM, Montgomery AB: Aerosolized pentamidine for treatment and prophylaxis of *Pneumocystis carinii* pneumonia: an update. Respir Care 33:676, 1988a.

Corkery K, Luce JM, Montgomery AB: Characteristics of nebulizers used in aerosolized pentamidine studies, Respir Care 33:916, 1988b (abstract).

Corkery K, Eckman D, Charney W: Environmental exposure of aerosolized ribavirin, Respir Care 34:1027, 1989 (abstract).

Corkery KJ et al: Airway effects of aerosolized pentamidine isethionate, Am Rev Respir Dis 141:A152, 1990 (abstract).

Dally MB, Kurrle S, Breslin ABX: Ventilatory effects of aerosol gentamicin, Thorax 33:54, 1978.

Davey RT Jr et al: Digital necrosis and disseminated *Pneumocystis carinii* infection after aerosolized pentamidine prophylaxis, Ann Intern Med 111:681, 1989.

Demers RR et al: Administration of ribavirin to neonatal and pediatric patients during mechanical ventilation, Respir Care 31:1188, 1986.

Dickie KJ, de Groot WJ: Ventilatory effects of aerosolized kanamycin and polymyxin, Chest 63:694, 1973.

Dolovich M, Chambers C, Newhouse M: Characterization of 3 systems used to deliver pentamidine (P) aerosol, Am Rev Respir Dis 141:A153, 1990 (abstract).

Driks MR et al: Nosocomial pneumonia in intubated patients given sucralfate as compared with antacids or histamine type 2 blockers, N Engl J Med 317:1376, 1987.

Eisenberg RS, Oatway WH: Nebulization of amphotericin B, Am Rev Respir Dis 103:289, 1971.

Fahy JV et al: Effect of aerosolized pentamidine prophylaxis on the clinical severity and diagnosis of *Pneumocystis carinii* pneumonia, Am Rev Respir Dis 146:844, 1992.

Fallat RJ, Kandal K. Aerosol exhaust: escape of aerosolized medication into the patient and caregiver's environment, Respir Care 36:1008, 1991.

Fine JM, Gordon T, Sheppard D: The roles of pH and ionic species in sulfur dixoide and sulfite-induced bronchoconstriction, Am Rev Respir Dis 136:1122, 1987.

Hall CB et al: Aerosolized ribavirin treatment of infants with respiratory syncytial viral infection, a randomized double-blind study. N Engl J Med 308:1443, 1983.

Hall CB et al: Ribavirin treatment of respiratory syncytial viral infection in infants with underlying cardiopulmonary disease, JAMA 254:3047, 1985.

Harrison R et al: Assessing exposures of health-care personnel to aerosols of ribavirin—California. Morbid Mortal Weekly Rep 37:560, 1988.

Hart CC: Aerosolized pentamidine and pancreatitis, Ann Intern Med 111:691, 1989 (letter).

Hata JS, Fick RB Jr: *Pseudomonas aeruginosa* and the airways disease of cystic fibrosis, Clin Chest Med 9:679, 1988.

Hodson ME: Antibiotic treatment, aerosol therapy, Chest 94(suppl):156S, Aug. 1988.

Hodson ME, Penketh ARL, Batten JC: Aerosol carbenicillin and gentamicin treatment of *Pseudomonas aeruginosa* infection in patients with cystic fibarosis, Lancet 2:1137, 1981.

Kacmarek RM: Ribavirin and pentamidine aerosols: Caregiver beware! Respir Care 35:1034, 1990 (editorial).

Kacmarek RM, Kratohvil J: Evaluation of a double-enclosure double-vacuum unit scavenging system for ribavirin administration, Respir Care 37:37, 1992.

Kun P, Landau LI, Phelan PD: Nebulized gentamicin in children and adolescents with cystic fibrosis, Aust Paediatr J 20:43, 1984.

Leoung GS et al: Aerosolized pentamidine for prophylaxis against *Pneumocystis carinii* pneumonia, N Engl J Med 323:769, 1990.

Levine SA, Niederman MS: The impact of tracheal intubation on host defenses and risks for nosocomial pneumonia, Clin Chest Med 12:523, 1991.

Levine SJ, White DA: *Pneumocystis carinii*, Clin Chest Med 9:395, 1988.

Littlewood JM et al: Nebulised colomycin for early *Pseudomonas* colonisation in cystic fibrosis, Lancet 1:865, 1985.

Martin MA et al: A comparison of the effectiveness of three regimens in the prevention of *Pneumocystis carinii* pneumonia in human immunodeficiency virus-infected patients, Arch Intern Med 152:523, 1992.

Martinez CM et al: Spontaneous pneumothoraces in AIDS patients receiving aerosolized pentamidine, Chest 94:1317, 1988 (letter).

Mathewson HS: Antiviral drugs for acute respiratory infections, Respir Care 31:46, 1986.

Mathewson HS: *Pneumocystis carinii* pneumonia: chemotherapy and prophylaxis, Respir Care 34:360, 1989.

Montgomery AB et al: Aerosolized pentamidine as sole therapy for *Pneumocystis carinii* pneumonia in patients with acquired immunodeficiency syndrome, Lancet 2:480, 1987.

Montgomery AB et al: Selective delivery of pentamidine to the lung by aerosol, Am Rev Respir Dis 137:477, 1988.

Montgomery AB et al: Second hand exposure to aerosol pentamidine (AP), Am Rev Respir Dis 139:A149, 1989 (abstract).

Neu HC: Quinolones: a new class of antimicrobial agents with wide potential uses, Med Clin North Am 72:623, 1988.

Newman SP et al: Evaluation of jet nebulisers for use with gentamicin solution, Thorax 40:671, 1985.

Newman SP, Pellow PGD, Clarke SW: Choice of nebulisers and compressors for delivery of carbenicillin aerosol, Eur J Respir Dis 69:160, 1986.

Nicholson KG: Antiviral therapy: respiratory infections, genital herpes, and herpetic keratitis, Lancet 2:617, 1984.

O'Riordan TG, Smaldone GC: Exposure of health care workers to aerosolized pentamidine, Chest 101:494, 1992.

Pugin J et al: Oropharnygeal decontamination decreases incidence of ventilator-associated pneumonia: a randomized, placebo-controlled, double-blind clinical trial, JAMA 265:2704, 1991.

Quieffin J et al: Aerosol pentamidine-induced bronchoconstriction: predictive factors and preventive therapy, Chest 100:624, 1991.

Reines ED, Gross PA: Antiviral agents. Med Clin North Am 72:691, 1988.

Riley RL, Nardell EA: Clearing the air: the theory and application of ultraviolet air disinfection, Am Rev Respir Dis 139:1286, 1989.

Rodriguez WJ et al: Environmental exposure of primary care personnel to ribavirin aerosol when supervising infants with respiratory syncytial virus infection, Antimicrob Agents Chemother 31:1143, 1987.

Ruiz-Santana S et al: ICU pneumonias: a multiinstitutional study. Crit Care Med 15:930, 1987.

Smaldone GC, Perry RJ, Deutsch DG: Characteristics of nebulizers used in the treatment of AIDS-related *Pneumocystis carinii* pneumonia, J Aer Med 1:113, 1988.

Smaldone GC et al: Detection of inhaled pentamidine in health care workers, N Engl J Med 325:891, 1991.

Smith DW et al: A controlled trial of aerosolized ribavirin in infants receiving mechanical ventilation for severe respiratory syncytial virus infection, N Engl J Med 325:24, 1991.

Stead RJ, Hodson ME, Batten JC: Inhaled ceftazidime compared with gentamicin and carbenicillin in older patients with cystic fibrosis infected with *Pseudomonas aeruginosa*, Br J Dis Chest 81:272, 1987.

Steinkamp G et al: Long-term tobramycin aerosol therapy in cystic fibrosis, Pediatr Pulmonol 6:91, 1989.

Stockley RA, Hill SL, Burnett D: Nebulized amoxicillin in chronic purulent bronchiectasis, Clin Ther 7:593, 1985.

Stoutenbeek CP et al: The effect of oropharyngeal decontamination using topical nonabsorbable antibiotics on the incidence of nosocomial respiratory tract infections in multiple trauma patients, J Trauma 27:357, 1987.

Vinciguerra C, Smaldone G: Treatment time and patient tolerance for pentamidine delivery by Respirgard II and AeroTech II, Respir Care 35:1037, 1990.

Wall MA et al: Inhaled antibiotics in cystic fibrosis, Lancet 1:1325, 1983.

Wanner A, Rao A: Clinical indications for and effects of bland, mucolytic, and antimicrobial aerosols, Am Rev Respir Dis 122:79, 1980.

Waskin H: Toxicology of antimicrobial aerosols: a review of aerosolized ribavirin and pentamidine, Respir Care 36:1026, 1991.

Williams MH Jr: Steroid and antibiotic aerosols, Am Rev Respir Dis 110:122, 1974.

Wilson FE: Acute respiratory failure secondary to polymyxin-B inhalation, Chest 79:237, 1981.

Wright BD, Lee TS, Tseuda K: Pulmonary aspergillosis treated with nystatin aerosol, Respir Care 24:150, 1979.

13

Anti-Infective Agents

A variety of respiratory infections are seen in the pneumonias, acute and chronic bronchitis, bronchiectasis, sinusitis, and cystic fibrosis. Such infections are caused by bacterial, fungal, protozoal, and viral organisms. Antibiotics and other anti-infective agents are used to treat respiratory and other types of infections. The goal of this chapter is to provide a general perspective of antibiotic and anti-infective pharmacology, including fundamental terms and concepts and major drug groups. The following major topics are considered:

- Basic terms and concepts
- β-lactam antibiotic groups
- Aminoglycosides, tetracyclines, fluoroquinolones, and miscellaneous antibiotics
- Chemical anti-infective agents
- Antifungal drugs
- Antituberculosis drugs
- Antiviral agents

TERMS AND CONCEPTS

Antibiotics have proved to be one of the most useful, as well as most used, class of drugs in modern therapeutics.

Antibiotic: Substance produced by microorganisms (bacteria, fungi, molds) that is capable of inhibiting or killing bacteria and other microorganisms.

The classic discovery of penicillin by Fleming in 1928 led to further research for the isolation and identification of additional antibiotics. The definition above was offered by Waksman in 1941. Since then, antibiotics have been produced synthetically in the laboratory, as is the case with most drugs, which requires some expansion of the original definition to include the laboratory origin of antibiotic substances.

Modes of Action of Antibiotics

The following mechanisms by which antibiotics inhibit or kill microorganisms have been identified or postulated.

Inhibition of Cell Wall Synthesis

Bacteria possess rigid cell walls, unlike many other cells that have only a membrane. These walls are needed to protect the bacterial cells because of high internal osmotic pressures. Without this protection, in the *relatively* hypotonic environment of the body, such cells would explode.

Examples of antibiotics that inhibit cell wall synthesis include the following:

Penicillins
Bacitracin
Cephalosporins
Vancomycin
Cycloserine

Inhibition of Cell Membrane Function

The cytoplasmic membrane that encloses a cell is a very selective, functional, and active filter that keeps certain proteins and nucleotides within the cell and allows other substances to enter the cell for metabolism. Disruption of the membrane function upsets the necessary flow and storage of cell material required for growth or life. The membranes of certain bacteria and fungi are especially susceptible to particular antibiotics such as polymyxins (polymyxin B, colistin).

Inhibition of Protein Synthesis

Protein synthesis is crucial to a cell's growth and function, as amino acids are linked to produce protein for structural enlargement, energy storage, or enzymes. Many antibiotics interfere with the ribosome's ability to synthesize needed proteins. The following are examples:

Chloramphenicol
Tetracyclines
Erythromycin
Lincomycin
Aminoglycosides

Streptomycin
Kanamycin
Gentamicin

Inhibition of Nucleic Acid Synthesis

Deoxyribonucleic acid (DNA) synthesis is the heart of cellular activity and life, acting as the master code for cell function and structure. Certain antibiotics will attach to the DNA strands and block further DNA replication or formation of messenger ribonucleic acid. Examples are as follows:

Actinomycin
Mitomycins
Rifampicin

Terms Describing Antibiotic Activity

In general, antibiotics can be either *bactericidal* or *bacteriostatic*, depending on the particular drug and mode of action. Examples include the following:

Bactericidal Antibiotics	Bacteriostatic Antibiotics
Penicillins	Chloramphenicol
Cephalosporins	Erythromycin
Cycloserine	Tetracyclines
Vancomycin	Lincomycin
Bacitracin	
Streptomycin	
Kanamycin	
Polymyxins	

Antibiotics are also distinguished as *broad-spectrum* or *narrow-spectrum.* Broad-spectrum antibiotics are useful against a wide range of organisms, both gram-positive and gram-negative bacteria. Narrow-spectrum antibiotics are useful against only a few organisms. Examples of each spectrum of activity include the following:

Broad-Spectrum Antibiotics	Narrow-Spectrum Antibiotics
Chloramphenicol	Penicillin
Tetracyclines	Streptomycin
Kanamycin	Erythromycin
Cephalosporins	Lincomycin
Ampicillin	Polymyxin B
	Vancomycin

Sensitivity and Resistance

Antibiotics are tested for use in therapy through sensitivity and resistance studies (S & R). Various antibiotics are impregnated onto disks of filter paper and placed in dishes, with each dish heavily inoculated with a different bacterial agent (Fig 13–1). If the organism is susceptible, or sensitive to, the antibiotic on a particular disk, then a clear zone of inhibited bacterial growth will occur around the disk.

A laboratory report (S & R report) can then be given to aid the clinician in choosing an antibiotic effective against the bacteria causing a particular infection. If the bacteria is not known, or cannot be cultured, or if time and the patient's health do not permit culturing and sensitivity studies before treatment, a broad-spectrum antibiotic may be employed to begin rapid management of the infection.

One aspect of the use of antibiotics that is disturbing is the development of bacterial strains that are resistant to particular antibiotics. The following example, which is qualitative and not meant to represent actual data, can clarify the potential of this problem. In a colony of staphylococcal species, most individual bacteria originally may be vulnerable to an antibiotic such as penicillin. However, perhaps 1% of the colony is resistant to penicillin through genetic variations. The penicillin will effectively quell the infecting colony by inhibiting growth in 99% of the bacteria, the number of organisms is reduced

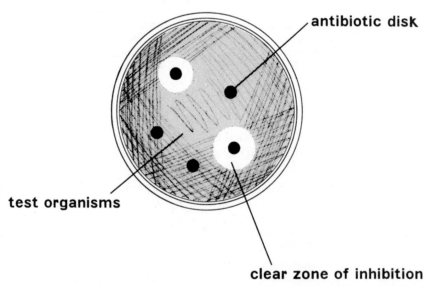

antibiotic disk

test organisms

clear zone of inhibition

FIG 13–1. Illustration of a test dish of organisms, with inhibition of growth around two disks.

to a safe level, and the infected host will clear of symptoms (e.g., fever, inflammation). Nonetheless, the remaining 1% of bacteria will continue to grow and reproduce, so that ultimately an essentially new population of bacteria exists that is resistant to the penicillin. This antibiotic is no longer effective against the mutant strain of staphylococcal species.

In reality this has occurred in the clinical use of antibiotics. The more widespread and indiscreet the use of antibiotics, the more rapid the development of resistant mutant strains is likely to be. The search for new, powerful antibiotics must keep pace with the growth of resistant strains that make currently effective antibiotics obsolete. For this reason too, antibiotic therapy is instituted in patients only when specifically indicated. In a patient with chronic lung disease, maintenance with continual antibiotic therapy is not considered useful, because the patient may acquire infection with resistant strains of bacteria. Generally, antibiotics are used at the first sign of infection in patients with chronic obstructive lung disease.

Major categories of drugs used to manage respiratory infections include the penicillins, the cephalosporins, and the aminoglycosides. A helpful review of antibiotic therapy, with emphasis on pulmonary applications, is found in Segreti and Trenholme (1986) and in Kuriyama and Panosian (1986).

β-LACTAM ANTIBIOTICS

The first four groups of antibiotics described are β-lactam agents. The β-lactam antibiotics include the penicillins, the cephalosporins, the carbapenem (imipenem), and the monobactam (azatreonam). An excellent review of these important drug groups is given by Donowitz and Mandell (1988).

The term β-*lactam* describes a common structure in the four groups of antibiotics listed above. This structure is the four-membered β-lactam ring connected to a second ring. In Figure 13–2, the β-lactam ring is labeled as A for the penicillin, cephalosporin, carbapenem, and monobactam structures.

The β-lactam antibiotics are bactericidal, through inhibition of bacterial cell wall synthesis. These antibiotics attach to and inactivate receptors known as penicillin-binding proteins on the inside of the bacterial cell membrane. This serves to block cell actions needed in the assembly of the cell wall.

Bacterial resistance to the β-lactam antibiotics can occur through the action of an enzyme, β-lactamase, produced by bacteria. β-lactamase is also known as penicillinase. β-lactamase hydrolyzes the cyclic amide bond of the β-lactam ring at the point illustrated for the penicillin structure in Figure 13–2. β-lactamase can be produced by a number of gram-positive and gram-negative bacteria. By disrupting the β-lactam ring, penicillin is inactivated to penicilloic acid and is unable to inhibit bacterial growth.

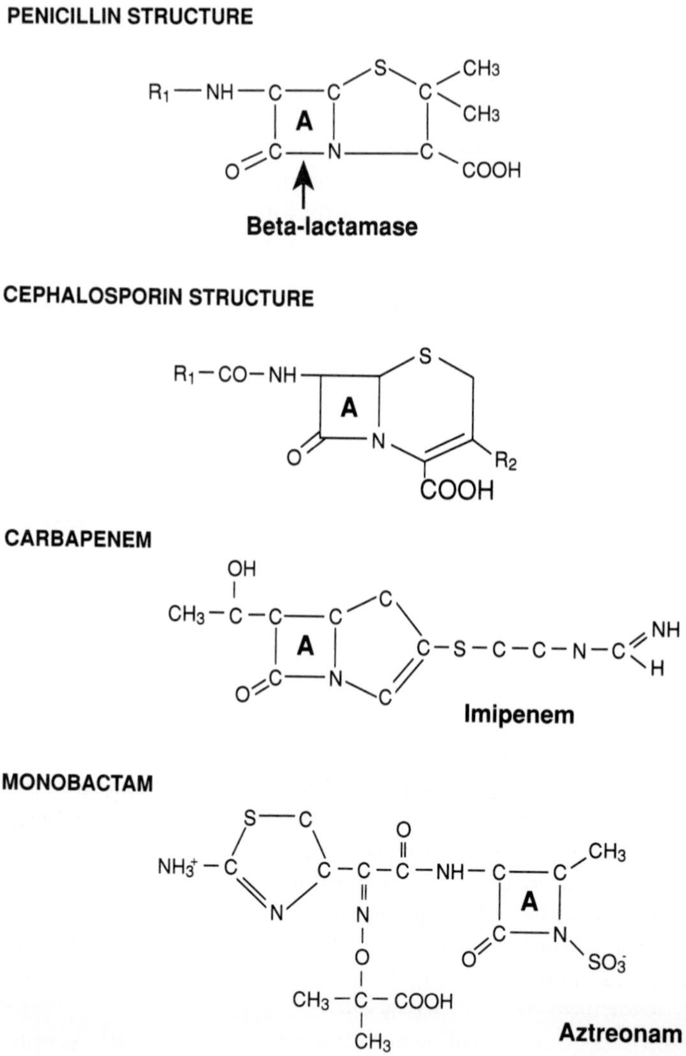

PENICILLIN STRUCTURE

R$_1$—NH—C—C —S—C CH$_3$ / CH$_3$
A
O=C—N—C COOH

Beta-lactamase

CEPHALOSPORIN STRUCTURE

R$_1$—CO—NH S
A
O N R$_2$
COOH

CARBAPENEM

OH
CH$_3$—C—C—C—C
A
O=C—N—C —S—C—C—N—C NH / H

Imipenem

MONOBACTAM

S—C O
NH$_3^+$—C C—C—C—NH—C—C CH$_3$
N N A
O O=C—N SO$_3^-$
CH$_3$—C—COOH
CH$_3$

Aztreonam

FIG 13-2. Structures of β-lactam antibiotics, showing the β-lactam ring *(A)* and the site of inactivation *(arrow)* by β-lactamase (penicillinase).

Penicillins

The penicillins, which represent one of the oldest classes of antibiotics, include natural and semisynthetic penicillins. Examples of penicillins include the following:

Penicillin G
Penicillin V

Oxacillin (Prostaphlin)
Cloxacillin (Tegopen)
Methicillin (Staphcillin)
Ampicillin (Omnipen)
Amoxicillin (Polymox)
Carbenicillin (Geopen)
Ticarcillin (Ticar)

The penicillin group is divided into three subgroups: the natural penicillins (e.g., penicillin G), penicillinase-resistant agents (e.g., methicillin or oxacillin), and the broad- or extended-spectrum penicillins such as ampicillin, carbenicillin, and ticarcillin.

Mode of Action.   Penicillins act by inhibition of an enzyme involved in synthesizing cell wall structure.

Resistance.   The mechanism of bacterial resistance to penicillin was previously described. β-lactamase (penicillinase) is produced by most strains of *Staphylococcus aureus* and by *Bacillus* species, *Escherichia coli, Enterobacter aerogenes, Proteus* species, *Pseudomonas aeruginosa,* and *Mycobacterium tuberculosis.* There are penicillinase-resistant penicillins (e.g., methicillin, nafcillin, oxacillin, and cloxacillin) that are effective against penicillinase-producing *S. aureus.*

Clavulanic acid is a β-lactamase inhibitor whose structure resembles penicillin. It can protect penicillin-type antibiotics by binding to and inactivating β-lactamase. Clavulanic acid is combined with ticarcillin as the product Timentin and with amoxicillin as Augmentin.

Penicillin Allergy.   Hypersensitivity reactions to penicillin drugs can occur and are more likely to occur with parenteral rather than oral administration. Such reactions are manifested by anaphylactic shock, urticaria, and various skin rashes, among other symptoms.

Uses.   Various penicillins are used in managing infections due to streptococcal species, staphylococcal species, *Haemophilus influenzae,* and gonococcal and syphilis-causing organisms.

Cephalosporins

The cephalosporin group of antibiotics was originally derived from a fungus, *Cephalosporium acremonium,* in 1948 and is said to be the most prescribed group of antibiotics in the United States. This group is categorized according to generations, based on their spectrum of activity. The first generation is active against gram-positive and a few gram-negative organisms. The second and third generations have better activity against gram-negative organisms. Examples of cephalosporins include the following:

First Generation
    Cephalexin (Keflex)
    Cefadroxil (Duricef)
    Cephalothin (Keflin)
    Cephradine (Velosef)
    Cephapirin (Cefadyl)
    Cefazolin (Ancef)

Second Generation
    Cefamandole (Mandol)
    Cefoxitin (Mefoxin)
    Cefonicid (Monocid)
    Cefaclor (Ceclor)
    Cefmetazole (Zefazone)
    Cefotetan (Cefotan)
    Cefuroxime (Zinacef)

Third Generation
    Cefoperazone (Cefobid)
    Cefotaxime (Claforan)
    Ceftizoxime (Cefizox)
    Ceftazidime (Fortaz)
    Ceftriaxone (Rocephin)
    Moxalactam (Moxam)

Mode of Action.   Cephalosporins act by inhibition of bacterial cell wall synthesis (same as penicillin).

Toxicity and Hazards.   Nephrotoxicity is a serious effect that can occur with use of the cephalosporins, resulting in acute tubular necrosis. Intravenous administration can cause thrombophlebitis, and intramuscular injection can be painful.

Uses.   Cephalosporins are important in clinical use for their broad-spectrum activity against many of the common pathogenic gram-positive cocci and some of the gram-negative organisms. However, they lack efficacy against *P. aeruginosa, Bacteroides fragilis,* and to some extent against *H. influenzae.* They are active against the *Klebsiella* species.

Carbapenem

The only product in this group is imipenem-cilastatin (Primaxin). Imipenem is formulated with cilastatin, which inhibits the metabolism of imipenem in the kidney by the enzyme dehydropeptidase-1, thereby decreasing possible renal toxicity. The carbapenem group is included as one of the β-lactam antibiotics.

Monobactam

The only product in the monobactam group is aztreonam (Azactam). This is a synthetic bactericidal and a member of the general β-lactam class. It is effective against a wide range of gram-negative aerobic organisms.

AMINOGLYCOSIDES

The aminoglycosides are a group of chemically similar agents derived from different species of *Streptomyces*. Their structure consists of amino sugars with glycosidic linkages, giving the name aminoglycoside. Examples of aminoglycosides include the following:

Streptomycin
Gentamicin (Garamycin)
Tobramycin (Nebcin)
Kanamycin (Kantrex)
Amikacin (Amikin)
Neomycin (Neosporin)
Netilmicin (Netromycin)

Mode of Action. The aminoglycosides act by prevention and distortion of bacterial protein synthesis, although this does not explain why the group is bactericidal.

Use. Gentamicin, tobramycin, netilmicin, and amikacin are used for treating gram-negative bacillary pneumonias, with the exception of *Haemophilus*. There is a possibility that the aminoglycosides do not reach a sufficient level in bronchial secretions to be completely effective in gram-negative pneumonia when given systemically. β-lactam agents (penicillins, cephalosporins) may be needed, and both endobronchial and inhaled administration of aminoglycosides has been practiced. Inhalation of aminoglycosides is commonly used to control *Pseudomonas* infection in cystic fibrosis (see Chapter 12).

Streptomycin is used in treating *M. tuberculosis,* and neomycin is used for topical wound irrigation.

Toxicity.   The most noteworthy side effect of aminoglycosides is damage to renal tubules (nephrotoxicity). Ototoxicity can also occur and is manifest by dizziness and nausea. These agents can produce mild neuromuscular blockade and increase the blockade of neuromuscular paralyzing agents (curare, succinylcholine). Because of their effect on neuromuscular function, aminoglycosides should be used cautiously in myasthenia gravis.

TETRACYCLINES

The tetracyclines are derived from *Streptomyces* species. Examples of tetracylines are as follows:

Tetracycline (Achromycin)
Oxytetracycline (Terramycin)
Demeclocycline (Declomycin)
Methacycline (Rondomycin)
Doxycycline (Vibramycin)
Minocycline (Minocin)

Mode of Action.   The tetracyclines can be bacteriostatic or bacteridicidal, depending on dosage. They act by interfering with bacterial protein synthesis.

Toxicity and Hazards.   Side effects with the tetracyclines include gastrointestinal irritation with nausea, vomiting, and diarrhea; bone marrow depression; and hypersensitivity reactions manifested by skin rashes or acute anaphylaxis. They can also cause oral or vaginal candidiasis or fulminating diarrhea, all due to superinfections. Tetracyclines are incorporated temporarily in the liver and kidneys and therefore should be used with caution, if at all, in the presence of liver or renal disease. Their use in children with developing teeth results in tooth discoloration caused by deposition of a tetracycline-calcium-orthophosphate complex in tooth enamel. Tetracyclines also affect skeletal bones and retard skeletal growth, a permanent effect.

Uses.   Tetracyclines should be taken before eating and with an empty stomach to promote absorption. An exception is doxycycline, which may be taken with food or milk. Tetracyclines are useful for managing mycoplasmal and other atypical pneumonias, as well as acute infections superimposed on chronic bronchitis. Mycoplasmal organisms do not respond to antibiotics that act by inhibiting cell wall synthesis. Resistant organisms are especially troublesome in the hospital environment.

FLUOROQUINOLONES

The fluoroquinolones, or quinolones, are synthetic quinolone derivatives with broad-spectrum antibacterial activity. The fluorine molecule provides increased potency against gram-negative organisms and broadens the spectrum of activity to include some gram-positive organisms. Agents in this group include the following:

Ciprofloxacin (Cipro)
Norfloxacin (Noroxin)
Ofloxacin (Floxin)
Enoxacin (Penetrex)
Lomefloxacin (Maxaquin)

Uses.   These agents are useful in infections associated with chronic bronchitis and cystic fibrosis. They have strong activity against *H. influenzae, Legionella pneumophila, Mycoplasma pneumoniae, Neisseria meningitides, Bordetella pertussis,* and especially important in cystic fibrosis, against *P. aeruginosa.* A particular feature of these drugs that makes them useful in respiratory infections is the lung bioavailability when taken orally (i.e., oral administration gives suitably high lung tissue levels). Although this makes them attractive for use in managing chronic infection with *P. aeruginosa* in cystic fibrosis, their use should be limited to several weeks to avoid bacterial resistance (Neu, 1988).

MISCELLANEOUS ANTIBIOTIC AGENTS

The following individual antibiotics do not constitute a related group but are briefly characterized for the clinician.

Vancomycin (Vancocin)

Vancomycin is an antibiotic obtained from an actinomycete. The drug has a bactericidal effect produced by interference with bacterial cell wall synthesis. It has been used to manage staphylococcal respiratory infections resistant to methicillin. Ototoxicity is a possible hazard with the drug.

Chloramphenicol (Chloromycetin)

Chloramphenicol represents another antibiotic produced by an actinomycete that has broad-spectrum bacteriostatic activity caused by prevention of bacterial protein synthesis. Although it is effective against organisms such as salmonellae, penicillinase-producing *S. aureus*, *Klebsiella pneumoniae*, and *H. influenzae*, this agent has a risk of causing aplastic anemia, and its use in respiratory infections is limited to severe cases with resistance to less toxic antibiotics.

Erythromycin (Erythrocin, Ilotycin)

Another antibiotic derived from an actinomycete is erythromycin, which acts by inhibition of protein synthesis in bacteria. This agent is bacteriostatic in low dosages and bactericidal in higher dosages. It is given orally or intravenously and is relatively safe with respect to side effects. This drug is useful as an alternative for penicillin-allergic patients with pneumococcal pneumonia, and in the management of legionnaires' disease.

Erythromycin is termed a macrolide antibiotic based on its chemical structure. Other macrolide antibiotics include the following agents:

Azithromycin (Zithromax)
Clarithromycin (Biaxin)
Troleandomycin (Tao)

Polymyxins

There are two antibiotics included under the general term polymyxin: polymyxin B and polymyxin E. The polymyxins are polypeptide antibiotics; their structure consists of peptide-linked amino acids, and they are derived from *Bacillus polymyxa*.

Polymyxin B is very effective against *Pseudomonas* and other gram-negative bacteria. It has been used topically for infections (eye, ear, skin), and because it is not absorbed from the gastrointestinal tract, it can be given orally to manage infections in the intestine. It is also given intravenously, since intramuscular injections are very painful. Polymyxin B has been used as an aerosolized antibiotic (see Chapter 12). Polymyxin E is known as colistin and is similar to polymyxin B.

Bacitracin

Bacitracin is another polypeptide antibiotic originally obtained from the organism *Bacillus subtilis*. The particular culture used was taken from the wound of a young trauma victim named Tracy, and the name bacitracin commemorates the source of the drug. It is often used for topical management of infections of the mouth, nose, eye, or skin. Like the polymyxins, it is not well absorbed from the gastrointestinal tract for systemic use.

Clindamycin (Cleocin) and Lincomycin (Linococin)

Clindamycin is a derivative of lincomycin, which inhibits bacterial protein synthesis. Clindamycin is similar to erythromycin against pneumococci and group A streptococci, and it is active against *S. aureus* and gram-positive and gram-negative anaerobes such as *B. fragilis*. Its pulmonary use is with aspiration pneumonia as an alternative to penicillins. Clindamycin can cause severe diarrhea and associated colitis.

Metronidazole (Flagyl, Metizole)

Metronidazole is active against anaerobic infections, whether pulmonary, intraabdominal, or gynecologic. There has been concern over the drug's carcinogenic effect in animals, but a long-term study of 771 women showed no notable increase in cancer development (Beard et al., 1979).

SYNTHETIC (NONANTIBIOTIC) ANTI-INFECTIVE AGENTS

Sulfonamides

The sulfonamide group was the first effective group of chemotherapeutic agents used to treat systemic bacterial infections. *They are not classed as antibiotics.* Before antibiotics such as penicillin became available, these drugs were the main line of antibacterial defense. Their use has declined with the availability of the many natural and semisynthetic antibacterial agents currently used. The generic term *sulfonamide* refers to derivatives of sulfanilamide, the prototype chemical investigated in 1935. Examples of sulfonamides include the following:

Sulfisoxazole (Gantrisin)
Sulfamethoxazole (Gantanol)
Sulfadiazine
Sulfacytine (Renoquid)
Sulfamethizole (Thiosulfil)

Mode of Action. The sulfonamides are bacteriostatic and act by competitive antagonism to prevent the use of *p*-aminobenzoic acid by bacteria, an effect that ultimately prevents bacterial growth.

Uses. The sulfonamides may be used in the management of intestinal (bacillary dysentery) and urinary tract infections. They are not generally used any longer in managing gonococcal, staphylococcal, or streptococcal infections. The most recent interest in sulfonamides has been a combination of trimethoprim with sulfamethoxazole (discussed below).

Trimethoprim-Sulfamethoxazole

The drug combination trimethoprim-sulfamethoxazol was previously discussed in Chapter 12 as an anti-infective agent for use with *Pneumocystis carinii* pneumonia in patients with the acquired immunodeficiency syndrome (AIDS). The agent is a compound of two synthetic antibacterial drugs, trimethoprim and sulfamethoxazole, the latter representing a sulfonamide. The compound is not an antibiotic but a laboratory-produced chemical agent. The compound is an attractive antibacterial agent because the two drugs potentiate each other. Trimethoprim acts on the same metabolic sequence in bacteria as the sulfonamides. The compound is bactericidal, and the potentiating effect lowers the concentration of each drug ingredient necessary for its action. The compound is commonly used to manage acute and chronic urinary tract infections and also respiratory infections. It is the drug of choice for management of *P. carinii* in AIDS patients, although the incidence of side effects such as rash, fever, or leukopenia is increased, and failure to respond may occur.

Nitrofurantoin (Furadantin)

Nitrofurantoin is another synthetic antibacterial agent that is not an antibiotic. It is effective against many gram-positive and gram-negative organisms, including many urinary tract pathogens such as *E. coli,* and species of *Proteus, Pseudomonas, Klebsiella,* and *Enterobacter.* The drug is relatively nontoxic and is primarily used in the management of urinary tract infections. Of interest to respiratory care clinicians is the report of pulmonary side effects, including pleural effusion and pulmonary infiltrates, with use of the drug (Rosenow, 1972; Cooper et al., 1986).

ANTIFUNGAL AGENTS

The body harbors certain potentially pathogenic fungi such as *Candida albicans,* which is normally found in the mouth, sputum, stools, or vagina. The presence of such fungi does not cause disease or local inflammation unless the balance of resident bacterial flora is suppressed by broad-spectrum antibiotics or inhaled corticosteroid aerosols. The latter can cause fungal opportunistic growth in the oropharynx by *Candida* (recall hazards with corticosteroids, Chapter 10), which is termed oral candidiasis. Other fungi that can lead to pulmonary infections include *Aspergillus* species, *Histoplasma capsulatum*, *Coccidioides* species, and *Cryptococcus neoformans*. Some of the major antifungal drugs are amphotericin B, nystatin, and griseofulvin.

Amphotericin B

Amphotericin B is a relatively toxic drug obtained from an actinomycete *(Streptomyces nodosus)*. Its fungicidal action is due to its ability to increase fungal cell membrane permeability, an effect that allows leakage of ions and small molecules from the cell. This may also account for its toxic effects, which include nephrotoxocity and which are dose related. The effect of the drug on the renal system can lead to loss of bicarbonate, resulting in a metabolic acidosis.

Nystatin

Nystatin is another antifungal antibiotic that is effective against yeastlike infections, such as *C. albicans*. It is applied topically to the skin, vulva, or mouth for treatment of *Candida* and may be recognized by its brand name Mycostatin.

Griseofulvin

Unlike nystatin, griseofulvin is effective systemically by mouth but not by topical application. This drug is used in treating tinea (ringworm) infections, which usually occur on the hands, head, fingernails, toenails, or groin; it is fungistatic. Side effects are minor.

Other Antifungal Agents

In addition to the three agents profiled, other drugs intended for management of fungal infections have been released and include the following:

Flucytosine (Ancobon)
Miconazole (Monistat)
Ketoconazole (Nizoral)
Fluconazole (Diflucan)
Itraconazole (Sporanox)

ANTITUBERCULOSIS AGENTS

Management of Tuberculosis

Effective management of tuberculosis began with the discovery of streptomycin in 1944. Previously, tuberculosis was "managed" by quarantine and isolation. However, the use of streptomycin alone was quickly found to lead to resistant strains of the bacillus *M. tuberculosis.* This necessitated the use of multiple-drug therapy, which is standard practice today and which was made possible by development of other chemotherapeutic agents active against *M. tuberculosis.* In 1949, *p*-aminosalicyclic acid was identified for use in tuberculosis, although generally this agent is no longer used. In 1952, isoniazid was shown to be effective and remains a standard antituberculosis drug. Originally, two- or three-drug regimens were used for periods of 18 to 24 months to manage tuberculosis. In the 1960s, rifampin was introduced, and shorter treatment periods of 6 to 9 months with two or three drugs became possible. A good review of antituberculosis therapy is given by Davidson and Hanh (1986). The February 1985 Supplement of *Chest* is devoted to management of tuberculosis and should be consulted for details. The following discussion is based on these sources.

Since infection in humans is by way of the respiratory tract through inhalation of the organism, tuberculosis and its management is of special interest to clinicians in respiratory care. Diagnosis of tuberculosis infection is aided by means of the tuberculin reaction, which is a delayed, lymphocyte-mediated immune reaction. For example, purified protein derivative is used in a skin test; if a person has been infected with *M. tuberculosis* and had developed an immunity to the capsule of the tubercle bacillus, then an inflammatory reaction would occur at the skin site where purified protein derivative was injected.

The two basic principles of drug therapy for tuberculosis are (1) concomitant administration of at least two drugs to which the patient's organisms are susceptible, and (2) treatment should continue beyond sputum conversion and symptomatic improvement. Management of the disease is considered effective in the United States and Canada only if the relapse rate is less than 5%.

9-Month Treatment

A standard approach to managing tuberculosis today consists of multiple-first-line drugs for 9 months. Isonizid and rifampin are given for 9 months. In an initial period of 2 to 8 weeks, these two drugs are supplemented with one of the following: ethambutol, streptomycin, or pyrazinamide. With these combinations, a relapse rate of only 0% to 4% has been seen. Efforts are also being made to reduce the 9-month period to 6 months, with use of *four* drugs (isoniazid, rifampin, pyrazinamide, and either ethambutol or streptomycin) for

2 months followed by 4 months of isoniazid and rifampin. Initial results are reported to be excellent. Each of these drugs is briefly characterized below.

Streptomycin

Streptomycin was the first drug available for effective management of tuberculosis and has been previously identified in this chapter as an aminoglycoside. The route of administration is intramuscular injection, which is inconvenient for patients and staff, although treatment is thus well controlled.

Isoniazid

Isonicotinic acid hydrazide, or INH, was found in the early 1950s to be an effective tuberculostatic agent that was superior to streptomycin. It has remained a primary drug in managing tuberculosis and is easily absorbed from the gastrointestinal tract with oral administration. There is a risk of severe or even fatal hepatitis with isoniazid, and this risk increases with age. While isoniazid is effective with all clinical forms of tuberculosis, resistance to the drug by the bacillus can develop. An interesting application of pharmacogenetics is the genetic control of the metabolism of isoniazid, dividing the population into "rapid" and "slow" inactivators of the drug. Slow inactivators, which lack an acetylating enzyme, maintain higher blood levels of the drug and may respond better, although there is increased potential for side effects.

Rifampin

Rifampin, or rifampicin, is a semisynthetic derivative of the antibiotic rifamycin. Its primary role is the management of mycobacterial infections, and it is often used in conjunction with isoniazid. Rifampin is usually given by mouth, is best absorbed on an empty stomach, and should therefore be taken before eating. The drug may cause the urine and sputum to have a brownish-red stain, and there is an increased risk of hepatoxoicity with preexisting liver diseases.

Ethambutol

Ethambutol is a synthetic tuberculostatic agent, but only the dextrorotatory isomer is active. Resistance of tubercle bacilli to this drug can occur rapidly, and it is used together with other tuberculostatic agents. The drug is taken orally and is fairly safe. However, it may impair vision by reducing visual sharpness or color discrimination, an effect that reverses with discontinuance of the drug.

Pyrazinamide

Pyrazinamide is a synthetic analogue of nicotinamide, whose mechanism of action is not well understood. The drug is taken orally in tablet form. The most common side effect is liver injury.

Other Agents

In addition to the above-mentioned drugs, certain agents are considered as second-line in managing tuberculosis. These agents include the following:

Ethionamide
Cycloserine
Capreomycin
Kanamycin
Viomycin

Clinicians should be aware of three other aspects of tuberculosis. First, exposure to the organism or a positive tuberculin reaction even without a positive sputum is often managed with prophylactic use of isoniazid. The drug is given for 1 year in a daily dosage. Second, persons who are positive for the human immunodeficiency virus (HIV) seem to be at greater risk for tuberculosis (Rieder and Snider, 1986), even prior to the diagnosis of AIDS. Third, the emergence of drug-resistant strains of *M. tuberculosis*, even with multiple-drug therapy, gives the prospect of an increase in this formerly controllable disease.

ANTIVIRAL AGENTS

The process of viral infection and the difficulties this process poses for drug therapy of viral infections were briefly summarized in Chapter 12 when discussing ribavirin. Some viral illnesses are mild and self-limiting, such as colds. Others, such as poliomyelitis, can be prevented with a vaccine. However, diseases such as AIDS have no successful vaccine to date and lead to death. Even influenza or respiratory syncytial viral pneumonia can be fatal in a compromised subject. The development and improvement of antiviral drug therapy continues in the effort to manage such illnesses.

Table 13–1 lists the relatively small group of antiviral agents currently available in the United States, along with their intended use.

Mode of Action.   The mode of action by which antiviral agents exert their effect on viruses is not completely known for every agent in use. However, many of the antiviral drugs structurally resemble nucleoside precursors of the nucleotide building blocks of DNA strands. This was discussed and illustrated for ribavirin in Chapter 12. As an example, ribavirin resembles the nucleoside guanosine. Phosphates attach to nucleosides to form nucleotides, which assemble to form DNA strands. Each nucleotide has one of four bases, which form the pairs when DNA strands pair: adenine, guanine, cytosine, and thy-

TABLE 13–1.

Antiviral Agents and Their Labeled Use in the
United States

Drug	Use*
Acyclovir (Zovirax)	HSV 1 and 2
Amantadine (Symmetrel)	Influenza A
Didanosine, ddl (Videx)	HIV
Foscarnet sodium (Foscavir)	CMV retinitis in AIDS
Ganciclovir (Cytovene)	CMV retinitis
Idoxuridine (Herplex)	HSV eye infections
Ribavirin (Virazole)	RSV respiratory infection
Rimantadine (Flumadine)	Influenza A
Vidarabine (Vira-A)	HSV encephalitis, occular infection
Zalcitabine, ddC (Hivid)	HIV
Zidovudine, AZT (Retrovir)	HIV

*HSV, herpes simplex virus; CMV, cytomegalovirus; RSV, respiratory syncytial virus.

mine. Antiviral drugs that are nucleoside analogues (e.g., ribavirin, zidovudine, didanosine, vidarabine, acyclovir, ganciclovir, and zalcitabine) substitute for natural nucleosides and interrupt the process of viral gene development and replication.

Management of HIV Infection.   The management of HIV infection continues to evolve. It is important to distinguish between drugs used to manage the many opportunistic infections (not necessarily viral) that occur with AIDS and management of the HIV organism itself with an antiviral agent. Foscarnet sodium and ganciclovir are used for infections associated with AIDS (i.e. cytomegalovirus retinitis) but are not targeted directly at the AIDS virus. Trimethoprim-sulfamethoxazole and pentamidine isethionate (aerosol and parenteral formulations) are used to manage *P. carinii* pneumonia, a nonviral infection. Didanosine, ddI (Videx); zalcitabine, ddC (Hivid); and zidovudine, AZT (Retrovir) are targeted directly at the AIDS virus.

At the time of this edition, there are over 60 potential drugs in various phases of clinical trials for use in AIDS, including vaccines, immunomodulators, and antiviral agents.

BIBLIOGRAPHY

Beard CM et al: Lack of evidence for cancer due to use of metronidazole, N Engl J Med 301:519, 1979.

Cooper JAD Jr, White DA, Matthay RA: Drug-induced pulmonary disease. II Noncytotoxic drugs, Am Rev Respir Dis 133:488, 1986.

Davidson PT, Hanh LQ: Antituberculosis drugs, Clin Chest Med 7:425, 1986.

Donowitz GR, Mandell GL: Beta-lactam antibiotics, N Engl J Med 318:419 (Part 1), 490 (Part 2), 1988.

Kuriyama S, Panosian C: Antibiotics II: aminoglycosides, polymyxins, vancomycin, trimethoprim-sulfamethoxazole, and pentamidine, Clin Chest Med 7:413, 1986.

Neu HC: Quinolones: a new class of antimicrobial agents with wide potential uses, Med Clin North Am 72:623, 1988.

Rieder HL, Snider DE: Tuberculosis and the acquired immunodeficiency syndrome, Chest 90:489, 1986 (editorial).

Rosenow EC: The spectrum of drug-induced pulmonary disease, Ann Intern Med 77:977, 1972.

Segreti J, Trenholme GM: Antibiotics I: Beta-lactam antibiotics, the tetracyclines, chloramphenicol, erythromycin, clindamycin, metronidazole, and the quinolones. Clin Chest Med 7:393, 1986.

14

Cold and Cough Agents

Chapter 14 reviews classes of drugs used to relieve symptoms of the common cold:

- Sympathomimetic (adrenergic) decongestants
- Antihistamine drying agents
- Expectorants to aid mucus clearance
- Antitussives to control cough

The combination of these classes in cold products are reviewed, and recommendations for use with colds are given.

INTRODUCTION

There are bewildering and in some cases irrational numbers of compounds, both prescription and over-the-counter (OTC), available for treating symptoms of the common cold.

The term *common cold* refers to nonbacterial upper respiratory tract infections usually characterized by a mild general malaise and a runny, stuffy nose. More specific symptoms include sneezing, a sore throat, cough, and possibly some chest discomfort.

Allergic rhinitis is *not* included in this discussion nor are serious illnesses such as influenza, acute bronchitis, or infections of the lower respiratory tract. Influenza, or the "flu," is associated with symptoms of fever, headache, general muscle ache, and extreme fatigue or weakness. Onset of symptoms is usually rapid. The fever and systemic symptoms with influenza distinguish this affliction from a common cold.

Four classes of agents can be distinguished in cold remedies, used singly or in combination:

Sympathomimetics: for decongestion.

Antihistamines: to reduce (dry) secretions.

Expectorants: to increase mucous clearance.

Antitussive: to suppress the cough reflex.

These four classes of cold and cough medications target the primary symptoms caused by the cold virus in the respiratory tract. This is illustrated conceptually in Figure 14–1.

Each class will be discussed briefly, with representative agents listed. In addition to these four types of ingredients, an analgesic such as acetaminophen may be included, as in Sinutab, which consists of the following ingredients: 30 mg pseudoephedrine (decongestant) and 325 mg acetaminophen (analgesic).

SYMPATHOMIMETIC (ADRENERGIC) DECONGESTANTS

Sympathomimetics were discussed in Chapter 5 for use as bronchodilators, and the general effects of sympathetic stimulation were outlined in Chap-

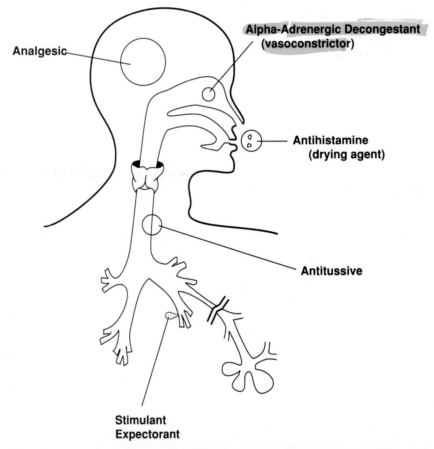

FIG 14–1. Cold and cough medications include four classes of drugs that are targeted at the symptoms produced by the common cold.

ter 4. In cold remedies, sympathomimetics are intended for a *decongestant* effect, which is based on their alpha-stimulating property and resultant vaso-constriction.

Sympathomimetics such as phenylephrine are found under the trade names Coricidin and Neo-Synephrine and can be used in topical sprays or taken orally. Generally, topical applications require lower doses than that for oral use. Problems can exist with either route of administration.

Topical Application

Although onset of action is faster with topical application than with oral use, repeated application of these sprays or drops can cause swollen mucosa, the exact problem being treated. Discontinuing this type of drug can also result in a rebound nasal congestion. Sympathomimetic decongestants should be used for short periods only, of a day or so. Some of the agents such as oxymetazoline (Afrin) can actually create tolerance and physical withdrawal symptoms.

Systemic Application

Systemic application has the advantage over topical of giving more extensive decongestant effects that involve deeper blood vessels. However, producing nasal vasoconstriction through systemic routes will often lead to other systemic effects of sympathomimetics, such as a rise in blood pressure and increased heart rate.

The following agents are classed as nasal decongestants in the sympathomimetic group of cold remedies:

Phenylephrine (Neo-Synephrine, Coricidin)
Epinephrine
Pseudoephedrine (Sudafed)
Ephedrine (Va-tro-nol)
Phenylpropanolamine (Propadrin)
Xylometazoline (Otrivin)
Naphazoline (Privine)
Tetrahydrozoline (Tyzine)
Oxymetazoline (Afrin)

ANTIHISTAMINE DRYING AGENTS

Histamine

Histamine occurs naturally in the body and is contained in tissue mast cells and blood basophils. The role of the mast cell in releasing histamine with allergic asthma was discussed in Chapters 10 and 11.

Effect of Histamine

Histamine is one of the chief mediators of local inflammatory responses. Some idea of its effect can be realized from the fact that stinging nettles produce their burning pain because of a high concentration of histamine and acetylcholine. Histamine can cause smooth muscle contraction, increased capillary permeability and dilatation, itching, and pain.

Scraping a tongue depressor or blunt pencil across the sensitive skin of the inner arm can illustrate a local inflammatory reaction at least partly mediated by histamine. The result is a wheal and flare reaction, also called a triple response (local redness, welt formation, and a reddish-white border). The redness and wheal (welt) are caused by dilatation and leakage of plasma proteins from skin capillaries. The exudation of plasma causes the swelling. The flare, or reddish-white area surrounding the wheal, is probably due to local axon reflexes from sensory fibers causing dilatation of neighboring arterioles.

Histamine Receptors

Histamine produces its inflammatory effects by stimulating specific cell surface receptors. There are two types of histamine receptors distinguished (Simons and Simons, 1991):

H_1 receptors: located in the bronchopulmonary region, and on blood vessels; these receptors are involved in inflammation and allergic reactions.

H_2 receptors: located in the gastric region; these receptors regulate gastric acid secretion, as well as feedback control of histamine release.

A third type of histamine receptor, H_3, has been discovered. This receptor is involved in modulation of cholinergic neurotransmission in the airway, in central nervous system (CNS) functioning, and in feedback control of histamine synthesis and release (Simons and Simons, 1991).

The typical antihistamine found in cold medications is an H_1-receptor antagonist. Examples of these include pyrilamine or chlorpheniramine. H_1-receptor antagonists block the bronchopulmonary and vascular actions of histamine, to prevent rhinitis and urticaria. H_2-receptor antagonists are exemplified by cimetidine (Tagamet) or ranitidine (Zantac), which are used to block gastric acid secretion when treating ulcers.

Antihistamine Agents and Effects

All of the antihistamines considered in this chapter are H_1-receptor antagonists. These antihistamine agents are further classified into six major groups (Table 14–1). The first five groups are found in cold preparations. Some trade names given may be familiar from OTC preparations, which are readily available in drugstores. Others are found in combination products, discussed and listed subsequently.

TABLE 14-1.

Major Groups of Antihistamines

Generic Names	Trade Name
Ethanolamine derivatives	
Diphenhydramine HCl	Benadryl
Carbinoxamine	Clistin
Clemastine	Tavist
Ethylenediamine derivatives	
Pyrilamine	—
Tripelennamine HCl	Pyribenzamine
Piperidine	
Cyproheptadine	Periactin
Azatadine	Optimine
Diphenylpyraline	Hispril
Phenindamine	Nolahist
Phenothiazine derivatives	
Promethazine HCl	Phenergan
Trimeprazine tartrate	Temaril
Methdilazine	Tacaryl
Propylamine derivatives	
Chlorpheniramine maleate	Chlor-Trimeton
Brompheniramine maleate	Dimetane
Triprolidine	Actidil
Dexchlorpheniramine maleate	Polaramine
Nonsedating long-acting	
Terfenadine	Seldane
Astemizole	Hismanal

Effects of Antihistamines

Antihistamines have three major classes of effects: antihistaminic, sedative, and anticholinergic activity.

The antihistaminic activity blocks the increased vascular permeability, pruritus, and bronchial smooth muscle constriction caused by histamine. These actions are the reason antihistamines are used to treat allergic disorders such as rhinoconjunctivitis, allergic rhinitis, and urticaria.

The sedative effect of antihistamines is thought to be caused by penetration of the agents into the brain, where inhibition of histamine N-methyltransferase and blockage of central histaminergic receptors occur. There is also antagonism of other CNS receptors, such as serotonin and acetylcholine (Simons and Simons, 1991). The effect of drowsiness with the classic (older) antihistamines can be a major hazard if alertness is required, such as in operating heavy machinery (e.g., a car) or monitoring a patient.

Finally, the anticholinergic effect produces considerable upper airway drying, just as would occur with an antimuscarinic agent such as atropine sulfate. The duration of action of the older antihistamines is generally 4 to 6 hours. However, development of newer agents, which are termed *nonsedating long-acting antihistamines,* has led to products that are effective for up to 12 hours, depending on dose, and that lack the sedating and anticholinergic effects. These newer agents are exemplified by terfenadine (Seldane) and astemizole (Hismanal).

Structure-Activity Relations

H_1-receptor antagonists were first discovered in 1937 (Woodward, 1990). The chemical structure of histamine, the general structure of the H_1-receptor antagonists, and two examples of H_1 antagonists are given in Figure 14–2. Chlorpheniramine is an antihistamine found in many cold remedies and represents one of the older, classic H_1-receptor antagonists. Terfenadine is a newer, nonsedating H_1-receptor antagonist.

The resemblance between histamine and the general formula for the H_1-

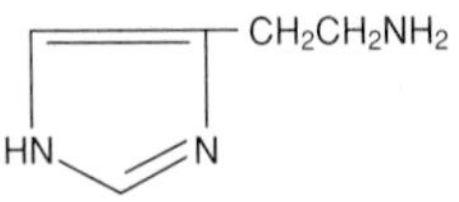

Histamine

General Structure,
H_1 Receptor Antagonists

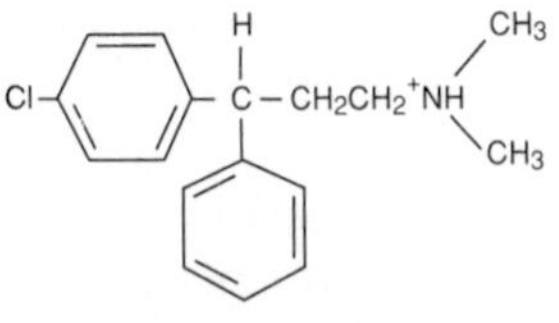

Chlorpheniramine

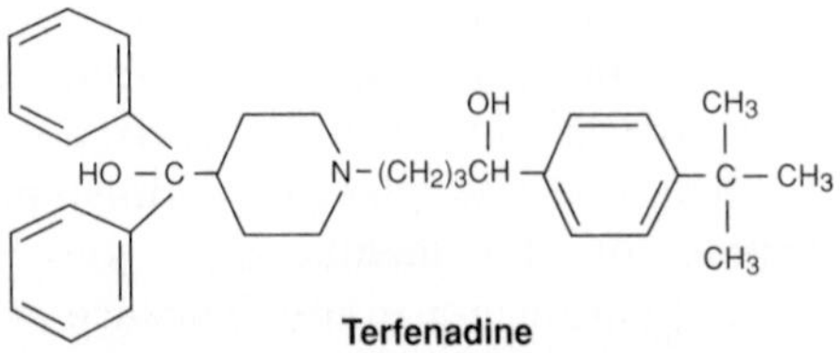

Terfenadine

FIG 14–2. The structure of histamine, an inflammatory mediator; the general structure of H_1-receptor antagonists; and the structure of two antihistamines, chlorpheniramine and terfenadine, are shown. R_1 to R_4 indicate the sites of attachments, with R_1 and R_2 being ring structures in most H_1 antagonists.

blocking agents can be seen in the structures shown. In the older agents, exemplified by chlorpheniramine, the R_1 and R_2 attachments are usually a ring structure connected to an ethylamine (C–C–N) group. The presence of the ring structures, and other substitutions on the structure, make the older antihistamines lipophilic. As a result, the classic antihistamines readily penetrate into the CNS and produce the effect of sedation and drowsiness previously discussed. The newer, nonsedating agents such as terfenadine do not readily cross the blood-brain barrier and therefore do not block central H_1 receptors (Woodward, 1990).

Use With Colds

One of the beneficial effects of antihistamine use with a cold is the drying of upper airway secretions, which lessens the rhinitis and accompanying sneezing. There is some question whether the drying of secretions is due to histamine antagonism or to the anticholinergic effect with these agents. How much histamine release occurs with colds is debated. In allergic rhinitis, there is no question that histamine causes much of the inflammatory response, and in fact the newer long-acting agents are particularly helpful with this condition.

Regardless of the exact effect, the drying of runny nasal secretions is welcomed by cold sufferers, and this coupled with drowsiness can be useful to produce needed rest and sleep at night. Secretions, however, are a defense mechanism with an upper airway viral infection. Around-the-clock antihistamines may be more harmful, because of suppressed secretion clearance, than a single nighttime dose. Adequate hydration with a cold is always helpful, with or without the use of antihistamines.

Other uses of antihistamines include the treatment of symptoms seen with motion sickness and the control of nausea.

EXPECTORANTS

Expectorants are defined as agents that facilitate removal of mucus from the lower respiratory tract. A distinction was made in Chapter 8 between the following types of expectorants:

Mucolytic expectorants: Agents that facilitate removal of mucus by a lysing, or mucolytic, action. EXAMPLE: acetylcysteine.

Stimulant expectorants: Agents that increase the production and therefore presumably clearance of mucous secretions in the respiratory tract.

Generally, the expectorants considered here are stimulant, although the action does not always allow clear distinction. An example is guaifenesin, which is thought to reduce the adhesiveness and surface tension of mucus, and thus increase mucokinesis, that is, movement and clearance of the secretion. Another term used with these agents is *mucoevacuant.*

Efficacy and Use

There is controversy over the effectiveness and use of expectorants. The issue is clouded by the following:

1. Difficulty in assessing the effectiveness of expectorants, and in particular, lack of objective criteria to demonstrate effectiveness.
2. In conjunction with the first point, who would benefit from use of expectorants? In particular, should expectorants be included in treatment of cold symptoms if a cold involves the upper respiratory tract?

Use in Chronic Bronchitis

Petty (1990) reported the results of a national study evaluating the use of the expectorant iodinated glycerol (Organidin). The subjects had chronic bronchitis, quite different from a common cold. Petty concluded that in chronic obstructive bronchitis, iodinated glycerol was safe and effective. Its use improved cough symptoms, chest discomfort, ease in bringing up sputum, and sense of well-being. The duration of acute exacerbations of chronic bronchitis was decreased. It is reasonable that, in bronchitis, symptoms and airflow will improve, and further infection will be reduced if mucus clearance can be improved.

Mode of Action

Stimulant expectorants are thought to work by a variety of means, depending on the agent. These mechanisms include the following:

1. Vagal gastric reflex stimulation.
2. Absorption into respiratory glands to directly increase mucus production.
3. Topical stimulation with inhaled volatile agents.

Guaifenesin, also known as glycerol guaiacolate, is classified as Category I, which is safe and effective (Covington, 1991). Ziment (1989) has reviewed the mechanisms of action with iodides, such as iodinated glycerol. Other agents, such as terpin hydrate, sodium citrate, ammonium chloride or menthols, have no demonstrated efficacy (Covington, 1991).

Since mucus incorporates water as it is produced, an adequate intake of plain water or other nondiuretic liquids (milk, fruit juices) can help preserve mucus viscosity and clearance, especially with a simple cold.

Expectorant Agents

Table 14–2 lists available expectorant agents. Some of these are sold with no particular trade name, as with terpin hydrate. Major agents or groups of agents are briefly characterized below.

Iodides

Potassium iodide is an old agent that has been used as an expectorant in asthma and chronic bronchitis (Alstead, 1939). It has a direct mucolytic effect in sufficient concentrations. It also has an indirect effect on mucus viscosity by stimulating submucosal glands to produce new, lower viscosity secretions.

The exact mechanism of action with iodinated glycerol (Organidin) is unclear. It is broken down into iodide and glycerol after absorption into the bloodstream. Iodide appears to distribute to mucous glands, where it is secreted along with increased mucus. Iodide also stimulates the gastropulmonary reflex, has a mucolytic effect, and can stimulate ciliary activity (Ziment, 1989).

Iodides are associated with hypersensitivity reactions in some individuals, and a case of pulmonary edema has been reported with its use (Huang and Peterson, 1981).

Guaifensin (Glyceryl Guaiacolate)

Guaifenesin by inhalation is also considered to be an emollient. In experimental animals, doses larger than those used in humans caused an increase in bronchial secretions. Guaifenesin taken orally is thought to reduce the adhesiveness and surface tension of mucous secretions, thereby enhancing mucus clearance. It is considered safe and effective by the Food and Drug Administration.

TABLE 14–2.

Major Expectorant Agents

Generic Name	Trade Names
Guaifenesin	Robitussin, Naldecon Senior EX, Humibid L.A.
Terpin hydrate	Various
Iodinated glycerol	Organidin
Potassium iodide (SSKI)	Various

Ipecac

Ipecac is usually limited to its use as an emetic, often in drug overdoses which are recent enough that marked gastric absorption has not occurred and the overdose victim is of course still conscious, with no danger of aspiration. There is some question as to whether ipecac simply increases salivation, common with nausea and vomiting, or actually stimulates increased respiratory secretions. A subemetic dose would have to be used with this agent. It is not commonly used as an expectorant.

Bromhexine

Bromhexine, a synthetic derivative of the alkaloid vascicine, not available in the United States, has been reported by Thomson et al. (1974) to increase the rate of mucociliary clearance when taken orally. Other researchers have indicated an increase in sputum volume with an accompanying decrease in viscosity (Brogan et al., 1974; Hamilton et al., 1970).

Other Expectorants

Ziment (1982) suggests that chicken broth flavored with garlic and curry may serve as a tasty and effective mucus stimulant via the gastric reflex. The major constituent of garlic is allicin, which has a structure similar to S-carboxymethylcysteine, discussed previously as a mucolytic (see Chapter 8). Other spices that could have the same potential are pepper sauce (Tabasco), horseradish, and mustard.

Topical Agents

This category usually evokes memories of the heated humidifier (vaporizer) with clouds of steam scented with camphor, menthol, or even in the past choloroform. These agents may still be found in use, but efficacy as an expectorant has not been shown. The burn risk of a hot vaporizer should preclude its use with the young or the old and debilitated.

Pavia et al. (1978) showed that so-called bland aerosols of saline do increase sputum volume, possibly through reflex irritation of the bronchi and with increased secretion clearance due to coughing. Certainly any particulate suspension can function as an irritant to the upper airways.

Parasympathomimetics

The use of parasympathomimetics will stimulate mucous gland secretion, but the effect on other muscarinic receptors is too diffuse for practical use as an expectorant. For this reason, a drug such as pilocarpine is not used as an expectorant. Likewise, stimulation of the medulla can increase respiratory tract secretions, but stimulation of the CNS is hazardous (see Chapter 16).

COUGH SUPPRESSANTS (ANTITUSSIVES)

A fourth category of drugs used with colds and cold symptoms is the cough suppressant. Coughing is a defense mechanism to protect the upper airway from irritants, such as dust particles, or aerosols, liquids, and other foreign objects. This mechanism is a reflex, coordinated by a postulated cough center in the medulla. Chapter 6 dealt briefly with the concept of a vagal reflex arc in bronchospasm, due to stimulation of subepithelial cough receptors. Here the focus is the cough itself, not bronchial smooth muscle constriction. Stimulation of vagal sensory endings (afferent fibers) in the larynx and bronchi, and even in the stomach, can cause the cough reflex. The strongest cough reflex is caused by stimulation of the laryngeal and tracheal vagal sensory fibers. Coughing that occurs during or just before vomiting is thought to be caused by stimulation of abdominal vagal receptors. Stimulation of vagal sensory receptors, whether during vomiting or "tickling" of the trachea also tends to increase bronchial secretions, which are under vagal control.

Agents and Mode of Action

Cough suppressants act by depressing the cough center in the medulla. Narcotics (see Chapter 16) possess powerful depressant effects on the medullary centers, including the CO_2 chemoreceptors, and are often used for this purpose. Common agents are codeine or hydrocodone. A common nonnarcotic is dextromethorphan.

Benzonatate (Tessalon), a nonnarcotic chemically related to tetracaine, has a local anesthetic effect with topical application. This would act upon the sensory (afferent) vagal receptors in the upper airway. It is also thought to inhibit the transmission of the afferent impulse to the motor nerves through the medulla. Diphenhydramine (Benadryl), available in a syrup, may be an effective cough suppressant.

A number of cough suppressants, or antitussives, contain codeine. In a dose below 15 mg, codeine does not produce analgesia in the adult. In the 10 to 20 mg range, there is an antitussive action. Above 30 mg, codeine produces analgesia. Hydrocodone produces an antitussive effect with a dose of approximately 5 mg. Table 14–3 lists agents and compounds containing either codeine, hydrocodone, or dextromethorphan. Both dextromethorphan and codeine are available in OTC preparations. These two agents are considered to be preferred cough suppressants based on both safety and efficacy. Diphenhydramine and noscapine are secondary OTC agents (Covington, 1991). The need for a prescription antitussive is unusual, especially in a cold, with the availability of OTC preparations.

TABLE 14–3.

Major Cold and Cough Medications by Agent

Trade Name	Dose of Agent
Codeine	
Calcidrine	8.4 mg/5 ml
Actifed with Codeine Cough Syrup	10 mg/5 ml
Dimetane-DC Cough Syrup	10 mg/5 ml
Novahistine DH	10 mg/5 ml
Tussi-Organidin Liquid	10 mg/5 ml
Pediacof Syrup	5 mg/5 ml
Robitussin A-C	10 mg/5 ml
Nucofed	20 mg/5 ml
Hydrocodone	
Entuss-D Liquid	5 mg/5 ml
Triaminic Expectorant DH	1.67 mg/5 ml
Hycodan (syrup)	5 mg/5 ml
Hycomine Syrup	5 mg/5 ml
Tussionex (liquid)	10 mg/5 ml
Dextromethorphan	
Triaminic-DM Cough Formula	10 mg/5 ml
Formula 44D Decongestant Cough Mixture	10 mg/5 ml
Dimetane-DX Cough Syrup	10 mg/5 ml
Rondec DM Syrup	15 mg/5 ml
Trind DM	7.5 mg/5 ml
Nyquil Nighttine Colds Medicine Liquid	5 mg/5 ml
Tussi-Organidin DM Liquid	10 mg/5 ml
Robitussin-DM	15 mg/5 ml
Tylenol Cold Tabs	15 mg tab
Tylenol Cold and Flu Powder	30 mg/packet
Theraflu Powder	20 mg/packet
Nyquil LiquiCaps	15 mg/cap
Dimetapp DM	10 mg/5 ml
Humibid DM Tabs	30 mg tab

Use of Cough Suppressants

Several principles apply to the use of antitussives.

1. They are helpful and indicated to suppress dry, hacking, nonproductive, irritating coughs, especially if the coughing causes sleep loss. Furthermore, a constant nonproductive cough can cause irritation of the trachea, which leads to more coughing.

2. Do not suppress the cough reflex in the presence of copious bronchial secretions, which need to be cleared. This includes situations of cystic fibrosis and other chronic obstructive lung diseases such as bronchitis. Excess mucous secretions from the lower respiratory tract are not present in an uncomplicated cold (see the definition of common cold) and indicate the need for further evaluation and possible treatment with an antibiotic.

3. The combination of an expectorant and an antitussive in a cold medication is questionable. This amounts to suppressing the clearance mechanism while stimulating secretions to be cleared. Use of a single-entity cough preparation such as Benylin DM (dextromethorphan 10 mg/5 ml) or Robitussin Pediatric (dextromethorphan 7.5 mg/5 ml) to treat a dry, irritating cough is recommended.

The combination of expectorant and antitussive is based on the rationale that a dry, hacking, frequent cough can be better replaced by a less frequent but productive cough. Unfortunately, the preexisting combination of expectorant and antitussive in many compounds does not allow tailoring of medication to individual need. Also, most cold compounds combine an antihistamine to dry secretions with the expectorant to stimulate mucus production. The rationale for this is open to question.

COLD COMPOUNDS

A list of cold remedies, with the classes of agents included in the compounds, is given in Table 14–4. Table 14–4 includes single-ingredient products, such as Neo-Synephrine, as well as compounds with multiple drug classes, such as Dimetapp DM. Some of the preparations in elixir form use substantial amounts of alcohol as a solvent. For example, Vicks Formula 44M Cough and Cold Liquid, produced by Richardson-Vicks, contains pseudoephedrine, chlorpheniramine, dextromethorphan, acetaminophen, and 20% alcohol. Nyquil Nighttime Cold/Flu Liquid contains 25% alcohol, and a terpin hydrate-dextromethorphan liquid has over 40% alcohol. No doubt some subjective sense of improvement reminiscent of the "hot toddy" may be found with such compounds. Another aspect of cold remedies that adds to their

TABLE 14–4.

Categories of Ingredients in Some Representative Cold Remedies

Trade Name	Sympathomimetic	Antihistamine	Expectorant	Antitussive
Sudafed Tablets	pseudoephedrine (30, 60 mg tab)			
Neo-Synephrine	phenylephrine (1% solution)			
Chlor-Trimeton		chlorpheniramine (4-mg tab)		
Robitussin (liquid)			guaifenesin (100 mg/5 ml)	
Vicks Formula 44				dextromethorphan (15 mg/5 ml)
Actifed 12-Hour Capsules	pseudoephedrine (120 mg)	triprolidine (5 mg)		
Dimetapp DM	phenylpropanolamine (12.5 mg)	brompheniramine (2 mg)		dextromethorphan (10 mg)
Novahistine Expectorant	pseudoephedrine (30 mg)		guaifenesin (100 mg)	codeine (10 mg)
Pediacof Syrup	phenylephrine (2.5 mg)	chlorpheniramine (750 μg)	potassium iodide (75 mg)	codeine (5 mg)

Product				
Robitussin-CF	phenylpropanolamine (12.5 mg)		guaifenesin (100 mg)	dextromethorphan (10 mg)
Robitussin-DAC	pseudoephedrine (30 mg)		guaifenesin (100 mg)	codeine (10 mg)
Robitussin-DM			guaifenesin (100 mg)	dextromethorphan (15 mg)
Triaminic Cold Tablets	phenylpropanolamine (12.5 mg)	chlorpheniramine (2 mg)		
Triaminic-DM Cough Formula	phenylpropanolamine (12.5 mg)			dextromethorphan (10 mg)
Triaminic Nite Light	pseudoephedrine (15 mg)	chlorpheniramine (1 mg)		dextromethorphan (7.5 mg)
Triaminic Expectorant	phenylpropanolamine (12.5 mg)		guaifenesin (100 mg)	
Triaminic Expectorant DH	phenylpropanolamine (12.5 mg)	pyrilamine (6.25 mg)	guaifenesin (100 mg)	hydrocodone (1.67 mg)
Humibid DM Tablets			guaifenesin (600 mg)	dextromethorphan (30 mg)

confusion is the variation in ingredients, all under the same basic trade name with suffixed initials to indicate substituted or deleted ingredients. For example, with Robitussin-CF, Robitussin-DM, and Robitussin-DAC, the ingredients vary as seen in Table 14–4. Since these compounds change fairly rapidly, no list remains current long, in terms of what is on the market. However, the basic principle of the typical four classes of ingredients remains, and new compounds can be evaluated for particular uses by considering the effects of these four classes of agents.

Many of these compounds are available as OTC preparations and thus require no prescription. The possibility of overdose and abuse is very real by combining prescribed compounds and OTC compounds. Often OTC preparations have the same classes of ingredients but in lower concentrations.

Treating a Cold

There is no cure for the common cold, and the four classes of drugs used in cold remedies treat only symptoms. Furthermore, their potentially undesirable effects as described below should be considered.

Sympathomimetics.   Tremor, tachycardia, and increased blood pressure can be seen especially when used orally. Rebound congestion can occur if used for longer than a day.

Antihistamines.   Antihistamines can cause drowsiness and impaired responses. Drying of secretions, whether due to antimuscarinic or antihistamine action, may suppress a needed defense reaction of the airways. Nocturnal use may be more indicated than around-the-clock use.

Expectorants.   Expectorants have questionable efficacy. The best expectorant, especially with colds, is plain water and juices, avoiding caffeinated beverages, such as tea or colas, and beer or other alcoholic mixtures.

Antitussives.   Antitussives are useful in the presence of an irritating, persistent, nonproductive cough. However, productive coughs should not be suppressed, and the logic therefore of an expectorant-antitussive combination is questionable.

A combination of all four classes of drugs in one compound does not allow short-term or occasional use of the sympathomimetic for decongestion, nocturnal use of antihistamines, and separate use of an expectorant or antitussive as indicated by symptoms. Single-entity cold medications, such as Sudafed for decongestion or Vicks Formula 44 for cough suppression, are available to treat specific symptoms. Fluids and rest remain a basic and rational approach to surviving colds.

BIBLIOGRAPHY

Alstead S: Potassium iodide and ipecacuanha as expectorants, Lancet 2:932, 1939.

Brogan TD et al: The effects of bromhexine on sputum from patients with chronic bronchitis and asthma, Br J Dis Chest 68:28, 1974.

Covington TR: OTC cough suppressants/expectorants, Facts and Comparisons Drug Newsletter 10:4, Jan 1991.

Hamilton WFD, Palmer KNV, Gent M: Expectorant action of bromhexine in chronic obstructive bronchitis, Br Med J 3:260, 1970.

Huang T, Peterson GH: Pulmonary edema and iododerma induced by potassium iodide in the treatment of asthma, Ann Allergy 46:264, 1981.

Petty TL: The national mucolytic study. Results of a randomized, double-blind, placebo-controlled study of iodinated glycerol in chronic obstructive bronchitis, Chest 97:75, 1990.

Simons FER, Simons KJ: Second-generation H_1-receptor antagonists, Ann Allergy 66:5, 1991.

Thomson ML et al: Bromhexine and mucociliary clearance in chronic bronchitis, Br J Dis Chest 68:21, 1974.

Woodward JK: Pharmacology of antihistamines, J Allergy Clin Immunol 86:606, 1990.

Ziment I: Expectorants in chronic bronchitis, Respir Care 27:1398, 1982.

Ziment I: Inorganic and organic iodides. In Braga PC, Allegra L, eds: Drugs in bronchial mucology, New York, 1989, Raven Press.

15

Skeletal Muscle Relaxants (Neuromuscular Blocking Agents)

Chapter 15 presents the neuromuscular blocking agents, also termed *muscle relaxants*. The two types of blocking agents are nondepolarizing, exemplified by tubocurarine, and depolarizing, with succinylcholine the only agent in this class. These agents are used to facilitate intubation and surgery, and less frequently for intubation and management of ventilation in intensive care. The following topics are presented:

- History and development
- Use of neuromuscular blocking agents
- Physiology of the neuromuscular junction
- Types of blocking agents
- Use with patients on ventilators

HISTORY AND DEVELOPMENT

The class of drugs known as neuromuscular blocking agents has a long and fascinating history. Some of the most notable events in their development for modern clinical use indicate the wealth of interesting detail available. Curare is a generic name for a variety of closely related agents, almost all of which were originally used by South American Indians as arrow poisons. The paralyzing effect of curare on skeletal muscle ensured food even if the quarry was not killed outright by the arrow itself. Curare become known to Europeans soon after the discovery of the American continents, and late in the sixteenth century, actual samples of native preparations were taken to Europe by explorers.

349

Curare can be extracted from several plants, one of which is *Chondroden-dron tomentosum,* a source of ᴅ-tubocurarine. The structure of ᴅ-tubocurarine was elicited by King and reported in 1935. The semisynthetic derivative of ᴅ-tubocurarine is dimethyl tubocurarine, which is approximately three times as potent as ᴅ-tubocurarine in man.

Griffith and Johnson in 1942 reported the first trial use of curare as a muscle relaxant in general anesthesia.

Further research on curarelike drugs led to the discovery of gallamine, reported in 1949, and to the methonium compounds (hexamethonium, a ganglionic blocker, and decamethonium [Syncurine], a neuromuscular blocker) in 1948 and 1949.

Another neuromuscular blocker with a mode of action different from that of curare, and of great clinical use for surgery today, is succinylcholine (Anectine, Quelicin). It is interesting that this drug was used experimentally as early as 1906, but since research workers used *curarized* animals for testing succinylcholine, the muscle relaxant abilities of succinylcholine were not noticed until nearly 40 years later!

USE OF NEUROMUSCULAR BLOCKING AGENTS

The primary clinical uses of neuromuscular blocking agents are to facilitate endotracheal intubation; for muscle paralysis during surgery, particularly of the abdomen; and to facilitate mechanical ventilation in certain patients.

These agents are usually given intravenously, and their effects are dose related (i.e., a small dose will not necessarily cause total paralysis). In the operating room, they are administered as part of anesthesia induction prior to endotracheal intubation. They are used in the intensive care unit (ICU) for elective intubation and management of mechanical ventilation.

A brief review of the physiology of the myoneural junction is given before the discussion on the neuromuscular blocking agents.

PHYSIOLOGY OF THE NEUROMUSCULAR JUNCTION

One of the branches of the peripheral nervous system, the somatic, or skeletal muscle, controls striated muscle, as opposed to smooth muscle found in bronchioles, myocardium, or arterioles, which are under the influence of the autonomic branch. Examples of skeletal muscle include the biceps, triceps, and diaphragm, and all are responsible for motor functions such as lifting or breathing. In addition, these motor functions are under conscious cerebral control, which is not true of autonomically controlled smooth muscle.

Nerve impulses to stimulate skeletal muscle are carried via large myelinated nerve fibers. The interface of nerve fiber and skeletal muscle is termed the *neuromuscular* or *myoneural junction* (Fig 15–1). Here a single ending of the motor neuron, termed the *sole foot,* which is one branch of the entire neuron's end plate, is seen to invaginate the muscle membrane. Acetylcholine is the neurotransmitter at the neuromuscular junction, analogous to its function at autonomic ganglia and parasympathetic neuroeffector sites. When the nerve impulse reaches the end of the motor neuron, acetylcholine (which has been synthesized and stored in vesicles) is released into the synaptic cleft, contacts receptor sites on the muscle fiber membrane, and within approximately 2 ms diffuses out of the synaptic gutter where it is then inactivated within milliseconds by *cholinesterase* stored around the border of the gutter.

During the short time that acetylcholine is in contact with the muscle fiber membrane, it can cause an *action potential,* which consists of a depolarization and repolarization phase. In the *depolarization* phase, the muscle membrane becomes permeable to sodium ions, and the sodium influx reverses the negative internal and positive external polarity, resulting in a rise in membrane potential. When the critical threshold is reached, a muscle action potential occurs, stimulating and contracting the muscle fiber. In the subsequent *repolarization* phase, the membrane potential returns to its previous level: sodium conductance is blocked once again, and there is a potassium-

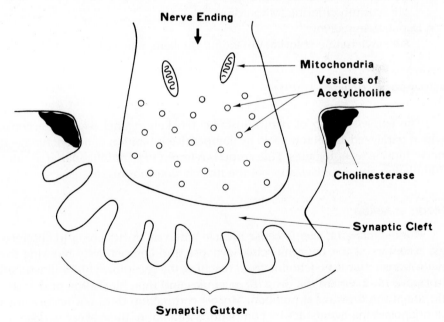

FIG 15–1. Basic description of the neuromuscular junction.

sodium exchange. The muscle fiber can now be restimulated by another nerve impulse.

On the basis of the myoneural function just described, two avenues become apparent for interruption of normal neural stimulation of skeletal muscles:

1. Blockade of the receptor sites usually reached by acetylcholine through competitive inhibition—this is the action of nondepolarizing agents.
2. Stimulation and prolonged depolarization of the postsynaptic receptors—this is the action of depolarizing agents. A list of both types of neuromuscular blocking agents includes the following:

- Nondepolarizing (Competitive) Agents
  Tubocurarine chloride
  Metocurine iodide (Metubine Iodide)
  Gallamine triethiodide (Flaxedil)
  Pancuronium bromide (Pavulon)
  Atracurium besylate (Tracrium)
  Vecuronium bromide (Norcuron)
  Pipecuronium bromide (Arduan)
  Doxacurium chloride (Nuromax)
  Mivacurium chloride (Mivacron)
- Depolarizing Agent
  Succinylcholine chloride (Anectine, Quelicin, Sucostrin)

NONDEPOLARIZING AGENTS

The earliest group of neuromuscular blocking agents were curariform, which paralyzed skeletal muscle by competitive inhibition of acetylcholine at nerve-muscle receptor sites. This group is referred to as nondepolarizing since stimulation and depolarization of the muscle does *not* occur.

Mode of Action

Nondepolarizing agents cause muscle paralysis by attaching to cholinergic receptors at the neuromuscular synapse and competitively blocking the neurotransmitter acetylcholine from reaching the receptor. This is illustrated in Figure 15–2, where the drug *(D)*, occupies and then blocks the postsynaptic site at the myoneural junction. Muscle contraction does not occur. Since nondepolarizing agents act by competitive inhibition, their effect is dose related: larger doses block more receptors. Likewise, this blockade can be re-

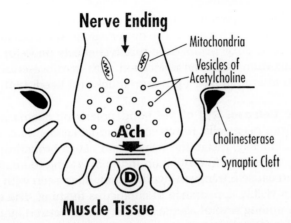

FIG 15–2.   Illustration of competitive blockade by a nondepolarizing drug *(D)* at the nerve-muscle junction. *Ach,* acetylcholine.

versed by making more acetylcholine available to compete for receptor sites.

Nondepolarizing neuromuscular blocking agents are ionized as quaternary ammonium drugs and are poorly absorbed from the gastrointestinal tract. They must be given parenterally, and the intravenous route is preferred for absorption and rapid onset.

Intravenous injection of curare causes reaction within 1 to 2 minutes: haziness of vision, drooping eyelids, relaxation of the jaw, inability to raise the head, paralysis of the legs and arms, and finally loss of respiratory muscles (intercostals, diaphragm) ensues. Maximal paralyzing effect is reached between 2 and 10 minutes. Recovery is in reverse order, with recovery of the diaphragm and respiratory muscles occurring first. In contrast with the depolarizing agent succinylcholine, which is discussed next, the nondepolarizing agents have a relatively long duration of action. In usual doses, the maximal paralyzing action of curare preparations lasts from 35 to 60 minutes, and complete recovery may take several hours. Metocurine, pancuronium, and gallamine have durations of action similar to tubocurarine. Atracurium, vecuronium, and mivacurium are metabolized more rapidly and have shorter durations than tubocurarine. Pipecuronium and doxacurium are both long acting.

Adverse Effects and Hazards

Cardiovascular Effects.   Because the nondepolarizing blocking agents competitively block acetylcholine receptors at autonomic ganglia and the adrenal medulla, they can produce effects on heart rate and blood pressure. Generally, there is a vagolytic effect, which causes tachycardia, and an increase in mean arterial pressure, which may be caused by excess sympathetic activity (Buck and Reed, 1991).

Tubocurarine and pancuronium both cause these cardiovascular effects, and gallamine causes tachycardia. The newer agents, vecuronium, atracurium, pipecuronium, and doxacurium have minimal effects on heart rate or blood pressure. Mivacurium has been associated with cardiovascular changes, including a drop in arterial blood pressure (Buck and Reed, 1991).

Histamine Release.   All of the nondepolarizing agents provoke histamine release from mast cells. However, individual agents differ in the degree of this effect. Clinically, histamine release can cause bronchospasm and increased airway resistance to ventilation in the operating room or the ICU. Vasodilatation can cause a transient hypotension, often seen with these agents. This may give a visible appearance of cutaneous flushing. The degree of histamine release among several agents relative to that caused by pancuronium was quantified by Galletly (1986):

Pancuronium: 1
Tubocurarine: 172
Atracurium: 52
Vecuronium: 1.1

The histamine-releasing property of metocurine seems to be similar to that of pancuronium and vecuronium, both of which have minimal release (Buck and Reed, 1991).

Inadequate Ventilation.   Muscle paralysis of the diaphragm and the intercostal muscles results in total apnea. Adequate airway control and ventilatory support are required until muscle recovery is adequate for spontaneous ventilation. With patients on ventilators in the ICU, close patient and machine monitoring are essential to prevent hypoventilation and hypoxemia.

Reversal of Nondepolarizing Blockade

Muscle paralysis caused by nondepolarizing blocking agents can be reversed by use of cholinesterase inhibitors, or indirect-acting parasympathomimetics (see Chapter 4). This is illustrated in Figure 15–3, which shows neostigmine inhibiting the cholinesterase, which would normally inactivate the body's acetylcholine. This makes more acetylcholine available at the myoneural junction, to compete with the nondepolarizing blocker and reverse the muscle blockade. Cholinesterase inhibitors include physostigmine, neostigmine, pyridostigmine, and edrophonium. Physostigmine is more lipophilic and crosses the blood-brain barrier to reverse central anticholinergic symptoms, but it is less efficient in reversing neuromuscular blockade. Edropho-

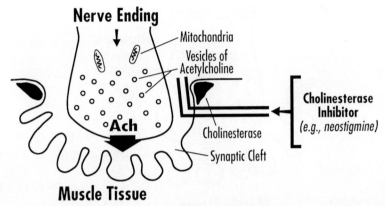

FIG 15–3. Mode of action of cholinesterase inhibitors, such as neostigmine, in reversing neuromuscular blockade caused by nondepolarizing agents. *Ach,* acetylcholine.

nium is quick acting but also is the shortest acting. Pyridostigmine is slower to act and is the longest acting. Neostigmine is intermediate in onset and duration of action.

Recommended doses for these agents are given in the review article of Buck and Reed (1991). Since these agents all produce cholinergic effects at parasympathetic end sites and at the neuromuscular junction, they are given with atropine to offset the muscarinic effect. The atropine will prevent possible bradycardia, increased salivation, and hyperperistalsis that would result from parasympathetic activity. The atropine does not block the reversing effect of the cholinergic drug at the neuromuscular junction, only the muscarinic effects at parasympathetic sites.

DEPOLARIZING AGENT

The depolarizing agent has a mode of action different from the curare group, are much shorter acting, and have no antidote for reversing blockade. The only currently used depolarizing agent is succinylcholine. With a usual dose of 1 to 1.5 mg/kg given intravenously, muscle paralysis occurs in 1 to 1.5 minutes and lasts from 10 to 15 minutes.

Mode of Action

The basic action of the depolarizing neuromuscular blocker is first to depolarize the postsynaptic muscle membrane in the same manner as acetylcholine, then to maintain it in a refractory state. This is illustrated in Figure 15–4, where the drug *(D)* attaches to and depolarizes the postsynaptic mem-

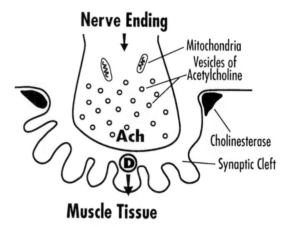

Nerve Ending

Mitochondria

Vesicles of Acetylcholine

Ach

Cholinesterase

Synaptic Cleft

Muscle Tissue

FIG 15–4. Illustration of the mode of action of the depolarizing agent succinylcholine *(D)* in causing neuromuscular blockade. *Ach,* acetylcholine.

brane. Further stimulation and contraction of the muscle fiber is not possible until the drug is metabolized. *Unlike* curare, there is an initial muscle contraction, referred to as *fasciculation,* a classic sign of the depolarizing agent succinylcholine (Anectine, Quelicin). This is followed by flaccid paralysis. With the depolarizing blocking agent, there is successive stimulation of vagal ganglia, which causes a fall in blood pressure and bradycardia, and then sympathetic ganglia, which in turn leads to transient hypertension and tachycardia. Succinylcholine produces histamine release, such as that seen with curare.

Normally, plasma cholinesterase will metabolize succinylcholine (a choline ester) within a few minutes. Generally, the depolarizing blocker is shorter acting than curare and its analogues.

Reversal

There are no effective antidotes to the depolarizing agent. Use of cholinesterase inhibitors (parasympathomimetics) here will result in even more prolonged depolarization, since the neuromuscular synapse is already being held in a depolarized state, and further stimulation will simply continue to cause depolarization, with no resumption of muscle activity.

Use of Hexafluorenium

Hexafluorenium bromide is a plasma cholinesterase inhibitor. As just described for such agents, this drug will not reverse blockade from succinylcholine but will in fact prolong the blockade.

Hexafluorenium (Mylaxen) is used as an adjunct with succinylcholine to prolong neuromuscular blockade during anesthesia, and to reduce the muscle fasciculation seen with succinylcholine. Its activity is limited to plasma esterases, and it does not act on intracellular cholinesterase. There is no effect on consciousness or pain awareness. Duration of action is approximately 20 to 30 minutes.

Adverse Effects and Hazards

Succinylcholine can cause a number of side effects, some of which would be of concern more with ICU patients on ventilators than with routine use in the operating room. Effects with both depolarizing and nondepolarizing agents have been summarized in a review of their use in the ICU by Isenstein and associates (1992).

Muscle Soreness. Muscle soreness can be caused presumably by the muscle fasciculation that accompanies the administration of succinylcholine. Some anesthesiologists use a prior dose of a nondepolarizing blocker to prevent this effect. Higher doses of succinylcholine may be needed for paralysis if this is done.

Serum Potassium Elevation. Succinylcholine can cause an efflux of potassium from cells, transiently raising the serum potassium level by 0.5 to 1.0 mEq/L (Buck and Reed, 1991). Muscle fasciculation can also cause a rise in serum potassium and creatinine phosphokinase levels. The resultant hyperkalemia can cause risk of cardiac arrhythmias or arrest. Hyperkalemia is also a risk in burn patients. Patients with spinal cord injuries, particularly upper motor lesions, are at risk for cardiac arrest or fibrillation.

Increased Intraocular Pressure. Succinylcholine can increase intraocular pressure, probably mediated by contractions of the extraocular muscles.

Increased Intracranial Pressure. Succinylcholine can also increase intracranial pressure, which is a risk in patients with cerebral edema and head trauma.

Malignant Hyperthermia. Succinylcholine can cause a hypermetabolic state, resulting in malignant hyperthermia, collapse, and death.

Sensitivity to Succinylcholine

There are two types of cholinesterase in the body: "true" or acetylcholinesterase found at parasympathetic nerve synapses and postsynaptic neuromuscular sites; and "pseudo-" or butyrylcholinesterase found in plasma.

The pseudocholinesterase in the plasma has no known metabolic function but it does catalyze the hydrolysis of succinylcholine; that is, it metabolizes succinylcholine (a choline ester) to an inactive form. A certain number of individuals have an atypical plasma cholinesterase of a different molecular species from the normal, an inherited abnormality.

As a result, such individuals will not rapidly hydrolyze the depolarizing neuromuscular blocker within minutes as usual, but will require hours of supported ventilation due to the prolonged paralysis of the respiratory muscles. Laboratory tests are available to determine atypical cholinesterases. One of these tests is based on a differential inhibition of the atypical and usual cholinesterase by the local anesthetic dibucaine. At a certain optimum concentration, dibucaine produces a much greater inhibition of the usual plasma cholinesterase than of the atypical enzyme. The percentage of inhibition of the cholinesterase enzyme by dibucaine is called the *dibucaine number*. The normal or usual cholinesterase has a number over 70, while the atypical cholinesterase gives a value below 30, at a specific concentration of dibucaine. Heterozygote individuals give values between 45 and 69, which distinguishes them from the normal and atypical homozygotes. Lehmann and Liddell (1969) give a clear discussion of the genetic variation of human cholinesterase and its detection.

Desensitization (Phase II) Block

In certain patients, a prolonged duration of action (1 to 4 hours instead of 2 to 4 minutes) occurs with succinylcholine that is *not* associated with inadequate plasma cholinesterase. In such cases, it has been theorized that a nondepolarizing block (phase II or dual block) follows the depolarizing block, possibly due to the first metabolic product of succinylcholine, which is succinylmonocholine. This may be seen with time and increasing dosages of succinylcholine. If this is the case, then a cholinesterase inhibitor should help reverse this secondary block and may further explain why such parasympathomimetics as neostigmine are occasionally helpful in reversing or antagonizing a prolonged depolarizing neuromuscular blockade. The occurrence of such a desensitization block must be considered as a possibility in the face of prolonged apnea with succinylcholine.

USE WITH PATIENTS ON VENTILATORS

The use of any agents that depress spontaneous ventilation must be used with caution or not at all in patients who have chronic or acute forms of ventilatory failure. These agents include sedatives, analgesics, and the neuromuscular blocking agents. In patients committed to mechanical ventilatory support, however, sedatives (lorazepam, diazepam, barbiturates) and analgesics (morphine) can be helpful for relaxation and pain.

The indication for use of neuromuscular blocking agents in ventilator management is to remove asynchronous spontaneous breathing efforts that "fight" the ventilator breaths and cause increasing intrathoracic pressure, decreased alveolar ventilation, and increased patient work. The desired goal with these drugs is improved ventilation and oxygenation and reduced ventilating pressures.

The most common uses clinically when muscle relaxation becomes necessary are ventilation in status asthmaticus and pressure control ventilation, especially with reversed inspiratory:expiratory ratios.

Precautions

Before subjecting a patient to neuromuscular blockade, ventilator malfunction must first be ruled out as the cause of patient agitation, otherwise muscle paralysis could cause death in the face of inadequate machine volume or oxygen delivery.

Paralysis of eyelid muscles can cause drying and abrasion of cornea and conjunctiva unless the eyelids are closed and lubrication is used.

Choice of Agents

The choice of a neuromuscular blocking agent is situation dependent: the depolarizing agent succinylcholine is well suited for intubation because of its rapid and short action. The nondepolarizing type of blocking agent is more suited for long-term ventilator use than is the depolarizing type. The kinetics of the nondepolarizing agents give a longer duration of action, needed for maintenance paralysis, and the blockade can be reversed with cholinesterase inhibitors such as neostigmine. The exact choice of agent involves clinical judgment and preference, but the following features of the different nondepolarizing agents offer a guide to selection for ventilator use.

Buck and Reed (1991) provide an excellent review of neuromuscular blocking agents for use with mechanical ventilation. As their review points out, most experience with these agents is in the operating room. Duration of effect and recovery may not be the same when these drugs are used for prolonged times with patients on ventilators. Hansen-Flaschen and associates (1991) reported that most physicians use pancuronium or vecuronium. Atracurium is not often used for paralysis of patients on ventilators. Pancuronium and vecuronium have advantages among other nondepolarizing agents for ventilator use. These two agents are intermediate acting compared with tubocurarine but longer acting than atracurium. They have the least amount of histamine release compared with that of the other nondepolarizing agents. Vecuronium has less effect than pancuronium on heart rate and blood pressure. Pipecuronium and doxacurium may offer alternative choices for use with patients on ventilators, because they are relatively long acting and have minimal cardiovascular effects.

The preferred route of administration is intravenous for rapid and complete onset and for dose adjustment to control paralysis. Pancuronium and vecuronium have recovery times of 10 to 30 minutes and are given either every 1 to 3 hours or by continuous infusion (Buck and Reed, 1991).

Interaction with Antibiotics

It should be noted that both nondepolarizing and depolarizing agents interact with certain antibiotic groups. Specifically, the following antibiotics can cause neuromuscular blockade as a side effect: the aminoglycosides (e.g., gentamicin), the tetracycline group, the polymyxins, clindamycin, and lincomycin. The dosage of a neuromuscular blocking agent may need to be reduced, or reversal of prolonged paralysis may be needed. With ventilator-dependent patients in critical care, including asthmatic patients, there is a likelihood of concomitant treatment with these antibiotics.

Use of Sedatives and Analgesics

While the neuromuscular blocking agents can cause muscle paralysis, they do not affect consciousness or the perception of pain. The classic experiment that established this was performed by the anesthesiologist Smith who in 1947 allowed himself to be paralyzed with tubocurarine. He reported full awareness during the paralysis, including sensations of choking while he was unable to swallow and shortness of breath even though he was being ventilated (Smith et al., 1947).

It is absolutely essential to provide sedation and analgesia for ventilator-dependent patients undergoing paralysis. Motor symptoms of pain, such as restlessness and moving about, are suppressed, removing such clues to pain from the clinician's perception. The experience of paralysis would also seem to be anxiety producing in the extreme, thus warranting sedation. In their survey, Hansen-Flaschen and others (1991) reported that the most commonly used drugs for sedation of patients on mechanical ventilation were morphine sulfate, lorazepam, and diazepam, in that order. The method of administration was intermittent intravenous injection. The drugs most commonly given for sedation by continuous intravenous infusion were midazolam hydrochloride (Versed), fentanyl citrate, and morphine. That survey also noted that diazepam is converted to metabolites that are slow to clear in the critically ill. Lorazepam would be a better sedating agent, although diazepam is cheaper and more familiar. Sedatives are also better given by intravenous injection, than by intramuscular or subcutaneous routes. Absorption and distribution are more erratic with intramuscular or subcutaneous injection, particularly in ICU patients, and such injections are unnecessarily painful to the patient. An intravenous line is almost invariably available, which removes the need for intramuscular or subcutaneous administration.

BIBLIOGRAPHY

Buck ML, Reed MD: Use of nondepolarizing neuromuscular blocking agents in mechanically ventilated patients, Clin Pharm 10:32, 1991.

Comer PB: The use of muscle relaxants in respiratory failure: a review of pharmacology, Respir Ther 7(3):31, 1977.

Foldes FF: The pharmacology of neuromuscular blocking agents in man, Clin Pharmacol Ther 1:345, 1960.

Froese AB, Bryan AC: Effects of anesthesia and paralysis on diaphragmatic mechanics in man, Anesthesiology 41:242, 1974.

Galletly DC: Comparative cutaneous histamine release by neuromuscular blocking agents, Anesth Intensive Care 14:365–369, 1986.

Griffith HR, Johnson GE: The use of curare in general anesthesia, Anesthesiology 3:418, 1942.

Hansen-Flaschen JH et al: Use of sedating drugs and neuromuscular blocking agents in patients requiring mechanical ventilation for respiratory failure. A national survey, JAMA 266:2870, 1991.

Hunt R, Taveau RM: On the physiological action of certain choline derivatives and new methods for detecting choline, Br Med J 2:1788, 1906.

Isenstein DA, Venner DS, Duggan J: Neuromuscular blockade in the intensive care unit, Chest 102:1258, 1992.

Kalow W, Genest K: A method for the detection of atypical forms of human serum cholinesterase. Determination of dibucaine numbers. Can J Biochem Physiol 35:339, 1957.

Katz RL: Clinical neuromuscular pharmacology of pancuronium, Anesthesiology 34:550, 1971.

King H: Curare alkaloids. I. Tubocurarine, J Chem Soc p 1381, 1935.

Lehmann H, Liddell J: Human cholinesterase (pseudocholinesterase): genetic variants and their recognition, Br J Anesth 41:235, 1969.

McIntyre AR: Curare: its history, nature, and clinical use, Chicago, 1947, University of Chicago Press.

Rumble L et al: Observations during apnea in conscious human subjects, Anesthesiology 18:419, 1957.

Smith SM et al: The lack of cerebral effects of D-tubocurarine, Anesthesiology 8:1, 1947.

Taylor DB, Nedergaard OA: Relation between structure and action of quaternary ammonium neuromuscular blocking agents, Physiol Rev 45:523, 1965.

16

Drugs Affecting the Central Nervous System

Joseph L. Rau, Ph.D., RRT, and John M. Holbrook, Ph.D.

Chapter 16 provides a survey of drugs affecting the central nervous system (CNS). The following topics are discussed:

- Function of the CNS
- Sedative-hypnotic agents
- General anesthetics
- Psychotherapeutic agents
- Narcotic and nonnarcotic analgesics
- Ventilatory stimulants

The drugs in the sedative-hypnotic group, the general anesthetics, many of the psychotherapeutic agents, and the analgesics are all CNS depressants. As such, they are capable of depressing the central respiratory centers of the medulla, thus decreasing the normal response to elevated CO_2 levels. This can produce hypoventilation or even apnea. An overdose of drugs in these categories is common in suicide attempts and necessitates ventilatory support and airway maintenance. Use of these drugs in patients on mechanical ventilation can depress the spontaneous level of ventilation, requiring changes in the level of ventilatory support or caution in weaning. The antidepressant drugs do not produce the same CNS depression, although certain agents can cause sedation or drowsiness.

In contrast to the CNS depressants, the CNS stimulants can cause ventilatory stimulation, and in fact certain agents are used as respiratory stimulants, for example, doxapram.

Before discussion of the individual groups of agents affecting the CNS, a brief, functional overview of the CNS itself is presented.

CENTRAL NERVOUS SYSTEM

The CNS is functionally divided into two components: the brain and spinal cord. The spinal cord consists of nerve fibers that transport information toward the brain and instructions from the brain to all body areas.

Organization of the Brain

The brain, which is responsible for all conscious and subconscious functions of the body, is subdivided into three areas: cortex, midbrain, and brainstem. Figure 16–1 provides a sketch of these structures.

Cortex

The cortex is a thin layer of cells that covers the entire cerebral hemispheres and is responsible for the integration of all body functions. The cortex is subdivided into specific areas that are responsible for functions such as skeletal muscle control, interpretation of sensations (heat, cold, touch, pressure, and pain), vision, hearing, speech, intellect, and memory. When cortical activity is depressed by drugs, the symptoms produced include sedation, ataxia, slurred speech, decreased mental functioning, and slowed reflexes.

Midbrain

The midbrain contains two major structures: the thalamus and the hypothalamus. The thalamus serves as a relay system for information traveling from

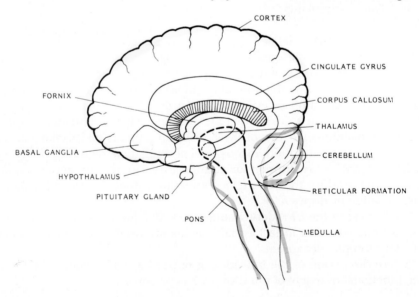

FIG 16–1. Major areas of the brain affected by CNS depressants and stimulants.

one brain area to another and from peripheral sites to the cortex. When the thalamus is depressed, the flow of specific stimuli to the cortex is decreased. For example, at least part of the activity of narcotic analgesics is related to their ability to interrupt transmission of sensory (pain) impulses between the thalamus and cortex. The hypothalamus is responsible for integration of functions of the autonomic nervous system, control of endocrine gland function, control of appetite, plasma glucose levels, and other related functions. When the hypothalamus is depressed, endocrine gland function is suppressed and vasomotor reflexes that are mediated via the autonomic nervous system are slowed, resulting in hypotension.

Medulla

The primary structure of the brainstem is the medulla. The medulla is responsible for maintaining blood pressure and ventilation and also contains the chemoreceptor trigger zone (CTZ), which is responsible for emesis. Depression of the medulla may result in death attributable to depression of the respiratory centers and/or collapse of the cardiovascular system.

Reticular Activating System

Scattered throughout the upper level of the spinal cord, the brainstem, and midbrain structures are nuclei that are collectively termed the *reticular formation*. A portion of the reticular formation, the reticular activating system (RAS), is located in the midbrain and performs two major functions: (1) stimulation of the cortex to maintain a state of wakefulness and (2) filtering of extraneous sensory information, which enhances the ability to concentrate. Examples of this function of the RAS include being able to sleep with a clock chiming on the quarter-hour or lack of conscious awareness of the pressure of a chair on one's legs and posterior. However, if a picture falls or a cat knocks over an object, such unexpected, new noises can immediately arouse a person to wakefulness. They are not filtered out; there is no adaptation to the stimulus. In its screening function, the reticular formation prevents sensory overload and allows conscious attention to less familiar stimuli. The noise of the clock chiming will not wake a person accustomed to it. The activating system "recognizes" the clock chime. However, a new noise *will* penetrate the higher areas of the brain and not be screened. Sleep, and the deeper state of anesthesia, can be caused by depressing the arousal mechanisms of the reticular formation to the point that stimuli do not cause excitation and arousal from unconsciousness.

Drug-induced depression of the RAS results in a decreased response to external stimuli (sedation), and if depression is sufficient, the result is hypnosis (sleep).

The RAS also serves as the mediator for the neurogenic drive state, which functions to regulate ventilation in response to variations in emotional states and activity levels. Thus, when the individual is asleep and stimulation of the RAS is minimal, the respiratory rate is lowered.

Limbic System

The limbic system consists of several associated structures and fiber tracts that are involved with the control and display of emotion. The basic limbic system structures form a ring around the brain stem and will not be named individually. Other structures associated with these limbic structures include the thalamus, frontal cortex, and hypothalamus. The anterior nucleus of the thalamus appears to be the relay nucleus for emotional activity. The frontal cortex is associated with aggressive or hostile behaviors, and the hypothalamus is involved with the display of emotion via the autonomic nervous system. Abnormality of limbic system function leads to disorders of emotion such as schizophrenia, depression, and mania. Drugs such as atropine, amphetamine, and steroids in large doses may adversely affect limbic system function to produce a state resembling a psychosis.

Extrapyramidal System

The brain also contains structures that are collectively termed the extrapyramidal system. These structures are responsible for the control of coordinated, fine muscle movement. Included in the extrapyramidal system are the cerebellum, which is responsible for balance, and the basal ganglia, which takes the information provided by the cerebellum and vestibular structures and uses this information to modify skeletal muscle movement. Many drugs that are used in the treatment of mental disorders such as the neuroleptics and antidepressants adversely affect extrapyramidal system function, which results in symptoms such as tremors and muscle rigidity.

CNS Drugs and Sleep States

Drugs that affect the function of the CNS do so in a dose-related fashion and usually in a descending manner from the cortex down to the brain stem and even into the spinal cord. Thus, small doses of a nonspecific CNS depressant affect only the cortex, producing sedation and ataxia. Larger doses initially depress the cortex, then depress the RAS to induce sleep. Very large doses may depress the medulla to produce a decrease in the function of the respiratory and cardiovascular reflex centers, which may lead to death. These same drugs may also alter normal sleep patterns, which are essential for appropriate mental and physical functioning.

Periods of sleep are required by man to allow the body to recuperate from both mental and physical activities. The time spent in sleep is divided into two states, which are categorized by measurement of electroencephalographic (EEG) brain patterns. These states are termed *slow wave sleep* and *rapid eye movement* (REM) sleep. REM sleep is characterized by desynchronous EEG patterns and by rapid, darting movements of the eyes. Dreaming occurs during REM sleep, and it is currently believed that REM sleep is required for normal emotional functioning.

Slow wave sleep is characterized by synchronized EEG patterns and is divided into four stages, corresponding to depth of sleep. Slow wave sleep is necessary to overcome physical fatigue.

During an individual's normal sleep period, a certain portion of the time is devoted to REM sleep (usually 25%) and the remainder is devoted to slow-wave sleep, with the slow wave sleep stages alternating with REM sleep. If a person is deprived of sleep for some reason, at the next normal sleep period, more than the usual amount of time will be spent in REM sleep. This is termed *REM sleep rebound* and emphasizes the importance of this type of sleep, because the body makes up for any lost REM sleep as rapidly as possible.

A number of the drugs discussed in this chapter have the ability to decrease REM sleep and thus have the potential for altering normal emotional functioning. Among these drugs are the sedative-hypnotics, neuroleptics, and antidepressants. Even though these agents all have the ability to produce sleep, the sleep is not entirely normal because the portion of sleep time devoted to REM sleep is reduced. When such drugs are discontinued, REM sleep rebound occurs and sleep patterns revert back to normal.

The benzodiazepine antianxiety agents also depress REM sleep but not to as great an extent as the previously mentioned drugs.

SEDATIVES AND HYPNOTICS

The sedative-hypnotic category is a broad grouping that includes barbiturate and nonbarbiturate CNS depressants. These agents are used for conscious sedation to relieve anxiety and as sleeping aids. The terms *sedative* and *hypnotic* can be thought of as differing in degree of relaxation and drowsiness produced. Hypnotic essentially refers to the ability of a drug to induce sleep, whereas sedation need not cause actual sleep but only relaxation. Other, more archaic terms for hypnotics are somnifacient and soporific. The minor tranquilizers, such as diazepam (Valium), can also induce sleep, but they are more often used for their sedative effect in the treatment of neuroses or anxiety states. Whether a given drug causes sedation or sleep (hypnosis) is dose dependent. The spectrum of activity ranges from mild sedation, through hypnosis (sleep), to full anesthesia (loss of reflexes, coma).

Barbiturates

Barbiturates are powerful hypnotics and are considered derivatives of barbituric acid. An interesting, although perhaps apocryphal, story persists describing the naming of barbituric acid, the chemical precursor of the barbiturate drugs. Barbituric acid results from the combination of urea and malonic acid and was first prepared by Adolph von Baeyer in 1864. At the time, von Baeyer was a research assistant to Kekulé, who is famous for his dream-inspired discovery of the cyclic carbon structures. Reputedly, von Baeyer celebrated his new discovery at a local tavern that catered to artillery officers, on the feast day of St. Barbara, the patron saint of artillery officers. Supposedly, in the subsequent rounds, Barbara came to be linked with urea, to produce barbituric, and the compound was so named.

The original barbiturate was barbital (Veronal), which was introduced to medical use in 1903 by Fischer and von Mering. Phenobarbital was introduced next in 1912 as Luminal and is the second oldest barbiturate. Of some 2500 barbiturates synthesized, approximately 50 have been marketed for general use, and currently around a dozen are in wide use.

Structure-Activity Relations, Metabolism, and Duration of Action

The structural formula of barbituric acid is given in Figure 16–2. Since the various barbiturates are theoretically derived from modifications to the structure of barbituric acid, a general formula for barbiturates can be constructed, with the selected sites of modification indicated by R_1, R_2, R_3, and X. By adding different substituents at these sites, different barbiturates can be produced. This is illustrated in Figure 16–2 for barbital and phenobarbital. For example, by substituting two ethyl groups for the hydrogens at R_1 and R_2, barbituric acid becomes diethylbarbituric acid, more commonly known as barbital. Other substitutions produce phenobarbital. General pharmacology texts offer tables indicating the substitutions required for all of the commonly used barbiturates, thus eliminating the need to reproduce drawings of each structural formula. The hypnotic activity of a barbiturate requires an alkyl or aryl group substitution at R_1 and R_2 on the carbon-5 position. The ethyl groups (C_2H_5) attached to the carbon-5 position in barbital exemplify an alkyl substitution, and barbital possesses strong hypnotic properties. If the oxygen at the carbon-2 position is replaced with a sulfur, thiobarbiturates are obtained. An example of a thiobarbiturate is thiopental (Pentothal), commonly used in the induction of general anesthesia.

The duration of action of a barbiturate is related to the rate of metabolism of the drug. Most barbiturates are metabolized in the liver, and the rate of metabolism depends on the ease with which their side chains can be oxidized. Generally, these agents are classified as long, intermediate, or short acting. Examples, with representative trade names, include the following:

- Long Acting (10 to 12 hours)
  Phenobarbital sodium (Luminal Sodium)
  Mephobarbital (Mebaral)
  Metharbital (Gemonil)

- Intermediate Acting (6 to 8 hours)
    Amobarbital (Amytal)
    Aprobarbital (Alurate)
    Butabarbital (Butisol)
    Talbutal (Lotusate)
- Short Acting (3 to 4 hours)
    Secobarbital (Seconal)
    Pentobarbital (Nembutal)

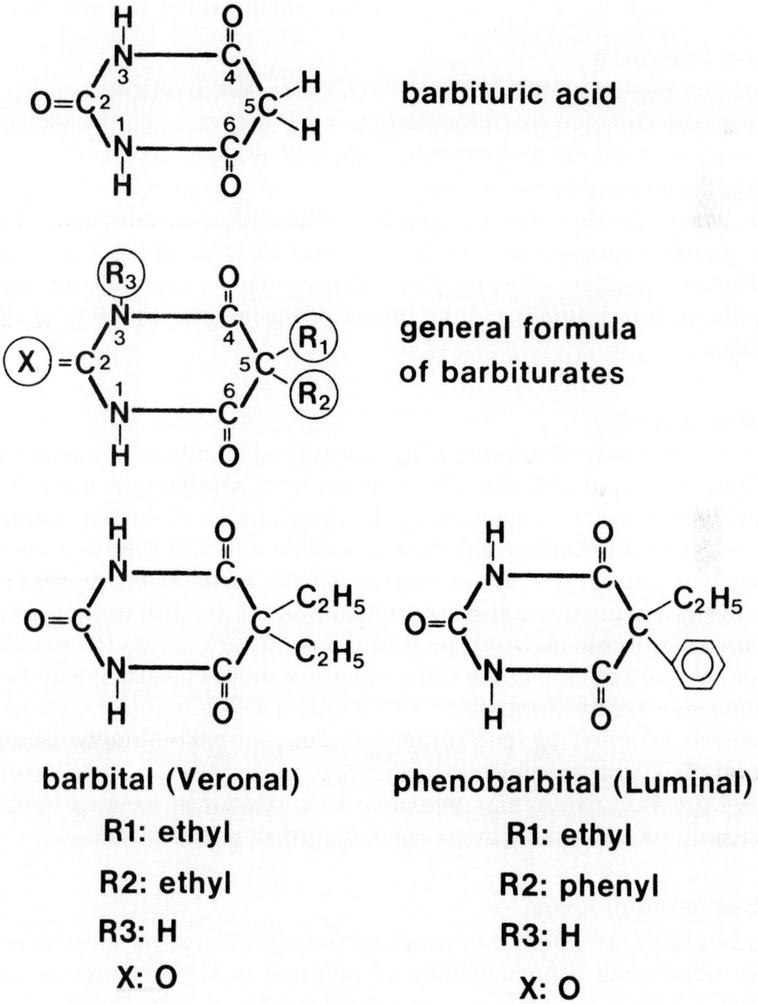

barbituric acid

general formula
of barbiturates

barbital (Veronal)

R1: ethyl

R2: ethyl

R3: H

X: O

phenobarbital (Luminal)

R1: ethyl

R2: phenyl

R3: H

X: O

FIG 16–2. General structure of barbiturates that are derived from barbituric acid by different attachments at the circled sites.

The plasma half-life of phenobarbital in man is greater than 20 hours, whereas thiopental has a plasma half-life of somewhat greater than 3 hours. The desired clinical effect, such as anesthesia with thiopental, can have a duration much shorter than the plasma half-life. The half-life simply indicates the rate of breakdown for the given barbiturate; the slower the rate, the longer will be the duration of clinical effects.

The metabolism and renal excretion of barbiturates are the basis for two of the clinically practical aspects of such drugs. The first is drug tolerance seen with repeated use, and the second is improved renal elimination of the drug by changing urine pH.

Drug Tolerance

Barbiturates are metabolized by microsomal enzymes in the liver. Repeated use or abuse of the drug leads to enzyme induction, or activation of the enzyme systems, as the body attempts to deal with increased amounts of the chemical presented to the liver. A vicious circle ensues in which increasing amounts of the drug are required to produce the desired effect, but which in turn causes increased enzyme activity, and so forth. There is also adaptation of nervous system receptors (pharmacodynamic tolerance) to the drug, so that tolerant individuals require higher doses for the induction of sleep or anesthesia.

Renal Excretion

In Chapter 1 the diffusion of drugs across cell membranes was discussed, and it was seen that diffusion depends on lipid solubility in the cell membrane, which in turn is influenced by the drug's pKa and degree of ionization in the ambient pH. Nonionized drug *is* soluble and will diffuse across cells; ionized drug will not dissolve or diffuse as well. Barbiturates are weak acids, which means they are less ionized in acidic urine (relative to their pKa) and more ionized in basic urine. To prevent diffusion back across the tubules and consequent reabsorption of the drug, the urine should be alkaline. If the urine is alkaline, more of the drug dissociates (ionizes), less is reabsorbed, and therefore more is excreted. In barbiturate overdose, intentional or accidental, reversal of effects can be improved with increased clearance and excretion of the drug, possibly shortening the time required for supported ventilation. There would be a disadvantage to allowing pH to become acidic.

Mechanism of Action

Barbiturates are thought to produce sedation, sleep, or anesthesia by reversibly depressing the excitability of neurons in the RAS, previously discussed.

The general view of barbiturate action is that barbiturates can reversibly depress excitable membranes, particularly those at nerve synapses. It is believed that the drugs interfere with chemical transmission across neuronal and neuroeffector junctions. While the CNS, especially the reticular formation and medulla, is sensitive to normal sedative doses of barbiturates, *sympathetic ganglia* can also be selectively depressed, accounting partly for the fall in blood pressure seen with concentrations of the drug used for anesthesia. With overdose and acute barbiturate intoxication, there will be impaired cardiac and circulatory function, presenting a typical shock syndrome. Because of the general mechanism of depressing excitable membranes in the nervous system, there are several clinical effects, or side effects, with barbiturates that are relevant to respiratory care. These include the following:

- Depression of respiratory drive
- Loss of blood pressure
- Potentiation of neuromuscular blocking agents
- Lack of analgesia

Although the last effect is really a lack of effect, it is important to realize that sedation is *not* the same as analgesia. In fact, in small doses, barbiturates may *increase* the response to pain (hyperalgesia) and may not be effective sedatives or hypnotics in the presence of pain. This is particularly helpful to realize when ventilator-dependent patients are sedated: If anxiety or restlessness is due to pain, then an analgesic would be more effective than a sedative, because the analgesic will provide relief from pain, as well as sedation.

The most important effect of barbiturates for respiratory care is the possible *loss of respiratory drive*. Barbiturates can depress the medullary respiratory centers and the reticular formation. As the dose of the drug increases, the medullary respiratory centers become increasingly unresponsive to carbon dioxide, the central respiratory stimulant in the normal nervous system. If intoxication increases, respiratory stimulation shifts to the more primitive peripheral receptor sites, the carotid and aortic bodies. Ultimately, hypoxic drive takes over as the last respiratory stimulant in barbiturate overdose. Since administration of oxygen will remove the hypoxic stimulus, supplemental oxygen *without supported ventilation* can hasten respiratory arrest in barbiturate overdose.

Barbiturates also depress the vasomotor centers of the medulla, which regulate blood pressure, and in addition produce sympathetic ganglionic blockade and direct depression of the myocardium. These effects all combine to cause a *fall in blood pressure* that is dose dependent. Because overdose can produce a shock syndrome of cardiovascular collapse, mean airway pressures during mechanical ventilation of such patients should be minimized.

In general, blood pressure and heart rate should be monitored during positive pressure ventilation for possible deterioration because of this effect of barbiturates.

Barbiturates can also *enhance the neuromuscular blocking effect* of nondepolarizing and depolarizing drugs. The same mechanism of depressing excitable membranes can act to reduce the sensitivity of the postsynaptic membrane at the skeletal neuromuscular junction. As a result, the postsynaptic membrane at the neuromuscular junction is less responsive to the depolarizing effect of acetylcholine, the neurotransmitter. A nondepolarizing block, for example by using curare, would therefore be prolonged and intensified because of the inhibited neuromuscular transmission. With a depolarizing agent such as decamethonium, the effect of acetylcholine is blocked at the same time the postsynaptic membrane is held in a refractory state, producing what seems to be a dual block. Both D-tubocurarine and decamethonium are potentiated by barbiturates.

Clinical Uses of Barbiturates

Barbiturates are used therapeutically to produce sedation, sleep, and anesthesia and for their anticonvulsant activity. Whether sedation, sleep, or anesthesia is produced is a function of drug dosage, with higher doses causing greater depression of the CNS.

Some barbiturates have been used to control convulsions, whether epileptic, electroconvulsions, or due to tetanus or analeptic drugs (see the section on respiratory stimulants in this chapter). The drugs act to prevent seizures by depressing brain activity. Phenobarbital is a good example of a barbiturate with specific anticonvulsant effects that are not related to its sedative actions. To have such an effect, a phenyl group at the carbon-5 or nitrogen site seems to be required (Fig 16–2). Both phenobarbital and mephobarbital have this group and have anticonvulsant activity. Phenobarbital is commonly used clinically for this effect.

Barbiturate Intoxication

An overdose of barbiturates may occur as an intentional suicide effort, or accidentally through a phenomenon known as *automatism*. This consists of taking the drug in the prescribed dose, but as drowsiness increases, additional doses are taken because the earlier dose has been forgotten.

The appearance of mild barbiturate intoxication is similar to alcoholic inebriation: slurred speech, disorientation, and "drunken" movements (cortical effects). With severe intoxication, there is respiratory depression, which causes respiratory acidosis and hypoxemia, loss of reflexes (coma), low blood pressure, cold and clammy skin, and ultimately dilated pupils, probably due to hypoxia. The general picture in severe cases of overdose is shock syndrome. Pupils may show constriction and reaction to light early in intoxication, with progression to a dilated appearance. The accurate differential diagnosis of a suspected barbiturate overdose is made by analysis of body fluids for presence of the barbiturate.

Treatment of barbiturate overdose after the diagnosis is made consists of the following general measures:

Ventilatory support
Circulatory support
Drug elimination
Prevention of dehydration, infection, and other complications

Ventilatory support is, as usual, indicated and modified as dictated by arterial blood gas values, clinical appearance (color, sensorium, responses), and other data such as vital signs, laboratory values, and chest radiographic findings. Endotracheal intubation will prevent pulmonary aspiration of stomach contents. If aspiration has already occurred, a respiratory distress syndrome may further complicate treatment and require positive end-expiratory pressure (PEEP), corticosteroids, and possible bronchoscopy. Generally, with acute overdose, airway pressures should be minimized to avoid impeded venous return superimposed on the drug-induced cardiovascular depression. Systemic acidosis should be avoided, to minimize reabsorption of this drug in the renal tubules (see the previous section on renal excretion). Renal function should be monitored with a creatinine clearance test to avoid renal failure, particularly if circulatory collapse occurs. Hemodialysis is an effective method of removing the drug, especially if long-acting agents have been taken. Emesis or gastric lavage will not be helpful in removing the drug if more than several hours have passed since ingestion. Circulation must be maintained with adequate fluid replacement and pharmacological agents if necessary. Avoidance of acidotic states also favors response of the circulation to vasopressor drugs, in addition to improved renal excretion of the barbiturate. Analeptics (respiratory stimulants) are not considered well advised in treating respiratory depression, because they are of relatively short duration and have toxic side effects. They may be used, however, in emergency situations when appropriate ventilatory equipment is not available.

Nonbarbiturate Sedatives and Hypnotics

The barbiturate sedative-hypnotics have a number of disadvantages, including the occurrence of physical dependence, abuse ("downers"), and a relatively low therapeutic index (median lethal dose/median effective dose ratio). A number of drugs have been developed to provide a sedative-hypnotic effect, as alternatives to the barbiturate class. Unfortunately, most of the nonbarbiturate sedatives share the drawbacks of the barbiturates with respect to respiratory depression, as well as the potential for dependence. They are generally nonselective CNS depressants. Examples of hypnotics include the following:

Zolpidem tartrate (Ambien)
Paraldehyde (Paral)
Chloral hydrate (Noctec)
Acetylcarbromal (Paxarel)
Glutethimide (Doriden)
Methyprylon (Noludar)
Ethchlorvynol (Placidyl)
Ethinamate (Valmid)
Propiomazine HCl (Largon)
Benzodiazepines
    Estazolam (ProSom)
    Flurazepam HCl (Dalmane)
    Temazepam (Restoril)
    Triazolam (Halcion)
    Quazepam (Doral)

These and several drugs not listed above, such as alcohol, are briefly characterized in the following sections.

Paraldehyde

Paraldehyde is primarily used as a preparation to cause sleep and is a safe drug for such use. There is little cardiac depression, and only large doses would cause respiratory depression. As a result, the drug has been useful as a sleeping agent with alcoholic patients, even during withdrawal phases. Unfortunately for the recipient, paraldehyde has a strong, distinctive odor and a very unpleasant taste. Given as a liquid, it is usually diluted with water to reduce irritation to the gastrointestinal tract. Although paraldehyde is an old drug, having been used therapeutically since 1882, surprisingly little is known concerning its pharmacological activity.

Chloral Hydrate

Chloral hydrate is another sleep-inducing preparation, and like paraldehyde, is an older drug predating the barbiturates as a hypnotic. In fact, chloral hydrate was the first and oldest member of the hypnotic group; its use dates back to 1869. As with the barbiturates, the drug is capable of causing a fall in blood pressure but probably not more so than that caused by equivalent doses of other powerful hypnotics. The drug has a disagreeable taste when given in liquid form. Its primary advantage is that, unlike most other sedative-hypnotic agents, in usual therapeutic doses it does not depress REM sleep, which is an essential part of normal sleep.

Glutethimide

Glutethimide is known by the trade name Doriden and is another hypnotic agent commonly prescribed for sleep. As with many of the depressants, an overdose can cause respiratory depression. It has been noted that the drug seems to create a relapse effect on ventilation in cases of overdose; an apparent recovery of respiratory reflexes may be followed by a relapse into respiratory depression. This effect necessitates close monitoring of volumes and rates, particularly if intermittent mandatory ventilation has been reduced to a low rate, or perhaps worse, if the patient is on a T-tube. Glutethimide differs from most other sedative-hypnotic agents in that it may produce death by cardiovascular collapse at doses that do not appear to severely depress respiratory reflexes.

Benzodiazepines

The benzodiazepines are largely used as antianxiety, or anxiolytic, agents and are referred to as minor tranquilizers. These will be presented in the section on psychotherapeutic drugs in this chapter. However, the benzodiazepine derivatives listed previously are used as aids to sleep when insomnia exists. The agent **triazolam** (Halcion) has been associated with amnesia after therapeutic doses. This may have been caused by too short a sleep period after taking the drug while traveling on business, and the use of alcohol may have added to this effect.

Methaqualone

Methaqualone is no longer available in the United States for therapeutic use because of its potential for abuse. This drug is better known by its proprietary name Quaalude. It is a hypnotic similar to the short-acting barbiturates. Toxic doses produce CNS depression, and fatalities have occurred in individuals combining alcohol and methaqualone.

Ethyl Alcohol

Ethyl alcohol should not be overlooked as a CNS depressant, since the CNS is the most sensitive of the body's systems to alcohol. Alcohol has a depressant effect on the higher functions of the brain, including the RAS. The effects are proportional to the concentration of alcohol in the blood. The first effects of alcohol, seen in loss of fine motor control and increased reaction time, occur with 20 to 30 mg/dl in the blood. Most subjects show gross drunkenness with 150 mg/dl, and a quantity of alcohol sufficient to produce 400 mg/dl or more in blood can dangerously depress the respiratory drive. Goodman, et al. (1985) noted that the amount of alcohol in *brains* of persons dying of intoxication varied from 300 to 600 mg/dl. Alcohol is uniformly distributed to all tissue and fluids of the body, so this concentration may reflect approximate blood levels.

Effects.   Alcohol can cool the skin through evaporation when topically applied. It can also redden and burn when rubbed into the skin (rubefacient). Alcohol has a strong irritant effect on mucous membranes of the gastrointestinal tract or the lung. It is for this reason that inhalation of nebulized alcohol can irritate the upper airway, and the concentration should be diluted to 30% or 50%, with discouragement of chronic use of inhaled alcohol aerosol. Furthermore, alcohol can cause depression of the ventilatory response to carbon dioxide, at concentrations below those causing general respiratory depression. Alcohol can also cause a feeling of euphoria, or mood elevation, and raise one's pain threshold. In having an analgesic effect, alcohol differs from the barbiturate hypnotics. There is cutaneous and peripheral vasodilatation, which produces the typical flushed appearance of the drinker and gives a feeling of increased warmth. Sweating may occur, with a more rapid loss of body heat due to peripheral vasodilatation in combination with sweating. Drinking alcohol to warm up in cold weather can lead to subjective feelings of warmth but dangerous loss of body heat. Concentrations of alcohol that cause mild inebriation do not increase cerebral blood flow, but larger amounts (300 mg/dl or more) can increase mean cerebral blood flow. The diuretic effect of alcohol is well known to those who participate in attitude-adjustment sessions after hours. Alcohol has a positive interaction with sedatives, hypnotics, tranquilizers, and some analgesics. When such drugs are taken with alcohol, the loss of motor coordination and judgment caused by the alcohol are much greater for a given amount of alcohol.

Metabolism.   Almost all ingested alcohol is oxidized ultimately to carbon dioxide and water. Unfortunately, in this process there are highly toxic intermediates formed, such as acetaldehyde, formaldehyde, and formic acid. The euphoria of intoxication inevitably gives way to the pain of sober recovery. Alcohol is somewhat peculiar in that the rate of oxidation is constant and does not change with concentration. For an average man this is approximately 12.5 ml/hr and is proportional to body weight.

GENERAL ANESTHETICS

General anesthetics are treated separately from the sedative-hypnotic drugs, although this group of drugs can be considered as one end of a single spectrum, with mild sedation at the other end, and hypnosis (sleep) in between the two extremes. The term *anesthesia* literally translates as without (an-) sensation (aisthesis). The degree of CNS depression produces stages of anesthesia. General anesthesia is commonly referred to as "being put to sleep." General anesthetics can cause CNS depression by producing total loss of consciousness and loss of reflexes, although particular drugs or low doses may produce lesser CNS depression. Drugs used for general anesthesia can be grouped into three categories as listed below:

- Barbiturates
    Thiopental sodium (Pentothal)
    Thiamylal sodium (Surital Sodium)
    Methohexital sodium (Brevital Sodium)
- Nonbarbiturate
    Ketamine HCl (Ketalar)
    Etomidate (Amidate)
    Midazolam HCl (Versed)
    Propofol (Diprivan)
    Droperidol (Inapsine)
    Fentanyl citrate and droperidol (Innovar)
- Anesthetic Gases
    Nitrous oxide
    Cyclopropane
    Ethylene
    Halothane (Fluothane)
    Methoxyflurane (Penthrane)
    Enflurane (Ethrane)
    Isoflurane (Forane)

Barbiturate Anesthetics

The barbiturates were previously considered as sedatives and sleeping aids. Certain ultrashort-acting barbiturates are used intravenously for induction of general anesthesia and as supplements to other anesthetic drugs during surgical procedures. The barbiturates listed previously produce a rapid and profound loss of consciousness in adequate doses. They have a high lipid solubility and quickly cross into the brain. They are rapidly redistributed from the brain, which causes a short duration of action. They produce *no* analgesia (control of pain).

Nonbarbiturate Anesthetics

The nonbarbiturates include a variety of drugs used either for general anesthesia, twilight anesthesia, or for conscious sedation during procedures (e.g., midazolam).

Ketamine is a rapid-acting general anesthetic that, unlike the barbiturates, does produce strong analgesia. It does not produce muscle relaxation. Ketamine can be used alone as an anesthetic for diagnostic procedures, or as an adjunct by intravenous administration with a low-potency anesthetic gas such as nitrous oxide.

Etomidate is a nonbarbiturate anesthetic that has no analgesic property. Intravenous administration can cause rapid hypnosis (sleep). It can be used for induction of anesthesia or as an adjunct with such agents as nitrous oxide.

Midazolam has become familiar to many respiratory care clinicians because of its widespread use with bronchoscopy. Midazolam (Versed) is used for other procedures as well and is a short-acting benzodiazepine CNS depressant. Intravenous doses of up to 2.5 mg can produce conscious sedation. Concomitant use of other CNS depressants, such as narcotics, may necessitate lower doses to avoid marked respiratory depression. Elderly patients may also require lower doses. Respiratory depression and arrest have occurred even with doses for conscious sedation. Depression of ventilation is greater in subjects with chronic obstructive pulmonary disease. Onset of sedation is within 3 to 5 minutes given intravenously and about 15 minutes by intramuscular administration. Although awake during a procedure such as bronchoscopy, some patients do not recall the examination when midazolam is used.

Propofol is a rapid and short-acting CNS depressant that produces loss of consciousness. It is given intravenously for the induction and maintenance of general anesthesia for surgery. After intravenous injection, patients are asleep within 40 seconds, and recovery following termination of the drug is within minutes. Propofol infusion can be used as an adjunct to nitrous oxide for maintenance of anesthesia. The drug does not provide analgesia.

Droperidol is a butyrophenone derivative that causes substantial sedation and a major tranquilizing effect, as well as an antiemetic effect. It is used as a surgical premedication to reduce anxiety and nausea or vomiting during surgical and diagnostic procedures. It is also used for the induction and maintenance of anesthesia. Droperidol is combined with the narcotic analgesic fentanyl as the brand Innovar. Since droperidol causes a tranquilizing effect, the combination can cause extreme relaxation and analgesia, without loss of consciousness.

Anesthetic Gases

The anesthetic gases are administered in a mixture with oxygen after the induction of hypnosis by one of the agents previously discussed and often after administration of a neuromuscular blocking agent to relax skeletal muscle for surgery. The first three gases, nitrous oxide, cyclopropane, and ethylene, exist in a gaseous state, while the remaining four agents are volatile liquids that evaporate into a gas state for inhalation. All have a rapid onset of action and depress the CNS to maintain a desired level of anesthesia. Nitrous oxide is a weak anesthetic that is usually used with other agents, as previously mentioned. Cyclopropane and ethylene are both explosive in oxygen and are rarely used.

PSYCHOTHERAPEUTIC AGENTS

Minor Tranquilizers

The minor tranquilizers, or anxiolytics, are perhaps best represented by drugs belonging to the benzodiazepine group. In contrast with the barbiturates, minor tranquilizers generally have two advantages: (1) lack of respiratory depression in sedative doses and (2) a higher therapeutic index.

Following is a list of the benzodiazepines and other agents used as minor tranquilizers in the treatment of anxiety and neuroses:

- Benzodiazepines
    - Oxazepam (Serax)
    - Prazepam (Centrax)
    - Lorazepam (Ativan)
    - Alprazolam (Xanax)
    - Chlordiazepoxide (Librium)
    - Diazepam (Valium)
    - Halazepam (Paxipam)
    - Chlorazepate dipotassium (Tranxene)
- Other agents
    - Meprobamate (Equanil, Miltown)
    - Buspirone HCl (BuSpar)
    - Hydroxyzine (Atarax)
    - Doxepin HCl (Sinequan)
    - Chlormezanone (Trancopal)
    - Droperidol (Inapsine)

Benzodiazepines

The benzodiazepine group seems to differ from barbiturates in their mechanism of action by not directly depressing the reticular formation. It has been suggested that these drugs instead shield the RAS in some manner and thus prevent stimuli from causing wakefulness.

As a general class, the minor tranquilizers have been used in the treatment of neuroses and the anxiety associated with such states. This use can be contrasted with the application of the major tranquilizers, such as phenothiazines, to the treatment of psychosis.

The benzodiazepines have the following effects:

Muscle relaxation
Antianxiety
Anticonvulsant
Sedative and hypnotic

In addition to uses based on the above effects, benzodiazepines have been used in the management of alcohol withdrawal syndromes. They appear to be useful in this respect because they substitute well pharmacologically for alcohol, decrease the likelihood of withdrawal seizures, and decrease anxiety associated with the withdrawal syndrome.

One of the attractive features of the benzodiazepine group is the minimal depression of the medullary respiratory center, even in overdose. Drowsiness and muscle weakness may occur, and fainting may be seen with normal doses, especially in older patients.

Other Antianxiety Agents

A drug not classed as a benzodiazepine, but also used in the treatment of anxiety states and neuroses, is meprobamate (Equanil, Miltown). The reduction of anxiety is based more on its muscle-relaxant properties than any sedative-hypnotic effect. This is caused by the drug's mode of action, which is the blockade of interneurons in the spinal cord. However, drowsiness can commonly occur as a side effect of the drug. Overdose can cause unconsciousness and coma, but an additional hazard at normal doses is the additive interaction of meprobamate with alcohol to cause loss of motor coordination and judgment. The drug is able to produce physiological dependence with repeated use or abuse, and termination of the drug will lead to physical withdrawal effects, for example convulsions.

Buspirone represents a nonbenzodiazepine anxiolytic that offers advantages over the benzodiazepine agents in the treatment of anxiety. Although its mode of action is unknown, buspirone differs from the benzodiazepines in not having anticonvulsant or muscle-relaxant effects. Its primary advantage is a lack of sedative effects seen with the traditional antianxiety agents (Seidel et al., 1985). Other miscellaneous agents used to treat anxiety include hydroxyzine (Atarax), doxepin (Sinequan), chlormezanone (Trancopal), and droperidol (Inapsine).

Antipsychotic Drugs

Antipsychotic is a general term denoting those drugs that are useful in alleviating the symptoms of major mental disorders such as schizophrenia, depression, mania, and organic brain syndrome. A partial listing of these drugs is as follows:

- Phenothiazines
    Thioridazine (Mellaril)
    Mesoridazine (Serentil)
    Chlorpromazine (Thorazine)*
    Promazine (Sparine)*
    Triflupromazine (Vesprin)
    Acetophenazine (Tindal)
    Perphenazine (Trilafon)
    Fluphenazine (Prolixin)
    Trifluoperazine (Stelazine)
    Prochlorperazine (Compazine)*
- Thioxanthenes
    Chlorprothixene (Taractan)
    Thiothixene (Navane)
- Butyrophenones
    Haloperidol (Haldol)
- Miscellaneous
    Loxapine (Loxitane)
    Molindone (Moban)
    Clozapine (Clozaril)
    Pimozide (Orap)

Neuroleptics

The term neuroleptic refers to drugs that modify psychotic behavior. Neuroleptic agents are used in the treatment of major mental disorders such as schizophrenia and organic brain syndrome. Under special conditions they may also be used for the treatment of mania and depression. Schizophrenia is characterized by a loss of touch with reality, hallucinations, and delusions. Neuroleptic agents do not "cure" schizophrenia but decrease or alleviate these symptoms in most patients.

The etiology of schizophrenia is unknown, but the current accepted theory proposes either that receptors for dopamine in the limbic system become hypersensitive or that the synthesis or release of dopamine in nerve terminals associated with these receptors is increased by some unknown mechanism. The end point of either of these mechanisms is excessive stimulation of dopamine receptor sites.

The neuroleptic agents all produce their antipsychotic effects by blocking dopamine receptor sites in the limbic system. Dopamine is also found as a

*Also used as antiemetics.

neurotransmitter in other areas of the brain such as the basal ganglia, the CTZ of the medulla, and the hypothalamus; therefore, the neuroleptics produce a number of other effects. Blockade of dopamine receptors in the basal ganglia results in extrapyramidal syndrome symptoms such as muscle rigidity and tremors. Blockade of dopamine receptors in the CTZ results in an antiemetic effect that is therapeutically beneficial in the treatment of nausea and vomiting. Blockade of hypothalamic dopamine receptors results in a decrease in the release of the pituitary hormones such as growth hormone.

The neuroleptics also produce a variety of other side effects. They block cholinergic receptor sites and thus produce tachycardia, dry mouth, blurred vision, constipation, urinary retention, and decreased respiratory secretions. They block peripheral alpha-adrenergic receptor sites, thus producing orthostatic hypotension and reflexive tachycardia.

The neuroleptics produce some effects that are related to nonspecific CNS depression and therefore are dose related. Their effects on the cortex include sedation and ataxia. At sufficiently high doses, they will depress respiration and produce death as a result of respiratory depression, cardiovascular collapse, or cardiac arrest.

Neuroleptic drugs have an extremely long therapeutic half-life, usually greater than 24 hours. With ingestion of toxic doses, emergency life support therapy requires maintenance of the airway and respiration and the cardiovascular system, possibly for several days.

Antidepressants

Depression occurs as one of two types: reactive depression, which is related to a traumatic event in life, and endogenous depression, which is thought to occur due to a neurotransmitter imbalance in the limbic system. The two neurotransmitters involved in depression are norepinephrine and serotonin, and a deficit of either of these will result in the occurrence of clinically noteworthy depression.

The categories of antidepressants and their agents are as follows:

- Tricyclic antidepressants
  - Amitriptyline (Elavil)
  - Imipramine (Tofranil)
    Doxepin (Sinequan)
    Trimipramine (Surmontil)
  - Nortriptyline (Aventyl)
    Desipramine (Norpramin)
    Protriptyline (Vivactil)
    Amoxapine (Asendin)

- Tetracyclic
    Maprotiline (Ludiomil)
- Monoamine oxidase inhibitors
    Isocarboxazid (Marplan)
    Phenelzine (Nardil)
    Tranylcypromine (Parnate)
- Miscellaneous
    Trazodone (Desyrel)
    Fluoxetine (Prozac)
    Sertraline (Zoloft)
    Bupropion (Wellbutrin)
    Paroxetine (Paxil)

Two distinct chemical categories of antidepressants are the tricyclic antidepressants, which produce their therapeutic effects by inhibition of the reuptake of norepinephrine and/or serotonin, and the monoamine oxidase (MAO) inhibitors, which increase levels of neurotransmitters. The tetracyclic category is a newly emerging category of antidepressants that are analogues of the tricyclic compounds.

Tricyclic and Tetracyclic Agents

The specific side effects of the tricyclic and tetracyclic antidepressants are related to their effects on the central and autonomic nervous systems. These compounds produce cholinergic receptor blockade peripherally and thus anticholinergic side effects, which are essentially the same as those seen with the neuroleptics. In addition, those compounds that inhibit norepinephrine reuptake may cause accumulation of this transmitter in cardiac tissue, resulting in life-threatening arrhythmias. The primary CNS side effects produced by these agents is sedation, which may be beneficial in depressed patients with a high level of anxiety.

Toxic doses of these antidepressants initially produce stimulation of the CNS, apparently due to increased levels of neurotransmitters. The initial stimulation may then be followed by a generalized CNS depression. Treatment of toxicity with these compounds is the same as for other nonspecific depressants.

Monamine Oxidase Inhibitors

MAO is an enzyme found throughout the gastrointestinal tract, liver, and in nerve endings that use norepinephrine as their transmitter. Drugs that inhibit the MAO enzyme increase the concentration of the monoamines such as epinephrine, norepinephrine, and serotonin. The increase in these neurotransmitters in the CNS is thought to be the basis for the antidepressant effect. The function of MAO in the gastrointestinal tract and liver is to destroy ingested substances such as tyramine and tryptophan, which are found in foods. These substances have sympathomimetic activity and, if not destroyed, would produce excessive stimulation of the sympathetic nervous system. The MAO found in nerve endings is responsible for the destruction of excessive amounts of norepinephrine found at sympathetic neuroeffector junctions. Since the effects of norepinephrine are terminated primarily by reuptake of norepinephrine back into the nerve terminal from which it was released, it would be expected that inhibition of MAO at the nerve terminal would have little effect on overall norepinephrine levels.

Toxicity associated with the MAO inhibitors is similar to that seen with the tricyclic compounds, in that stimulation of the CNS is followed by overt depression of all basic functions. Therapy is aimed toward maintenance of the respiratory and cardiovascular systems.

Hypertensive crisis is a serious side effect of MAO inhibitors that can be caused by excess norepinephrine. Patients should be warned against eating foods such as cheese and dairy products or meat and fish, which are high in tyramine. Inhibition of MAO can allow these foods to produce a hypertensive crisis, which can be fatal.

Lithium

Currently, the drug of choice for the treatment of manic-depressive psychosis is lithium carbonate. Manic-depressive psychosis is a mental disorder characterized by extreme mood swings that occur in a cyclic pattern.

Lithium is unique as a psychoactive agent in that it produces almost no adverse behavioral effects in the individual with normal mental status. However, it does produce a number of adverse physiological side effects including polydipsia, polyuria, tremors, exophthalmos, muscle weakness, slurred speech, nausea, vomiting, and diarrhea.

Symptoms such as polyuria, vomiting, and diarrhea, if they are allowed to continue for an extended period, can seriously affect electrolyte balance and fluid hemodynamics. This can in turn lead to cardiovascular changes and diminish or exaggerate the action of therapeutic agents. In addition, lithium decreases the pressor response to norepinephrine, which may be an important consideration in patients with compromised cardiovascular function.

ANALGESICS

Analgesics, previously identified as drugs used to provide relief from pain, are divided into two groups: narcotics and nonnarcotics. The narcotic group consists of the naturally occurring derivatives of opium such as morphine and codeine and a number of semisynthetic and synthetic agents that are termed *opioids*. The narcotic analgesics are useful for alleviating moderate-to-severe pain and produce their therapeutic effect by an action within the CNS.

The nonnarcotic analgesics are useful for the treatment of mild-to-moderate pain and may also possess antipyretic and anti-inflammatory activity. These analgesic agents alleviate pain by a twofold mechanism: (1) a direct effect on the CNS, possibly in the hypothalamus, to produce both analgesic and antipyretic activity; and (2) a peripheral effect at the site of tissue trauma to reduce inflammation and prevent the origin of pain impulses.

Differences among analgesic drugs and their use are related to the different types of pain. Generally, three types of pain are distinguished:

Superficial, cutaneous pain
Deeper joint or muscle pain and ache
Deep visceral pain

Pain is initiated as a sensation when pain receptors that lie within skin and body structures are stimulated. Such stimulation may occur as a result of compression, deformation, stretching, or cutting. This trauma induces the synthesis of prostaglandins, which cause the pain receptors to become sensitive to endogenous chemicals such as bradykinin or serotonin. The sensitized receptors then are stimulated by these chemicals and a pain impulse is initiated.

$$\text{Tissue Trauma} \rightarrow \text{Prostaglandin synthesis} \rightarrow \text{Pain receptors become sensitive to bradykinin} \rightarrow \text{Pain}$$

After its initiation, the pain impulse is transmitted through the spinal cord to the thalamus and from the thalamus to the sensory cortex where the impulse is actually perceived as pain. Nerve impulses are also transmitted from the thalamus to the limbic system where the emotional response to pain is produced. This emotional response almost always includes an increase in the activity of the sympathetic portion of the autonomic nervous system.

Narcotic analgesics appear to produce their therapeutic effects by combining with specific receptor sites found throughout the nervous system but in high concentrations in the limbic system, thalamus, and hypothalamus. These receptors seem to also be the receptors for several endogenous peptide substances that are termed *enkephalins* and *endorphins*. It has been theorized that these substances are endogenously produced analgesics and that the narcotic analgesics produce analgesia by mimicking the action of these drugs.

Narcotic Analgesics

Opioid refers to either natural or synthetic drugs with morphine-like pharmacological properties. Opium itself is obtained by powdering the dried milky exudate from the unripe seed capsules of the poppy plant (Papaver somniferum). By weight, powdered opium contains about 25% alkaloids, including the following:

Morphine: 10%
Codeine: 0.5%
Thebaine: 0.2%
Papaverine: 1%
Noscapine: 6%

Opium may well have been known to the ancient Sumerians circa **4000** BC, who had an ideograph for the poppy plant that consisted of hul (joy) and gil (plants). Of course one may argue that the appearance alone of poppies brings joy. There is clear reference in the writings of the third century BC Greek Theophrastus to poppy juice, and the word *opium* is from the Greek term for juice. Paracelsus is credited with compounding laudanum, a 10% opium compound containing 1% morphine, in the 16th century, and in 1803, the German pharmacist Serturner isolated morphine itself from opium. The drug was named after Morpheus, the Greek god of dreams. Codeine was subsequently discovered in 1832. Although drug abuse with opium existed prior to the twentieth century, the invention of the hypodermic needle and parenteral use of morphine led to a more severe variety of drug abuse.

Pharmacological Properties of Morphine

The major effects of morphine and its derivatives are on the CNS and the bowel. The narcotics depress CNS function, including ventilatory drives, and increase bowel tone to the point of constipation.

Morphine probably interacts with more than one neurotransmitter and with heterogeneous receptors in the CNS. In its effect on the CNS, morphine produces analgesia and drowsiness but, additionally, mood changes and mental clouding. The analgesic effect is due to elevation of the pain threshold, dissociation of pain perception (euphoria), and production of sleep or lethargy. The narcotic group provides better analgesia with dull constant pain than with sharp stabbing pain and can provide relief for visceral pain, unlike the antipyretics. An unwanted side effect of morphine analgesia is depression of the central medullary respiratory center, causing decreased responsiveness to arterial P_{CO_2} levels and a decreased respiratory rate. Large doses of morphine can cause irregular breathing and apnea by depressing the pontine and medullary rhythm centers. Other areas of the CNS that are affected by morphine or its derivatives include the following:

Oculomotor Nucleus: Pupillary constriction in the eye and the classic pinpoint pupil are seen with opioid overdose.

Cough Reflex: sensitive to morphine-like drugs. Codeine was often an ingredient in preparations to suppress dry, irritant coughs, and is now frequently replaced with synthetic nonnarcotic antitussives such as dextromethorphan.

CTZ: The area postrema of the medulla is stimulated, resulting in nausea and vomiting in a minority of subjects.

In its effect on the cardiovascular system, morphine causes peripheral vasodilatation, which is at least partly due to histamine release. Narcotic-induced hypotension is further enhanced by stimulation of the vagal center in the medulla, which slows the heart rate.

In the gastrointestinal tract, sphincter (pyloris, ileocecal, anal) tone is increased and peristaltic movement is decreased by morphine, probably because of a direct effect on the bowel wall that results in increased tone.

In the pulmonary system, morphine-induced release of histamine can cause increased airway resistance resulting from bronchoconstriction. In general, the use of narcotics for analgesia, or even sedation, is discouraged in subjects with hyperreactive airways, such as asthmatic patients. To summarize, the analgesic and cough suppressant effects of morphine, usually desirable, are combined with the effects of ventilatory depression, constipation, and sometimes nausea and vomiting. There is also the potential for addiction and abuse.

Therapeutic Uses of Narcotics

Sir William Osler called morphine "God's own medicine," and it has also been observed that, without the opioid drugs, few would be hard-hearted enough to practice medicine. The therapeutic uses of narcotics are directly related to the pharmacological properties of morphine and its derivatives. These uses include the following:

Relief of pain
Sedation
Cough suppression
Relief of dyspnea resulting from acute left ventricular failure
Antidiarrhea

The fourth use of morphine (i.e., relief of dyspnea), or the archaically termed *cardiac asthma,* is often seen with left ventricular failure. The mechanism by which morphine relieves such dyspnea, or what the therapeutic effect actually is, remains unclear but may involve several features. First, patients' reactions to impaired respiratory function may simply be altered. Second, there may be indirect reduction in myocardial work because of reduced fear and anxiety. Third, and perhaps most important, there is decreased peripheral vascular resistance and increased venous reservoir to reduce the work of the left side of the heart. This effect is similar to the clearing of pulmonary edema and reduced myocardial work seen with impeded venous return during treatment with PEEP. With pulmonary edema caused by left ventricular failure, an increased venous capacity, whether caused by PEEP or morphine, can be a beneficial side effect to allow recovery of cardiac function.

Use of narcotic compounds to alleviate diarrhea takes advantage of their effect on the gastrointestinal tract, which was previously mentioned. Diphenoxylate, which is combined with atropine as Lomotil (Searle), is a derivative of meperidine (Demerol) and is used as an antidiarrheal. Another frequently used agent is paregoric, which is an alcoholic solution (tincture) of opium.

Derivatives of Morphine

Following is a list of the major derivatives of morphine and drugs with morphine-like activity, as well as narcotic antagonists:

- Narcotic analgesics
  Opium (Pantopon, Paregoric)
  Morphine
  Codeine
  Oxycodone (Roxicodone)
  Oxymorphone (Numorphan)
  Levorphanol (Levo-Dromoran)
  Pentazocine (Talwin)
  Meperidine (Demerol)
  Methadone (Dolophine)
  Fentanyl (Sublimaze)
  Sufentanil (Sufenta)
  Alfentanil (Alfenta)
  Propoxyphene (Darvon)
  Butorphanol (Stadol)
  Nalbuphine (Nubain)
  Buprenorphine (Buprenex)
  Dezocine (Dalgan)
- Narcotic antagonists
  Naloxone (Narcan)
  Naltrexone (Trexan)

Codeine is the methyl ether of morphine and is an ingredient found in opium. It is commonly used in cough suppressants and in analgesic compounds such as Empirin with codeine, which is used for mild-to-moderate pain relief.

Heroin is not legally available in the United States for clinical applications, but it is commonly used by morphine addicts and is available as a street drug. There is a high addictive potential. In the body, heroin, which is a morphine ester, is converted rapidly to monocetylmorphine and then to morphine.

Oxymorphone (Numorphan) is a semisynthetic derivative of morphine, with five to ten times the analgesic activity of morphine. The narcotic antagonist naloxone is a chemical derivative of oxymorphone.

Pentazocine (Talwin) is a chemical relative to morphine with analgesic properties. Use of pentazocine for analgesia in patients with chronic obstructive lung disease has been studied. Doses capable of producing analgesia did not adversely affect arterial co_2 or o_2 tensions in the patients studied (Glass et al., 1970).

Synthetic analgesics have been developed with morphine-like activity, but which are chemically distinct from opium alkaloids. These include meperidine (Demerol); methadone (Dolophine), often used for maintenance of narcotic addicts during withdrawal; and propoxyphene (Darvon). Propoxyphene is structurally related to methadone, and only the dextro isomer has analgesic activity. The levorotatory form does have antitussive effect. The drug is one of the most commonly prescribed narcotic analgesics in the United States, ranked in the top fifty of filled prescriptions since 1966. Although many synthetic analgesics were developed in search of nonaddictive pain drugs, there is abuse of such drugs as propoxyphene. Overdoses of Darvon can produce the same clinical picture of pulmonary edema as heroin or morphine. Naloxone, as discussed below, can reverse intoxication and ventilatory depression caused by propoxyphene. The pulmonary effects of narcotics are well discussed in the October 1980 issue of *Seminars in Respiratory Medicine*, and details of pathological conditions can be found there.

Of the synthetic analgesics, meperidine differs most widely from others in the group. As an analgesic, it closely resembles morphine in its actions on the nervous and cardiovascular systems. It produces much less constipation than morphine and is not useful as an antidiarrheal agent. Its most striking difference from other narcotics is related to its ability to stimulate the CNS, producing tremors and even convulsions in high therapeutic doses. This stimulation cannot be reversed by narcotic antagonists and can be potentiated by other stimulant drugs.

Overdose of Morphine and Its Derivatives

The combination of pinpoint pupils, coma, and depressed ventilation is suggestive of opioid overdose. Since most patients with heroin intoxication have constricted pupils, this sign serves to distinguish opioid intoxication from barbiturate overdose, where pupils become dilated with cerebral hypoxia. The usual dose of morphine is 10 mg intramuscularly or subcutaneously in an adult, but even this dose may affect ventilatory drive. Doses above 100 mg may be fatal, and 300 mg is considered lethal, although morphine addicts have tolerated up to 5 g/d. In overdose with morphine, a deep sleep is caused, with depression of breathing, followed by periodic, irregular breathing of a Cheyne-Stokes pattern and eventual respiratory failure. Some patients are apneic or breathing only several breaths per minute. Needle tracks may be found on some portion of the anatomy in many cases. Intravenous overdose of heroin, a morphine ester, may result in acute pulmonary edema and a general adult respiratory distress syndrome: hypoxia, loss of compliance, pulmonary exudate, possibly caused by contaminants in the street-supplied heroin. Pulmonary complications include pneumonia and bronchiectasis. Arterial blood gases usually show hypoxemia, with varying degrees of hypercapnea. Support of opioid overdose is similar to that with any CNS depressant and includes airway maintenance, prevention of aspiration, supported ventilation, oxygenation, and cardiac function. Narcotic antagonists may be helpful with morphine overdose, and the renal excretion of morphine is increased in acidic urine, unlike barbiturates, which require alkaline urine.

Narcotic Antagonists

Therapeutic agents such as naloxone and naltrexone have the ability to nullify the effects of narcotic analgesics when administered to an individual who already has a narcotic in the system (antagonist effect). They are used in the clinical setting to counteract the ventilatory depression produced by morphine and related compounds.

Naloxone occupies the opiate receptors but stabilizes them in the inactive state so that narcotic actions are not seen, thus there is no depression of ventilation or analgesia produced. Naloxone can be used safely in patients with drug-related respiratory depression when the drug involved has not been identified. If the drug is a narcotic, the respiratory depression will be antagonized. If the drug is not a narcotic, naloxone will not add to the respiratory depression.

Because naloxone is a pure antagonist, when it is administered to an individual who is physically dependent on a narcotic drug, it will precipitate an immediate withdrawal syndrome and has been used for the purpose of identifying dependent individuals.

Naloxone is also used to reverse depressed ventilation in neonates whose mothers had been treated with narcotics to alleviate pain during the delivery process.

In using naloxone to reverse narcotic overdose or depression, repeated dosages are necessary because naloxone is rapidly metabolized and appropriate plasma naloxone levels must be maintained to effectively antagonize the narcotic effects. Doses of 0.4 to 0.8 mg intramuscularly or intravenously are used in adult patients.

Nonnarcotic Analgesics

Following is a list of the nonnarcotic analgesics:

- Salicylates
  Aspirin (acetylsalicylic acid)
  Sodium salicylate
  Salsalate (Amigesic, Disalcid)
  Diflunisal (Dolobid)
- Aniline derivative
  Acetaminophen (Tempra, Tylenol)
- Pyrazole Derivatives
  Phenylbutazone (Butazolidin)
  Oxyphenbutazone (Oxalid)
- Central Acting
  Methotrimeprazine (Levoprome)
- Nonsteroidal Anti-inflammatory Drugs (NSAIDs)
  Indomethacin (Indocin)
  Ibuprofen (Motrin)
  Ketoprofen (Orudis)
  Fenoprofen (Nalfon)
  Naproxen (Naprosyn)
  Sulindac (Clinoril)
  Tolmetin (Tolectin)
  Mefenamic acid (Ponstel)
  Meclofenamate (Meclomen)
  Piroxicam (Feldene)
  Flurbiprofen (Ansaid)
  Nabumetone (Relafen)
  Diclofenac (Voltaren)
  Etodolac (Lodine)
  Ketorolac (Toradol)
  Oxaprozin (Daypro)

The antipyretic analgesics were originally used to reduce elevated body temperature. In fact, the use of aspirin, or acetylsalicylic acid, which is derived from salicin found in willow tree bark, dates back to 1899. Today, both analgesia and control of body temperature are desired effects, with analgesia predominating, in the clinical use of the nonnarcotic analgesics.

Salicylates

The salicylates actually have a number of pharmacological effects, including analgesia, antipyresis, and anti-inflammation, as well as an undesirable inhibition of hemostasis. The analgesic and anti-inflammatory effects work together for the overall relief of pain. Analgesia and reduction of fever may both be mediated by action of the salicylate at the hypothalamus. The anti-inflammatory effect seems to be mediated by the ability of salicylates to inhibit prostaglandin synthesis in inflamed tissues. Both salicylates and indomethacin block the synthesis of prostaglandins from the precursor fatty acids by inhibiting prostaglandin synthetase. Prostaglandin E_1 and E_2 intensify the effect of such chemical mediators of inflammation as histamine, bradykinin, and serotonin (5-hydroxytryptamine or 5-HT).

When absorbed from the stomach, aspirin or other salicylates can cause ulceration of gastric mucosa and gastric bleeding. This hazard is worsened by cheap aspirin preparations that may clump and lead to highly concentrated sites of acetylsalicylic acid. Aspirin also affects hemostasis by platelet inhibition, and in large doses (6 g or more), by reducing plasma prothrombin levels. Aspirin blocks the adhesion of platelets to connective tissue or collagen fibers during the blood clotting process. For this reason aspirin is contraindicated in patients with hemophilia, with hepatic damage, or undergoing anticoagulant therapy. Aspirin interacts with the anticoagulant coumadin, competing for binding sites on plasma protein that coumadin usually occupies. Consequently, aspirin causes more free, unbound anticoagulant, which can also lead to clotting problems in patients on this particular anticoagulant.

Overdose of aspirin or salicylic acid leads to metabolic acidosis, which causes an attempted respiratory compensation, resulting in the familiar Kussmaul breathing, an example of hyperpnea (increased rate and depth).

An important therapeutic use of salicylates, not to be overlooked, is the treatment of rheumatoid arthritis. This use is based on the anti-inflammatory effect of the drug group.

An additional problem with aspirin is a sensitivity to the drug by certain asthmatic patients, particularly those with rhinitis and nasal polyps. Aspirin has caused bronchospasm in such patients, perhaps partially through inhibition of prostaglandins able to cause bronchodilatation, or through a direct release of chemical mediators such as histamine. Penna (1976) gives a good summary of hypotheses regarding aspirin-induced asthma.

Aniline Derivatives

The aniline derivatives include acetaminophen and phenacetin. These are alternatives to aspirin, having both analgesic and antipyretic effects but lacking the undesirable side effects of aspirin, such as interference with clotting mechanisms. However, overdose of acetaminophen can cause hepatotoxicity.

A minor but toxic metabolite of acetaminophen is usually metabolized in the liver by glutathione, which contributes a sulfhydril radical necessary for the breakdown of the metabolite to a nontoxic form. Urinary excretion then eliminates the substance. However, in overdose, the liver cannot supply enough glutathione, nor can glutathione be given effectively intravenously because glutathione will not cross the cell membrane into the liver where it is needed. Acetylcysteine, taken orally in large doses, will cross into liver cells and can supply the required sulfhydril, just as it does when interacting with mucus molecules, thus preventing hepatic toxicity due to binding of the metabolite to the liver cells (see Chapter 8).

Acetaminophen does not have a strong anti-inflammatory effect and is not useful in treating rheumatoid arthritis. It is very useful as an alternative analgesic for aspirin-sensitive patients with asthma, hemophilia, or ulcerated stomach mucosa.

Pyrazole Derivatives

The first pyrazole drugs were antipyrine and aminopyrine. These were followed by phenylbutazone and oxyphenbutazone, which are effective analgesics, antipyretics, and especially anti-inflammatory agents for use with rheumatoid patients. Toxicity with these drugs limits long-term use.

Nonsteroidal Anti-inflammatory Drugs

The NSAIDs resulted from a search for less toxic anti-inflammatory agents with fewer side effects. There has been a proliferation of these agents, which are listed previously. The NSAIDs have analgesic and antipyretic effects as part of their general anti-inflammatory action. Their uses reflect these effects: rheumatoid arthritis and osteoarthritis; mild-to-moderate pain associated with dental extraction or soft-tissue athletic injuries; primary dysmenorrhea; treatment of sunburn; and prophylaxis of migraine headaches, including those occurring with menstruation. The exact mode of action is unknown, but inhibition of prostaglandin and leukotriene synthesis is the basis for their therapeutic effect. Because of this, asthmatic patients may show sensitivity to these drugs in much the same way as with aspirin. Although there is a reduction in gastrointestinal side effects, patients should be watched for gastointestinal ulceration and bleeding, which can occur.

RESPIRATORY STIMULANTS

By contrast with the sedative-hypnotics, the analgesics, and the antipsychotic drugs, all of which are CNS depressants, there are CNS stimulants that can *increase* ventilation instead of depressing it. The more correct term for these agents would be *ventilatory* stimulants; however, much of the literature designates these drugs as respiratory stimulants. To prevent confusion, the latter designation will be used here. Most respiratory care personnel are aware of the distinction between ventilation and respiration. Drugs producing central stimulation as their predominant action are termed *analeptics*, or even convulsants, because they can cause convulsions in sufficient doses. By virtue of the general stimulation of the CNS, the central respiratory centers in the medulla are also stimulated. A respiratory stimulant should selectively affect only the respiratory control, but the analeptics in use are all general stimulants. Their toxicity and side effects result from this nonspecific stimulation. Side effects indicative of subconvulsive stimulation include: restlessness, sweating, hypertension, tachycardia, vomiting, and hyperpyrexia. Greater stimulation can produce convulsions.

Agents

Central nervous stimulants include the following:

- Analeptic
    Doxapram (Dopram)
- Xanthines
    Theophylline
    Caffeine
- Carbonic anhydrase inhibitors
- Salicylates
- Progesterone

Among four respiratory stimulants—doxapram, ethamivan, nikethamide, and pentylenetetrazol—doxapram had the greatest margin of safety between a dose giving ventilatory stimulation and a dose resulting in convulsions, and it remains available. Doxapram more selectively stimulates the peripheral chemoreceptors than the CNS receptors, unlike the other agents mentioned. The usual route of administration is intravenous, and effects on ventilation seldom last longer than 5 to 10 minutes with a bolus dose. Long-term effects require continuous infusion, which generally increases the risk of toxic side effects.

There are several groups of drugs used for various purposes that also have an effect on ventilatory drives. The xanthines, often used as bronchodilators, are ventilatory stimulants. Carbonic anhydrase inhibitors such as acetazolamide are usually used as diuretics. Because these drugs lead to an increase in arterial Pco_2 and a fall in pH, they can stimulate ventilation.

The salicylates, previously discussed under analgesics, are capable of producing increased ventilation, when taken in high doses. In the case of aspirin overdose, the Kussmaul breathing has been noted.

Progesterone, an ovarian hormone, has been noted to stimulate ventilation when given parenterally. Progestins, which is the term used for the class of hormones released by the ovaries, are usually used in contraception and to help regulate various abnormalities of the female reproductive system (e.g., uterine bleeding, dysmenorrhea, endometriosis).

Two older agents, which are no longer used clinically because of either toxicity or ineffectiveness, are picrotoxin and strychnine. Strychnine produces excitation of the entire CNS but has no demonstrated therapeutic value. Picrotoxin has a similar effect on the CNS and has been used for treatment of toxic doses of CNS depressants. However, ventilatory stimulation is only seen with doses approaching convulsion.

Clinical Use

Controversy has existed over the clinical application of respiratory stimulants. The analeptic doxapram is usually considered for increasing the ventilatory drive, as opposed to the other agents mentioned with the exception of progesterone, which may be useful for this effect. In any therapeutic application, doxapram is limited by two major factors: (1) short duration of action (5 to 10 minutes for a single dose) and (2) low margin of safety with general CNS stimulation. The second factor limits the use of continuous intravenous infusion required to solve the first problem of short-term duration. That is, cumulative levels can easily cause too much CNS stimulation in continuous infusion. The applications of CNS stimulants, or more particularly ventilatory stimulants, are discussed below.

Sedative-Hypnotic Overdose

The ease and relative safety of continuous ventilatory support presents a safer alternative than ventilatory stimulants. Around 1970, most of the literature was against use of CNS stimulants to counteract overdose with CNS depressants, whether barbiturate, alcohol, or narcotic.

Chronic Ventilatory Failure

Analeptics are unsuited to relieve chronic hypercapnea and hypoxemia because of their transitory effect.

Acute Ventilatory Failure

It is actually illogical to further stimulate a pulmonary system that is incapable of continuing the work of breathing in acute failure, whether due to pneumonia, adult respiratory distress syndrome, or other causes. The analogy would be that of flogging a dead horse. Also, aggressive therapy *before* ventilatory failure would be better aimed at supporting oxygenation while treating the causes of the respiratory distress. Although some may feel that doxapram can "buy time" and slow the onset of ventilatory failure by keeping a patient breathing to reduce hypercapnea and hypoxemia, it should be realized that an analeptic increases the work of breathing and oxygen consumption.

Acute-on-Chronic Ventilatory Failure

The argument has been advanced that analeptics such as doxapram may allow use of more oxygen in chronically hypercapneic patients without suppressing peripheral hypoxemic drives. However, well-controlled oxygen therapy is available in many centers. If a patient is unable to support spontaneous ventilation despite a return of oxygen tensions to the patient's usual baseline, then supported ventilation is required, not more oxygen. This is well exemplified by case studies, such as described by Riordan et al. (1974). One *might* envision a situation in outlying regions where a ventilatory stimulant such as doxapram could gain time for transport to a center where mechanical ventilation is possible. It should be realized that analeptics cause increased oxygen consumption and work of breathing, as previously mentioned. The desired effect of temporary stimulation pending transport may simply not be achievable in these patients. A good discussion of these advantages and disadvantages, although not recent, can be found in Pierson (1973). Moser et al. (1983) also provide a helpful discussion concerning use of doxapram in respiratory failure.

Postanesthetic Recovery

The same principle applies to postanesthetic recovery as with drug overdose: Temporary supported ventilation is safer than use of analeptics. Specific agents for reversal of neuromuscular blockers (such as neostigmine) and reversal of narcotics (such as naloxone) are better used than a general CNS stimulant.

Miscellaneous Applications

Doxapram and other analeptics have been used to reverse hypercapnea and hypoventilation in perinatal respiratory depression, in congenital central hypoventilation syndromes, and in obesity-hypoventilation syndromes.

BIBLIOGRAPHY

Adams JE, Hosobuchi Y, Linchitz R: The present status of implantable intracranial stimulators for pain, Clin Neurosurg 24:347, 1977.

Arens JF: Sedation for patients on long-term ventilatory care. Inhal Ther 15:150, 1970.

Bloom FE, Guillemin R: Stimulation of human periaqueductal grey matter for pain relief increases immunoreactive beta-endorphin in ventricular fluid, Science 203:279, 1979.

Brashear RE: Effects of heroin, morphine, methadone, and propoxyphene on the lung, Semin Respir Med 2(2):59, 1980.

Forster A, et al: Respiratory depression by midazolam and diazepam, Anesthesiology 53:494, 1980.

Gilman AG, Goodman LS, Rall TW, Murad F: Goodman and Gilman's The Pharmacological Basis of Therapeutics, 7th ed, New York, Macmillan Publishing Co., 1985.

Glass P, Sbar S, Cheema M: Talwin® as an analgesic in chronic obstructive lung disease, Am Rev Respir Dis 102:116, 1970.

Goldstein A: Enkephalins, opiate receptors and general anesthesia. Anesthesiology 49:1, 1978 (editorial).

Greenblatt DJ, Shader RI: The clinical choice of sedative-hypnotics. Ann Intern Med 77:91, 1972.

Gupta PK, Moore J: The use of doxapram in the newborn, J Obstet Gynaecol Br Comm 80:1002, 1973.

Houser WC, Schlueter DP: Prolonged doxapram infusion in obesity-hypoventilation syndrome, JAMA 239:340, 1978.

Hunt CE, Inwood RJ, Shannon DC: Respiratory and nonrespiratory effects of doxapram in congenital central hypoventilation syndrome, Am Rev Respir Dis 119:263, 1979.

Lugliami R, Whipp BJ, Wasserman K: Doxapram hydrochloride: a respiratory stimulant for patients with primary alveolar hypoventilation, Chest 76:414, 1979.

Moser KM et al: Respiratory stimulation with intravenous doxapram in respiratory failure, N Engl J Med 288:427, 1973.

Penna PM: Bronchial asthma induced by aspirin and other analgesics: review of incidence, mechanisms, and predisposing factors, Respir Care 21:1135, 1976.

Pierson DJ: Respiratory stimulants: review of the literature and assessment of current status. Respir Care 18:549, 1973.

Riordan JF, Sillett RW, McNicol MW: Response to a respiratory stimulant (doxapram) in severe respiratory failure, Br J Dis Chest 68:39, 1974.

Seidel WF et al: Buspirone: an anxiolytic without sedative effect, Psychopharmacology 87:371, 1985.

17

Cardiovascular Agents

Chapter 17 considers drugs that affect the cardiovascular system: the heart, circulatory vessels, and blood. The following major topics are discussed:

- Cardiovascular system
- Drugs affecting the heart
- Drugs affecting circulatory vessels
- Drugs affecting the blood

Agents in the cardiovascular group are used for many clinical situations, including congestive heart failure (CHF), cardiac arrhythmias, cardiopulmonary resuscitation, angina, myocardial infarction, hypertension, shock, and thromboembolism. Individual drugs are characterized briefly as outlined above. The emphasis is on identification of the agents and their primary use and mode of action. Details of prescription and clinical application are available in general pharmacology sources referenced in Chapter 1 and from manufacturers' literature.

CARDIOVASCULAR SYSTEM

The entire cardiovascular system functions as an interdependent set of units. This is illustrated in Figure 17–1. Such a visual outline is useful for understanding the site of action of a particular drug (e.g., heart, pulmonary circulation, arterial or venous circulation). It is also helpful in understanding how changes at one point (e.g., the venous return) can affect the rest of the system, such as the cardiac output.

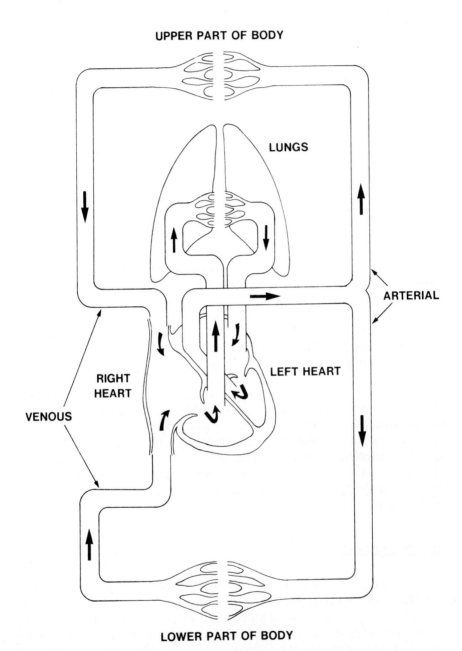

FIG 17–1. Simplified illustration of the integrated cardiopulmonary circuit.

Factors Affecting Blood Pressure

Blood pressure, or more accurately mean arterial pressure, exemplifies the interrelated nature of the cardiovascular system:

Mean arterial pressure = cardiac output × total peripheral resistance.

This equation, which relates the two primary factors determining blood pressure, is the basic pressure-flow-resistance relationship familiar from airway resistance: $P = \dot{V} \times R$, where P is pressure, $\dot{V}$ is gas flow, and R is resistance, defined by Poiseuille's law in laminar flow. As with gas flow, resistance with blood flow depends on viscosity, and more importantly, vessel radius. Hence, vasoconstrictors and vasodilators can markedly alter vascular resistance by influencing the radius, or size, of the blood vessel. Increased vessel size decreases resistance, and as the equation indicates, blood pressure falls if cardiac output does not compensate.

Just as resistance depends on more basic factors, so cardiac output is determined by blood volume, venous return, and contractile force of the heart. Figure 17–2 indicates the relationship of these factors to arterial pressure. The goal of adequate arterial pressure is tissue perfusion and oxygenation. Increasing blood pressure by severe vasoconstriction may actually impair tissue perfusion, although arterial pressure may be satisfactory.

In general, cardiac agents, both stimulants and antiarrhythmics, are aimed at promoting adequate pressure. Drugs targeted at the circulatory system are

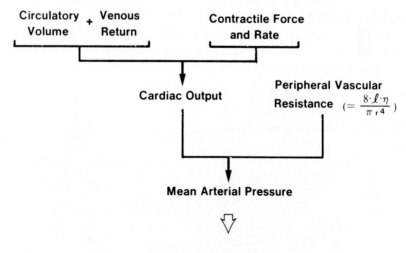

FIG 17–2.   Interrelationship of factors influencing mean arterial pressure necessary for tissue perfusion.

intended to alter peripheral resistance, the second term in the equation; they can lower blood pressure by increasing blood vessel radius (dilatation), or raise it by vasoconstriction. Vasoconstrictors, or vasopressors, are usually reserved for nonhypovolemic shock (i.e., acute hypotensive states when excess dilatation must be quickly reversed to maintain perfusion pressure.

The Heart

In identifying and briefly characterizing drugs that affect cardiac function directly, it is assumed that normal electrophysiology of the heart and basic cardiac arrhythmias are understood. Figure 17–3 illustrates the main cardiac events in a normal heart beat and their corresponding electrical counterparts seen on an electrocardiogram (ECG). The four major areas of the heart of importance for cardiac drugs are the sinoatrial (SA) node, the atrial muscle, the atrioventricular (AV) node, and the ventricular muscle. Normal conduction of the electrical pacemaker signal arising spontaneously from the SA node results in the ECG tracing with a P wave, QRS complex, and a T wave. The excitatory and conductive system of the cardiac muscle represents a particular application of the physiology of membrane and action potentials. The action potential of pacemaker cells in the SA node gives a different appearance from that of myocardial cells and Purkinje fibers. Pacemaker cells possess automatic depolarization and are more permeable to calcium ions than other myocardial cells. The automatic depolarization of SA node cells is largely a function of calcium influx, unlike other myocardial cells.

Action Potentials

Action potentials of both pacemaker and myocardial cells are illustrated in Figure 17–4. The action potential of myocardial cells is divided into five phases. *Phase 0* is the sudden and rapid depolarization when the membrane

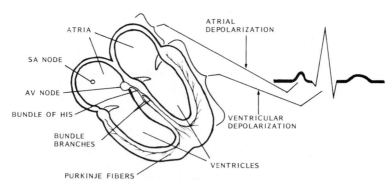

FIG 17–3. Basic cardiac structure and corresponding electrical activity seen on a normal ECG tracing.

ACTION POTENTIAL

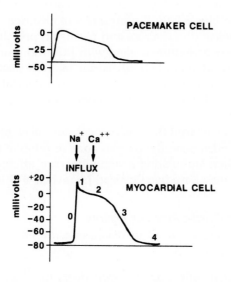

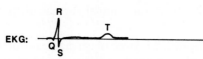

FIG 17–4. Action potentials of pacemaker and myocardial cells, with ion influx and five phases indicated.

is brought to threshold at the beginning of the action potential. There is a rapid inward flow of sodium ions termed the *fast response* associated with this sudden depolarization. In *phase 1*, there is an early, incomplete repolarization, which is stopped by the *phase 2* slow current influx of calcium ions. This second, slower influx of calcium is termed the *slow response* or *slow channel* influx. This depolarizing action of calcium influx overlaps the repolarization of the sodium pump and produces the plateau of phase 2. *Phase 3* consists of rapid repolarization, returning the myocardial cell to its resting state of *phase 4*. Figure 17–4 shows the ion influxes at their point of occurrence during an action potential, as well as the corresponding tracing of a surface ECG. The electrophysiology just presented is the basis for describing the mode of action of cardiac, especially antiarrhythmic, drugs, which are characterized as fast or slow channel inhibitors. Changes produced by drugs in depolarization (fast channel inhibitors) will cause changes in the QRS interval of the ECG, whereas drugs affecting repolarization during phase 3 cause alterations in the QT interval.

Basic Arrhythmias

Normal cardiac function also requires an adequate force of contraction resulting from the electrical depolarization recorded on the ECG. Failure to mechanically pump blood, *with* the presence of electrical activity, is referred to as *electromechanical dissociation,* and perfusion pressure falls.

The basic cardiac arrhythmias seen with ECG monitoring, and for which cardiac agents are used, include bradycardia, tachycardias (atrial, nodal, ventricular), premature beats (atrial, nodal, ventricular), atrial and ventricular fibrillation, asystole, and degrees of heart conduction block (first, second, and third degree).

It should be remembered that the myocardium itself requires oxygen, and the effect of cardiac drugs on the oxygen consumption of the heart is important to consider when stimulating a failing heart or attempting to correct an arrhythmia, which may have been caused by myocardial ischemia.

Terminology of Cardiovascular Agents

A number of terms are used in discussing the effects of cardiac agents and are defined for reference.

Chronotropic: Agent affecting the *rate* of cardiac contraction. Very low (<40) or high (>140) heart rates lower cardiac output and can cause other arrhythmias.

Inotropic: Agent affecting the *force* of cardiac contraction. Both calcium and digitalis are examples of positive inotropes (increased force). Sympathomimetics such as isoproterenol or epinephrine are both chronotropic and inotropic: They increase force and rate.

Preload: Load or tension on the cardiac muscle as it begins to contract. This is taken as the quantity of blood in the ventricle at the beginning of systole. Starling's law relates to the amount of blood in the heart at end diastole: *The more the heart fills and ventricular fibers stretch during diastole, the greater the cardiac work during systole.* Or, the greater the preload, the more work the heart will do. Some cardiac agents, such as digitalis, can decrease the work of the heart by improving contractile force and ventricular emptying, thereby decreasing the preload, in accordance with Starling's law.

Afterload: Amount of resistance against which the heart must pump. Increased afterload can increase ventricular contractile force and decrease stroke volume and cardiac output. Since peripheral vascular resistance can be an important factor determining afterload, drugs affecting circulatory resistance, such as vasoconstrictors or vasodilators, can affect afterload. *Venous* vasodilatation may affect and lower cardiac *preload.*

Central Venous and Pulmonary Artery Wedge Pressure

Filling pressures in the right and left sides of the heart are indicated by central venous pressure (CVP) and pulmonary artery wedge pressure (PAWP) respectively. While a normal CVP in young adults is 0 to 2 mm Hg, 3 to 6 mmHg is often considered acceptable in critical care units. CVP can be increased by a rise in blood volume, loss of right ventricular function whether or not secondary to left ventricular failure, and by increased systemic vasoconstriction that reduces peripheral storage capacity. A normal PAWP is 6 to 12 mm Hg; PAWP increases with left ventricular failure or with fluid overload. These terms and the concepts they represent are used to characterize the various cardiovascular agents presented.

DRUGS AFFECTING THE HEART

Cardiac Glycosides

The term *digitalis* is used to refer to the entire group of related substances called glycosides. Official digitalis is the dried leaf of the foxglove plant.

Digitalis Purpurea. The cardiac glycosides have their main effect on the myocardium, to increase the force of contraction, a positive inotropic action. The main sources of glycosides are the following:

Digitalis purpurea (foxglove): contains digitoxin, gitoxin, and gitaloxin.

Digitalis lanata (a foxglove species): contains digoxin.

Strophanthus gratus: contains another glycoside, ouabain.

Generally, ouabain has the most rapid onset of action and shortest duration, digoxin (Lanoxin) is intermediate in onset and duration, while digitoxin is the longest acting. For immediate, acute use, digoxin would be preferred to digitoxin.

Mode of Action

Digitalis inactivates the sodium pump and causes an increase in intracellular sodium, which is accompanied by an increased calcium influx. Calcium promotes an increased force of contraction by the actomyosin complex, resulting in a positive inotropic effect. There is also a decrease in heart rate because of vagal stimulation and impaired AV conduction, a direct effect on the conducting tissue. In fact, this effect constitutes a potential hazard of heart block with digitalis.

Clinical Use

The primary uses of digitalis, or the cardiac glycosides, are as a cardiotonic in CHF, and as an antiarrhythmic with atrial flutter or fibrillation. As a cardiotonic, digitalis increases cardiac output, decreases heart size and central venous pressure, and improves diuresis as a result of improved cardiac output. All of these effects are due to increased cardiac contractile force. The antiarrhythmic effect is caused by slowing AV conduction. With irregular and rapid atrial impulses, this slows the ventricular rate and increases force of contraction.

Amrinone (Inocor)

Amrinone is a unique cardiotonic agent with both positive inotropic and vasodilating effects. As a result of these effects, amrinone causes an increase in cardiac output. Preload and afterload are reduced by its relaxation of vascular smooth muscle. The drug improves left ventricular function in CHF without causing symptoms of myocardial ischemia.

The mechanism of action of amrinone is not fully understood. It is *not* a glycoside such as digitalis, nor a catecholamine such as a beta agonist. It inhibits phosphodiesterase activity in myocardial cells, causing increased cyclic AMP levels.

Use of this agent is for short-term management of CHF in patients who do not respond to digitalis, diurectics, or vasodilators.

Milrinone Lactate (Primacor)

Milrinone represents a new class of inotropic agents with phosphodiesterase-inhibiting activity. At suitable concentrations, milrinone inhibits phosphodiesterase enzyme in cardiac and vascular muscle. The drug is a positive inotrope and a vasodilator. In patients with CHF and depressed myocardial function, milrinone can increase cardiac output and decrease systemic vascular resistance. It can have a favorable inotropic effect in digitalized patients. Milrinone is not a glycoside nor a beta agonist. It is used as short-term intravenous therapy in CHF.

Antiarrhythmic Agents

Antiarrhythmic agents are classified into four groups, based on their effect on the action potential and electrophysiology of the myocardial cells. The four classes, with a brief description of each, are listed in Table 17–1, along with antiarrhythmic agents representing each class. Each drug is briefly described and its clinical use indicated. More detailed presentations of antiarrhythmic agents and their action based on electrophysiology of the heart can be found in Coodley et al. (1986), Podrid (1985), Singh et al. (1980), Mathewson (1982), Zipes (1981), and Nademanee and Singh (1982).

TABLE 17–1.

Classification of Antiarrhythmic Agents

Class	Agents
I	
Membrane stabilizing or local anesthetics that depress phase 0 (depolarization); prolongation of the action potential and QRS interval by most agents	Quinidine Procainamide (Pronestyl) Disopyramide (Norpace) Lidocaine (Xylocaine) Phenytoin (Dilantin) Tocainide (Tonocard) Mexiletine (Mexitil) Flecainide (Tambocor) Encainide (Enkaid) Moricizine (Ethmozine) Propafenone (Rythmol)
II	
Beta-adrenergic blocking agents	Propranolol (Inderal) Acebutolol (Sectral) Esmolol (Brevibloc) Sotalol (Betapace)
III	
Prolongation of phase 3 (repolarization), with an increase in action potential duration	Bretylium (Bretylol) Amiodarone (Cordarone)
IV	
Calcium (slow channel) blocking agents	Verapamil (Calan, Isoptin) Diltiazem (Cardizem)

Class I Antiarrhythmic Agents

Class I antiarrhythmic agents in general act by depressing the fast, inward sodium flow in myocardial cells, to depress their automaticity and to increase their resting potential. There are additional differences in the modes of action among agents in this group, which lead to further subdivisions within the Class I group, to Class IA, Class IB, and Class IC. A Class IA antiarrhythmic is represented by procainamide, a drug that lengthens the refractory period during phases 1 and 2 and decreases the resting potential. This effect on the action potential is illustrated in Figure 17–5 for the Class IA agent procainamide, only.

The net effect of the different types of Class I agents is a decrease in ex-

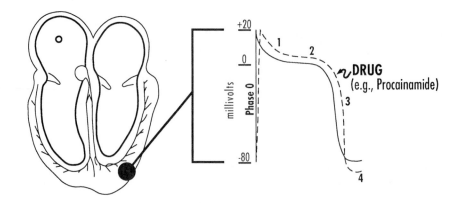

CLASS IA ANTIARRHYTHMIC

FIG 17–5. Effect of the Class IA antiarrhythmic drug procainamide on the action potential of the myocardial cell. The modes of action for Class IB and IC agents are not represented by this illustration.

citability of the myocardium, which makes these drugs useful for treating atrial and ventricular fibrillation, flutter, or premature ventricular contractions (PVCs).

Representative agents in this group are briefly characterized below.

Quinidine is the dextrorotatory isomer of quinine, which latter agent was found by Wenckebach to stop atrial fibrillation when used for treating malaria. Quinidine is more effective than quinine, however, with atrial fibrillation.

Uses: atrial fibrillation and flutter, paroxysmal atrial tachycardia (PAT), ventricular tachycardia, and PVCs.

Lidocaine (Xylocaine) is a local anesthetic, given intravenously for cardiac ventricular arrhythmias.

Uses: for control of PVCs or tachycardia, especially in cardiac surgery or with myocardial infarction.

Procainamide (Pronestyl) is the amide corresponding to the ester procaine and is more stable than the latter. It is given by mouth or intravenously.

Uses: to treat ventricular ectopic beats, ventricular tachycardia, and atrial arrhythmias.

Disopyramide (Norpace) is an antiarrhythmic agent that has parasympatholytic (anticholinergic) side effects such as dry mouth and urinary retention. In contrast to quinidine and procainamide, disopyramide has a *negative* inotropic effect and increases vascular resistance.

Uses: treatment of supraventricular arrhythmias such as PAT, atrial flutter and atrial fibrillation, as well as ventricular tachycardia.

Phenytoin (Dilantin) is a drug used for epileptic seizures and also has antiarrhythmic properties. It is used for atrial and ventricular arrhythmias, especially if caused by digitalis toxicity.

Uses: PAT and digitalis-induced ventricular ectopic rhythms.

Tocainide (Tonocard) is a congener of lidocaine and has similar side effects. Failure to respond to lidocaine usually indicates poor results with tocainide.

Use: control of PVC, and ventricular tachycardia.

Mexiletine (Mexitil) is another congener of lidocaine, given orally or intravenously.

Use: suppression of ventricular premature beats or tachycardia.

Flecainide (Tambocor) has local anesthetic activity, is a negative inotrope, and reduces left ventricular function, which can cause worsening of CHF.

Use: treatment of ventricular ectopy.

Encainide (Enkaid) has electrophysiologic effects similar to flecainide, *without* the negative inotropic effect or depression of left ventricular function. Encainide inhibits automaticity and reduces membrane excitability.

Use: sustained ventricular tachycardia.

Moricizine (Ethmozine) reduces the fast inward sodium current to stabilize the myocardial membrane. Moricizine also has local anesthetic activity. It can actually shorten phase 2 and 3 repolarization and the overall action potential duration.

Use: sustained ventricular tachycardia. Moricizine can promote arrhythmias as an adverse reaction.

Propafenone (Rythmol) has local anesthetic effects and directly stabilizes myocardial membranes. It prolongs the effective refractory period and depresses spontaneous automaticity.

Use: life-threatening sustained ventricular tachycardia.

Class II Antiarrhythmic Agents

Class II antiarrhythmic agents are beta-adrenergic blocking agents, or beta-receptor antagonists. These agents act by blocking β_1 receptors in the heart, to control arrhythmias. Their mode of action is illustrated in Figure 17–6. Some, but not all, of the beta-receptor antagonists are cardioselective in their blocking action. The beta-blocking agents used for arrhythmias are listed below by their receptor preference.

- β_1 selective
  Acebutolol (Sectral)
  Esmolol (Brevibloc)
- β_1 and β_2 antagonists
  Propranolol (Inderal)
  Sotalol (Betapace)

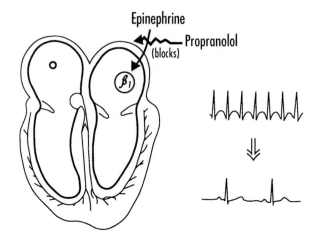

CLASS II ANTIARRHYTHMIC

FIG 17–6. Mode of action of Class II antiarrhythmic agents such as propranolol.

Many of the beta-blocking agents are used to control hypertension and will be reviewed in the section on antihypertensive agents. As antiarrhythmics, the blockade of cardiac beta receptors reduces heart rate, prolongs AV conduction, and reduces contractile force. Propranolol and esmolol are used to slow supraventricular tachycardias. Propranolol can be used for ventricular tachycardia. Acebutolol is used for PVCs and sotalol for sustained ventricular tachycardia.

A side effect of importance for respiratory care is the induction of wheezing and increased airway resistance with the nonselective beta blockers, such as propranolol, resulting from blockade of β_2 receptors in the airway (Patakas et al., 1983).

Class III Antiarrhythmic Agents

Class III antiarrhythmic agents act by prolonging the duration of phase 3 repolarization. This is illustrated in Figure 17–7. This causes an increase in action potential duration and the refractory period. There is an increase in the threshold for ventricular fibrillation. The two agents in this class, bretylium and amiodarone, are briefly characterized below.

Bretylium tosylate (Bretylol), because of the effects described for Class III agents, is used to prevent and treat ventricular fibrillation. Bretylium also inhibits norepinephrine release, causing a sympathetic blockade.

Amiodarone HCl (Cordarone) also prolongs the action potential duration and refractory period. In addition it produces alpha- and beta-adrenergic

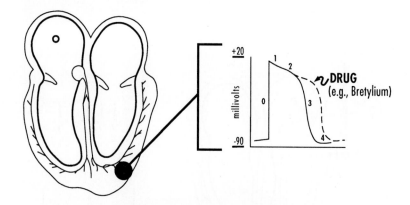

CLASS III ANTIARRHYTHMIC

FIG 17–7. Illustration of the effect of a Class III antiarrhythmic agent on the action potential of the myocardial cell.

inhibition. Amiodarone is used for recurrent ventricular fibrillation and to treat hemodynamically unstable ventricular tachycardia. A pulmonary toxic reaction consisting of pneumonitis has occurred in some patients.

Class IV Antiarrhythmic Agents

Class IV antiarrhythmic agents act by inhibiting the slow channel influx of calcium, both in the pacemaker cells and in the myocardial cells. The contraction of vascular smooth muscle also depends on the influx of calcium ions, and these agents are used for coronary artery vasodilation and for treating hypertension. The calcium channel blocking agents, which are also termed slow channel blockers and calcium antagonists, exert their antiarrhythmic effect by depressing the automaticity of atrial tissue and pacemaker cells and by slowing conduction velocity through the AV node. Their mode of action is illustrated in Figure 17–8.

The calcium channel blocking agents usually used for cardiac arrhythmias include the following:

Verapamil (Calan, Isoptin)
Diltiazem (Cardizem)

Verapamil, as well as diltiazem, are used for supraventricular tachycardia.

Other Antiarrhythmic Agents

Adenosine (Adenocard) is an endogenous nucleoside, previously mentioned when discussing the mode of action of xanthines (see Chapter 7). The

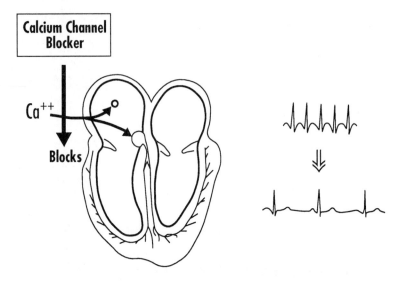

CLASS IV ANTIARRHYTHMIC

FIG 17–8. Conceptual illustration of the effect of Class IV, calcium channel blocking agents, on the heart.

drug slows conduction through the AV node and is used to treat paroxysmal supraventricular tachycardia.

Calcium Chloride is an agent used to provide calcium ions necessary for cardiac contractility. Calcium ions increase myocardial contractile force, producing an effect similar to digitalis preparations.

Use: to reverse electromechanical dissociation (electrical activity without mechanical pumping force) and increase cardiac output. Calcium is no longer recommended during cardiac resuscitation and for maintenance of cardiac output unless there is hyperkalemia, hypocalcemia, or calcium channel blocking toxicity.

Atropine is a parasympatholytic previously discussed as a bronchodilating agent (see Chapter 6). Vagal slowing of the sinus and AV nodes is *blocked* by atropine with its parasympatholytic effect; this results in an increased heart rate.

Uses: treatment of severe sinus bradycardia and perhaps AV block.

Cardiac Stimulants

Epinephrine

Epinephrine is an endogenous catecholamine classified as a sympathomimetic that stimulates both alpha and beta receptors. Because of its effect on both alpha and beta receptors, epinephrine causes a number of results in the cardiovascular system. The β_1 stimulation (cardiac receptors) increases heart rate and contractile force. Alpha stimulation can increase systemic vascular resistance, which together with increased cardiac performance can elevate the blood pressure. β_2 stimulation can cause bronchodilatation and dilatation of blood vessels to deep muscle.

Uses: to treat asystole or fine ventricular fibrillation prior to electrical countershock. It is also used in the presence of inadequate pump action in the heart.

NOTE: Intracardiac administration of epinephrine can cause bleeding and cardiac tamponade, or pneumothorax. Epinephrine is given intravenously during cardiopulmonary resuscitation or even by direct intratracheal instillation of a 1:10,000 solution.

Isoproterenol

Isoproterenol is classified as a potent beta-sympathomimetic agent, also previously discussed as a bronchodilator. Stimulation of β_1 cardiac receptors has a positive chronotropic and inotropic effect on the heart. However, the resulting increase in cardiac output is associated with an increased myocardial oxygen consumption, which can cause ischemia or extended infarction.

Uses: emergency control of severe bradycardia that does not respond to atropine and is resulting in inadequate cardiac output. Isoproterenol decreases systemic vascular resistance as a result of its β_2 effect.

Dobutamine (Dobutrex)

Dobutamine is a synthetic catecholamine that has a primary and preferential effect as a β_1 stimulant, with only slight indirect effects. The cardiovascular effect is inotropic: The contractile force of the heart is improved. Heart rate (chronotropic) response is less than with isoproterenol. In addition, dobutamine does not cause renal vasoconstriction. Total peripheral resistance is not substantially changed, making dobutamine an attractive agent for increasing cardiac output and supporting blood pressure without peripheral vasoconstriction, which would only increase afterload and myocardial work. Dobutamine is therapeutically used intravenously in CHF to counter depression of ventricular function. Dobutamine differs from dopamine in that dopamine will not only stimulate the heart to increase cardiac output, but will also change peripheral vascular resistance in a dose-dependent fashion. The drug is antagonized by beta-blocking agents such as propranolol.

DRUGS AFFECTING THE CIRCULATION

Circulatory System

The most important purpose of the circulatory system is to supply oxygen-saturated blood, and therefore oxygen itself, to the tissues. Because of the interdependent nature of the cardiovascular system, changes in vascular resistance can affect other parts of the system. For example, if the venous reservoir is increased with a sufficient dosage of vasodilator or with morphine, venous return *decreases,* along with cardiac preload, allowing the heart to contract with less work in the event it had been distended as in CHF. In such a case, cardiac output may even increase since the heart is functioning at a more efficient point on the Starling curve.

Agents that affect the tone of the circulatory system act by a variety of means to alter peripheral vascular resistance. They are used as vasodilators to treat hypertensive states, as coronary artery vasodilators to treat angina, and as vasoconstrictors to treat severe hypotension or shock.

Hypertension and Treatment

Adult hypertension is defined as blood pressure of 140/90 mm Hg, or higher. If there is no primary disorder such as aldosteronism, pheochromocytoma, neurological disorders, or anxiety states, this is referred to as *essential* hypertension. Ferguson and Vlasses (1986) give a good overview of hypertensive emergencies. A variety of drugs, as well as mechanisms of action, exist for lowering blood pressure. Table 17–2 classifies representative agents by these mechanisms of action. Each group of antihypertensive drugs will be discussed to clarify the mode of action, rather than presenting each drug separately. The treatment of essential hypertension follows a stepped approach

TABLE 17–2.

Classification of Antihypertensive Agents

Generic Name	Trade Name
Diuretics	
Thiazides (e.g., chlorothiazide)	Diuril
Indapamide	Lozol
Furosemide	Lasix
Amiloride	Midamor
Spironolactone	Aldactone
Antiadrenergic (central activity)	
Methyldopa	Aldomet
Clonidine	Catapres
Guanabenz	Wytensin
Guanfacine	Tenex

(Continued.)

Antiadrenergic (peripheral activity)
Reserpine	Serpasil
Guanethidine	Ismelin
Guanadrel	Hylorel
Prazosin	Minipress
Terazosin	Hytrin
Doxazosin	Cardura

Beta-adrenergic blockade
Metoprolol	Lopressor
Atenolol	Tenormin
Acebutol	Sectral
Nadolol	Corgard
Pindolol	Visken
Timolol	Blocadren
Propranolol	Inderal
Penbutolol	Levatol
Bisprolol	Zebeta
Carteolol	Cartrol
Betaxolol	Kerlone

Alpha- and beta-adrenergic blockade
Labetalol	Normodyne, Trandate

Vasodilators (direct acting)
Hydralazine	Apresoline
Minoxidil	Loniten

Angiotensin converting enzyme inhibitors
Captopril	Capoten
Enalapril	Vasotec
Lisinopril	Prinivil
Quinapril	Accupril
Ramipril	Altace
Fosinopril	Monopril

Calcium channel blocking agents
Verapamil	Calan, Isoptin
Nicardipine	Cardene

Emergency (acute) antihypertensives
Nitroprusside	Nipride
Diazoxide	Hyperstat
Trimethaphan	Arfonad
Nitroglycerin injection	Tridil

Miscellaneous agents
Mecamylamine	Inversine
Pargyline	Eutonyl

that uses a cumulative selection of agents from the groups in Table 17–2. In brief, the management of essential hypertension has usually involved the following ordered approach:

1. Nonpharmacologic control of weight, dietary sodium and alcohol restriction, smoking cessation, and exercise.

2. Use of a thiazide diuretic or beta blocker.
3. Addition of adrenergic inhibitors, calcium channel blockers, angiotensin converting enzyme inhibitors, or other types of antihypertensive agents.

It should be noted that this stepped approach is being less rigorously adhered to now than in the past. The choice of a particular type of antihypertensive agent depends on the presence and type of coexisting disease a person may have. For example, a combination of hypertension and angina may be best treated with a calcium channel blocking agent. Likewise, a beta blocker would be avoided in a hypertensive patient with asthma.

The mechanisms by which different groups of antihypertensive agents act are illustrated in Figure 17–9, which will be referred to as each group is presented. A good review of drug therapy in managing hypertension is found in O'Malley and O'Brien (1980).

Antihypertensive Drug Classes

Diuretics

A complete overview of the classes of diuretics will be presented in Chapter 18. A number of diuretics are used for management of hypertension, based partly on their diuretic effect, which increases sodium loss, and also on a pos-

ANTIHYPERTENSIVE MECHANISMS

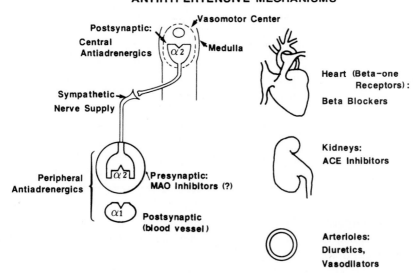

FIG 17–9. Conceptual illustration of the various mechanisms and sites of action for antihypertensive drugs.

sible direct effect on blood vessels, to lower vascular resistance. The thiazides, such as chlorothiazide, can reduce vascular resistance and are usually preferred for control of hypertension. The reduction of plasma volume, which will lower blood pressure, is not maintained with chronic administration of the diuretic, which reinforces the theory that the antihypertensive effect is not caused by diuresis alone. Other diuretics with antihypertensive properties include spironolactone, furosemide, and ethacrynic acid.

Centrally Acting Antiadrenergic Agents

The mechanism by which centrally acting antiadrenergic agents, or α_2 sympathetic agonists, lower blood pressure is based on the distinction between α_1 and α_2 receptors. This distinction was presented in Chapter 4 and should be reviewed if necessary. Alpha receptor subtypes are analogous to beta receptor subtypes. Just as β_1 receptors in the heart stimulate and excite, so α_1 receptors in peripheral blood vessels stimulate and cause constriction, which can raise blood pressure. Similarly, as β_2 receptors in bronchioles or blood vessels inhibit and cause relaxation, so α_2 receptors in the brain stem and other areas of the central nervous system inhibit and suppress sympathetic activity. Just as the differentiation of beta receptors was based on the different responses to beta stimulants (some excitatory [β_1] and some inhibitory [β_2]) such as isoproterenol, so alpha receptors were subdivided because of contradictory responses, some excitatory (α_1) and some inhibitory (α_2). For example, phenylephrine was identified in Chapter 4 as an alpha stimulant that causes vasoconstriction. However, clonidine is also an alpha stimulant, or alpha-adrenergic agent, but this agent causes a *lowering* of blood pressure, although there is a transient initial vasoconstriction. Because of these opposite effects, two distinct types of alpha receptors were postulated. The model of alpha receptor subtypes is slightly complicated by their location. In the *periphery*, α_1 receptors are located postsynaptically (e.g., on blood vessels), and α_2 receptors are thought to be presynaptic (e.g., on the terminal neuron membrane). *Centrally*, α_2 receptors are considered to be most likely postsynaptic, although a presynaptic location is still debated. This is seen in Figure 17–9 and is summarized as follows:

Peripheral α_1: postsynaptic and excitatory.

Central α_2: postsynaptic and inhibitory.

Agents in this group of antihypertensives act by stimulating central alpha-adrenergic (α_2) receptors in the vasomotor center of the central nervous system. This inhibits the cardioaccelerator and vasoconstrictor centers, and in general, inhibits sympathetic outflow activity to peripheral sympathetic sites. With clonidine, long-term therapy keeps peripheral resistance decreased while cardiac output can return to pretreatment values. It was previously thought that methyldopa acted by inhibiting the enzyme dopa-decarboxylase to prevent the formation of norepinephrine in peripheral sympathetic nerves.

However, its antihypertensive effect is probably due to its metabolism to alpha-methyl norepinephrine, which in turn stimulates central α_2 receptors to decrease sympathetic activity. A clear review of central alpha receptors is given in Hoffman and Lefkowitz (1980), Gross (1983), Kobinger (1983), and van Zwieten and Timmermans (1983).

Peripherally Acting Antidrenergic Agents

This group of antihypertensive agents generally act by interfering with peripheral sympathetic activity at the neuroeffector, or terminal, site (not the ganglia). The rauwolfia derivatives include reserpine, as well as deserpidine (Harmonyl), rescinnamine (Moderil), and alseroxylon (Rauwiloid). Rauwolfia alkaloid is obtained from the plant *Rauwolfia serpentina.* The rauwolfia group, as well as guanethidine and guanadrel, act by inhibiting norepinephrine release and depleting norepinephrine stores in postganglionic adrenergic nerve endings (Fig 17–9). This causes a relaxation of vascular smooth muscle and a decrease in total peripheral resistance, with a lowering of blood pressure. Prazosin, terazosin, and doxazosin cause essentially the same effect on vascular resistance by blocking postsynaptic α_1 adrenergic receptors. Although not in Table 17–2, phentolamine (Regitine), phenoxybenzamine (Dibenzyline), and metyrosine (Demser) are alpha-blocking agents that are mainly used to lower blood pressure in pheochromocytoma. This condition most often involves a tumor of the adrenal gland, which results in elevated catecholamine levels and hypertension.

Beta-Adrenergic Blockade

Drugs in the beta-adrenergic blockade group are identified in Table 17–2. The effect of these agents in lowering blood pressure is mediated chiefly by their blocking action at β_1-receptor sites in the heart. Both chronotropic and inotropic responses to beta-adrenergic stimulation are inhibited, cardiac output is lowered, and blood pressure decreases. This mechanism avoids side effects of orthostatic hypotension or sexual dysfunction. The β_2 blockade by the nonselective drugs such as propranolol or penbutolol can cause passive bronchial constriction, increased airway resistance, and a decreased response to exogenous beta agonists such as beta bronchodilators, an interaction of importance in respiratory care (Patakas et al., 1983).

Alpha- and Beta-Adrenergic Blockade

Labetalol acts to lower blood pressure by competitively blocking postsynaptic α_1 receptors, as well as beta receptors (both β_1 and β_2). This is a combination of the mechanisms seen in the preceding two groups of drugs.

Vasodilators

Hydralazine, minoxidil, and nitroglycerin (given intravenously) all lower blood pressure by a direct relaxation of vascular smooth muscle. Hydralazine acts primarily on arteriolar sites and may cause reflex tachycardia, necessitating an additional agent to block sympathetic activity (beta-adrenergic blocker or centrally acting alpha stimulant). The exact mechanism of minoxidil on vascular smooth muscle is not known; it may block calcium uptake needed for contraction.

Angiotensin Converting Enzyme Inhibition

The angiotensin converting enzyme inhibitors act by interference with the renin-angiotensin system, outlined in Figure 17–10. The converting enzyme that produces angiotensin II is peptidyl dipeptidase. Drugs such as captopril and enalapril inhibit this enzyme and hence inhibit the production of angiotensin II, blocking the potential for vasoconstriction and increased arterial pressure.

Acute Antihypertensive Agents

Sodium nitroprusside exerts a direct action on peripheral blood vessels, causing vasodilatation of both arterial and venous circulations. It is used for acute hypertensive emergencies, since its effect begins rapidly with intravenous administration and ends as infusion is stopped (Ziesche and Franciosa, 1977). The half-life of the drug is several minutes. Nitroprusside is metabolized to thiocyanate, with cyanide as an intermediate product. However, toxicity due to the cyanide is rare. Although not a diuretic, diazoxide is a chemi-

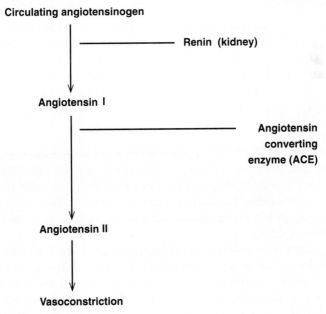

FIG 17–10. The renin-angiotensin system, showing the site of action for angiotensin converting enzyme (ACE).

cal relative of the thiazide diuretics, which has a potent peripheral vasodilator effect on precapillary smooth muscle. It is used intravenously in hypertensive emergencies to produce an immediate drop in blood pressure, which lasts for hours. Unlike diuretics, diazoxide causes water and sodium retention. Trimethaphan is a short-acting ganglionic blocking agent that blocks both sympathetic and parasympathetic ganglia. It also has a direct peripheral vasodilator action, causing peripheral blood pooling and a decrease in blood pressure.

Miscellaneous Agents

Mecamylamine is a potent ganglionic blocker taken orally. It primarily causes postural hypotensive effects and is less frequently used because of side effects. Pargyline is a monoamine oxidase (MAO) inhibitor. MAO was identified in Chapter 4 as one of the enzymes inactivating norepinephrine. MAO inhibitors were first used therapeutically to treat depression. However, such inhibitors are unexpectedly able to cause hypotension, an effect opposite to what would be expected. Their hypotensive effect is thought to be caused by accumulation of false transmitters or by accumulated norepinephrine inhibiting its own release. There are dangerous interactions between MAO inhibitors and foods such as cheese or wine, which contain tyramine; such interactions can lead to a hypertensive crisis.

Antianginal Agents

The antianginal agents are primarily used to treat angina pectoris, defined as a paroxysmal precordial pain with a feeling of suffocation. Angina is often triggered by exertion or excitement in coronary artery disease and is caused by inadequate blood flow through the coronary arteries to the myocardium. Table 17–3 lists examples of three categories of drugs used in the treatment of angina.

Nitrates

The nitrates are a collection of drugs that act as coronary and systemic vasodilators and are chiefly employed to relieve anginal pain. Nitrates relax vascular smooth muscle. Venous dilatation predominates with nitroglycerin, which decreases cardiac preload and oxygen consumption. Nitrates also redistribute coronary blood circulation along collateral channels, and large coronary arteries are dilated.

Nitroglycerin is probably the best known of the nitrate antianginal agents and is available in the most dosage forms, including intravenous, sublingual, translingual spray, transmucosal tablet (placed between the cheek and gum, or the lip and gum), a topical ointment, and a transdermal pad, as well as oral tablets and capsules. Amyl nitrate is inhaled from a crushed capsule

TABLE 17-3.

Categories of Antianginal Agents

Generic Name	Trade Names
Nitrates	
Amyl nitrite	—
Nitroglycerin	Nitrostat, Nitrogard, Nitroglyn, Minitran
Isosorbide mononitrate	ISMO
Isosorbide dinitrate	Isordil
Erythrityl tetranitrate	Cardilate
Pentaerythritol tetranitrate	Pentylan, Peritrate
Calcium Antagonists	
Nifedipine	Procardia
Diltiazem	Cardizem
Verapamil	Calan, Isoptin
Amlodipine	Norvasc
Bepridil	Vascor
Nicardipine	Cardene
Beta Adrenergic Blocking Agents	
Nadolol	Corgard
Propranolol	Inderal
Atenolol	Tenormin
Metoprolol	Lopressor

placed under the nose. Specific examples of nitrate agents used for angina are listed in Table 17-3.

Nitrates can cause methemoglobinemia, in a dose-related fashion, by oxidizing hemoglobin to methemoglobin. Clinically important methemoglobin is rare with conventional dose levels.

Calcium Channel Blocking Agents

Calcium channel blocking agents, or calcium antagonists, have been previously discussed as antiarrhythmic agents and as antihypertensive agents. They can also be used as antianginal agents. Calcium antagonists dilate coronary arteries and inhibit coronary artery spasm to increase myocardial oxygen delivery. They are used in vasospastic angina (Prinzmetal's variant), as well as stable, effort-associated angina. Calcium antagonists also dilate peripheral arterioles and reduce afterload, which reduces myocardial oxygen demand. They are useful if nitrates or beta-blocking agents are not tolerated. Hypotension is a potential side effect. Examples of these agents are given in Table 17-3.

Because of their potential for relaxing bronchial smooth muscle by inhibiting calcium influx, these agents have been investigated as possible bronchodilators and specifically as antiasthmatic drugs. Results with currently available agents, even delivered by aerosol, have been disappointing. However, the value of investigation with these drugs has been to point to newer generations of agents that are more bronchoselective and to elucidate the mechanisms of calcium activity in cell function. This may result in new modes of blocking calcium-induced bronchoconstriction and mediator release. Good reviews of calcium channel blockers in airway disease are in Mathewson (1985), Ahmed and Abraham (1985), and Middleton (1985). Rossi and Antman (1983) and Karlsberg (1981) review the use of calcium channel blockers as cardiac drugs.

Beta-Adrenergic Blocking Agents

Beta-adrenergic blocking agents are also used for treatment of angina. Specific examples of such agents are given in Table 17–3 also. Their use as antianginal drugs is based on their blocking effect on cardiac β_1 receptors. By blocking β_1-mediated increases in heart rate, systolic blood pressure, and cardiac contractile force, beta-receptor antagonists reduce myocardial oxygen demand.

Vasoconstricting Agents (Vasopressors)

Vasopressors are used in the treatment of shock, a condition caused by inadequate tissue perfusion. The following types of shock indicate the cause:

Hypovolemic: fluid loss.

Cardiogenic: cardiac dysfunction.

Septic: septicemia.

Blood flow obstruction: embolus, aneurysm.

Neurogenic: spinal injury or drug induced.

Anaphylactic: hypersensitivity reaction.

The primary goal of vasopressor therapy is the support of blood pressure until the underlying cause of shock can be reversed. There are two general mechanisms for increasing blood pressure: positive inotropic effect and vasostriction. The agents in this group range from positive inotropes (such as isoproterenol, dopamine, and dobutamine) to mixed inotropic and pressor effects (with epinephrine, norepinephrine, mephentermine, and ephedrine) to fairly pure vasoconstrictors (such as metaraminol, methoxamine and phenylephrine). Purcell (1982) provides an overview of this class.

Phenylephrine (Neo-Synephrine)

Phenylephrine is a relatively pure alpha-sympathomimetic similar to cyclopentamine, which causes vasostriction by stimulation of alpha receptors on peripheral or cutaneous blood vessels. A common use of this agent is as a nasal decongestant, to shrink swollen vasculature in the nasal passages.

Norepinephrine (Levarterenol, Levophed)

Norepinephrine has a predominant alpha-stimulating effect to cause peripheral vasoconstriction, as well as some beta effects to stimulate cardiac receptors and increase cardiac output. Norepinephrine differs from epinephrine in the degree of beta stimulation. Epinephrine will cause more vascular dilatation with increased cardiac output, so that *systolic* pressure will typically rise, whereas *diastolic* pressure may drop slightly, widening the pulse pressure. Norepinephrine will typically increase *both* systolic and diastolic pressure.

Norepinephrine is used with hypotension or cardiogenic shock, when there is a low peripheral vascular resistance with myocardial infarction. This agent is not useful with hypovolemic shock and may increase myocardial oxygen demand, a possible hazard with infarct and myocardial ischemia. In addition, norepinephrine constricts renal blood vessels, a disadvantage, impairing kidney function. However, norepinephrine gives a rapid response in blood pressure improvement, assuming cardiac function and volume are sufficient. A 0.2% solution is used intravenously for emergency situations with a dose of 16 mg.

Dopamine (Intropin)

Dopamine is both an alpha and beta, as well as a dopamine receptor, stimulant. Its effect on the heart and blood vessels varies with dose. As the dose increases, cardiac stimulation increases cardiac output, and then peripheral vasoconstriction occurs. This includes renal vasoconstriction. Dopamine is indicated in emergency cardiogenic shock and hypotension. Tachyarrhythmias may result with the drug, and small doses can actually decrease blood pressure by vasodilation.

Metaraminol (Aramine)

Metaraminol is used to treat hypotensive states, is a sympathomimetic amine, and causes an increase in blood pressure by both direct and indirect actions. Direct effects refer to direct stimulation of alpha and beta receptors; indirect refers to the release of endogenous norepinephrine by the agent, which in turn leads to stimulation of alpha receptors. If catecholamine stores are already depleted, such as in chronic heart failure, or if reserpine has depleted catecholamine stores, the effect of metaraminol is reduced. Metaraminol is given intravenously and is generally not considered superior to dopamine or norepinephrine.

Mephentermine (Wyamine)

Mephentermine is another amine with both a direct action on blood vessels and an indirect action as a result of norepinephrine release, causing a vasopressor effect. It is used for hypotensive states and increases cardiac output at the same time that vasoconstriction is produced.

Methoxamine (Vasoxyl)

Methoxamine is a vasopressor amine with relatively pure alpha-stimulating properties. Because of this, the rise in blood pressure is primarily due to vasoconstriction and not increased cardiac output, since there is little beta-receptor stimulation of the heart. Isoproterenol, dobutamine, epinephrine, and ephedrine (injectable) are other agents in this group whose actions have already been discussed in previous sections of this chapter.

Emergency Cart Drugs

Table 17–4 lists some of the drugs commonly found on resuscitation, or "crash," carts, with a brief indication of their effect and use in cardiorespiratory emergencies. This list represents agents from the cardiac and circulatory (vasopressor) groups.

TABLE 17–4.

Drugs Used in Resuscitation

Drug	Use
	Control of Cardiac Rhythm and Rate
Lidocaine	Raises fibrillation threshold with ventricular tachycardia or PVCs
Bretylium	Antiarrhythmic that raises the fibrillation threshold but also increases cardiac response to catecholamines as a positive inotrope
Propranolol	Beta-adrenergic blocking agent to control recurring supraventricular tachycardia
Atropine sulfate	Reverse bradycardia by vagal blockade
Isoproterenol	For asystole and cardiovascular collapse; blood pressure is improved initially by increased cardiac output
Verapamil	Slow channel calcium blocking agent for PAT
	Increase Cardiac Output and Blood Pressure
Epinephrine HCl (1 : 10,000)	For asystole and ventricular fibrillation; with positive inotropic and chronotropic action
Norepinephrine	Vasopressor action through alpha-receptor stimulation
Dopamine HCl	Positive inotropic effect and increase of blood pressure through alpha- and beta-receptor stimulation
Dobutamine HCl	Synthetic catecholamine with positive inotropic action, without increasing peripheral resistance

DRUGS AFFECTING THE BLOOD

Anticoagulant Agents

The anticoagulants that are common in clinical use, to manage thrombo-embolism, namely, heparin and the coumarin group, interfere with the prothrombin-thrombin system of fibrin and clot formation. Briefly, that system involves the sequence shown in Figure 17–11.

Other agents such as oxalic acid, sodium nitrate, and disodium edetate are effective inhibitors of coagulation in vitro (in tubes or glass containers) but are too toxic for use in vivo.

The two major types of drugs used for prevention of blood clotting in vivo are represented by heparin and dicumarol.

Heparin

Heparin has acidic properties and a strong electronegative charge. Heparin combines with antithrombin III (heparin cofactor) and the resulting complex inactivates factor X, and thus inhibits the conversion of prothrombin to thrombin, the substance that converts fibrinogen to fibrin to produce clotting. In larger doses, heparin interferes with thrombin's action on fibrinogen, preventing fibrin formation. Protamine is an antidote to heparin that neutralizes its negative charge.

Coumarin Group

The coumarin group includes dicumarol and warfarin. These anticoagulants are thought to work by an antagonist effect on vitamin K needed for the production of several clotting factors (factors II, IX, X, and VII). Factor X is common to both intrinsic and extrinsic clotting systems.

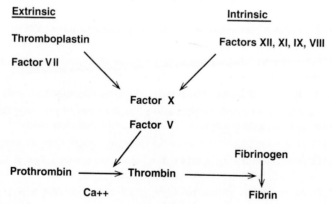

FIG 17–11. Prothrombin-thrombin system of fibrin and clot formation.

Anticoagulants are used to prevent clotting in arterial samples and are given to treat deep venous or arterial thrombosis and in pulmonary embolism. Hemorrhage is a hazard with such therapy.

Fibrinolytic Agents

Drugs considered to be fibrinolytic agents generally cause the conversion of plasminogen to plasmin, a substance that will initiate local fibrinolysis in a blood clot or thrombus. Exact mechanisms for conversion of plasminogen to plasmin differ among the specific agents.

Agents that have fibrinolytic activity include the following:

Alteplase (Activase)
Anistreplase (Eminase)
Urokinase (Abbokinase)
Streptokinase (Streptase)

Because of their fibrinolytic effect, these drugs are used to dissolve clots that occlude both coronary and pulmonary arteries (pulmonary thromboembolism).

BIBLIOGRAPHY

Ahmed T, Abraham WM: Role of calcium-channel blockers in obstructive airway disease, Chest 88(suppl):142S, Aug 1985.

Coodley EL, Ofstein M, Rick J: Cardiac arrhythmias. An update on identification and therapy, Postgrad Med 80:38, 1986.

Ferguson RK, Vlasses PH: Hypertensive emergencies and urgencies, JAMA 255:1607, 1986.

Gross F: Central alpha-adrenoceptors in cardiovascular regulation, Chest 83(suppl):293, Feb 1983.

Hoffman BB, Lefkowitz RJ: Alpha-adrenergic receptor subtypes, N Engl J Med 302:1390, 1980.

Karlsberg RP: Welcome—the calcium channel blockers, Chest 80:657, 1981.

Kobinger W: Central blood pressure regulation. Involvement of presynaptic or postsynaptic α_1 or α_2 adrenoceptors? Chest 83(suppl):296, Feb 1983.

Mathewson HS: Drugs for prevention of sudden death, Respir Care 27:1536, 1982.

Mathewson HS: Anti-asthmatic properties of calcium antagonists, Respir Care 30:779, 1985.

Middleton E Jr: Newer drugs in management: calcium antagonists, Chest 87(suppl):79S, Jan 1985.

Nademanee K, Singh BN: Advance in antiarrhythmic therapy: the role of the newer antiarrhythmic drugs, JAMA 247:217, 1982.

O'Malley K, O'Brien E: Management of hypertension in the elderly, N Engl J Med 302:1397, 1980.

Patakas D et al: Beta-blockers in bronchial asthma: effect of propranolol and pindolol on large and small airways, Thorax 38:108, 1983.

Podrid PJ: Antiarrhythmic drug therapy: benefits and hazards, Chest 88:452 (Part 1); 618 (Part 2), 1985.

Purcell JA: Shock drugs: standardized guidelines, Am J Nurs 82:965, 1982.

Rossi LP, Antman EM: Calcium channel blockers: new treatment for cardiovascular disease, Am J Nurs 83:382, 1983.

Singh BN, Collett JT, Chew YC: New perspectives in the pharmacologic therapy of cardiac arrhythmias, Prog Cardiovasc Dis 22:243, 1980.

van Zwieten PA, Timmermans PBMWM: Pharmacology and characterization of central α-adrenoreceptors involved in the effect of centrally acting antihypertensive drugs, Chest 83(suppl):340, Feb 1983.

Ziesche S, Franciosa JA: Clinical application of sodium nitroprusside, Heart Lung 6:99, 1977.

Zipes DP: New approaches to antiarrhythmic therapy. N Engl J Med 304:475, 1981.

18

Diuretic Agents

Chapter 18 describes diuretic drug groups, or drugs intended to increase urine output and water loss from the body. The following topics are reviewed:

- Renal structure and function
- Major diuretic groups

The main purpose of diuretics, or agents that increase urine output, is to eliminate excess fluid from the body.

Diuretic: Any substance that increases urine flow, and specifically an agent whose therapeutic purpose is to cause a net loss of water from the body.

The above definition excludes agents that promote urine output without a *direct* action on the kidney. For example, digitalis is not considered a diuretic, although it can increase urine output by restoring cardiac output, which improves circulation and renal perfusion.

Details of renal physiology must be assumed, although a brief review of elements essential for understanding the mechanisms of diuretic agents is presented.

RENAL STRUCTURE AND FUNCTION

The kidneys are paired retroperitoneal organs that are found on either side of the spinal cord at the level of the umbilicus. In the adult, each kidney weighs approximately 160 to 175 g and is 10 to 12 cm long. Perfusion of the kidney is via the renal artery, and approximately 21% of the cardiac output goes to the renal system. This is a perfusion of 1000 to 1250 ml/min in the healthy adult. Like the heart and brain, the kidney is an active organ (not a passive filter) with a high oxygen consumption. For this reason, impaired circulation can cause renal damage or failure.

Figure 18–1 gives a description of the kidney and its functional unit, the nephron, which is analogous to the alveolus as the functional unit in the lung. Each kidney contains around a million nephrons, 75% of which can be lost before problems arise. The nephron is made up of the glomerulus, proximal tubule, loop of Henle, distal tubule, and collecting tubule.

The renal artery branches into the afferent arteriole, which enters and forms the capillary tuft of the glomerulus. This blood flow then leaves in the efferent arteriole, which then forms the capillary network around the tubules and loop of Henle. This capillary network rejoins to form the renal vein.

The glomerulus is supported and surrounded by an epithelial-lined capsule, referred to as Bowman's capsule. The glomerular capsule is actually the beginning of the proximal tube, and filtration of fluid from the blood to the tubule occurs in the glomerulus. This fluid is the glomerular filtrate, which empties into the proximal convoluted tubule, goes through the descending and ascending loops of Henle, into the distal convoluted tubule and then the collecting duct, and finally empties into the ureter to be stored in the bladder.

Nephron Function

Beginning in the glomerulus, the nephron forms a protein and cell-free ultrafiltrate, which has the same ionic concentration (Na^+, Cl^-, HCO_3^-, etc.) as plasma. Of the blood going to the nephron, around one-fifth of the volume is filtered through the glomerulus, or about 130 ml/min. In the passage through the nephron, over 99% of the glomerular filtrate is reabsorbed in the tubules, and less than 1% of the fluid is excreted as urine. Out of the 130 ml/min filtered, 129 ml/min will be reabsorbed. *Diuretics interfere, in various ways, with the reabsorption of water in the tubules of the nephron.*

Usually, the nephron accomplishes the following:

- Keeps blood protein and cells out of the glomerular filtrate
- Maintains the alkaline reserve of the blood by bicarbonate reabsorption and hydrogen ion excretion, using bicarbonate, phosphate, and ammonia buffers
- Excretes nitrogenous wastes such as urea and uric acid
- Eliminates drugs and their breakdown products from the body

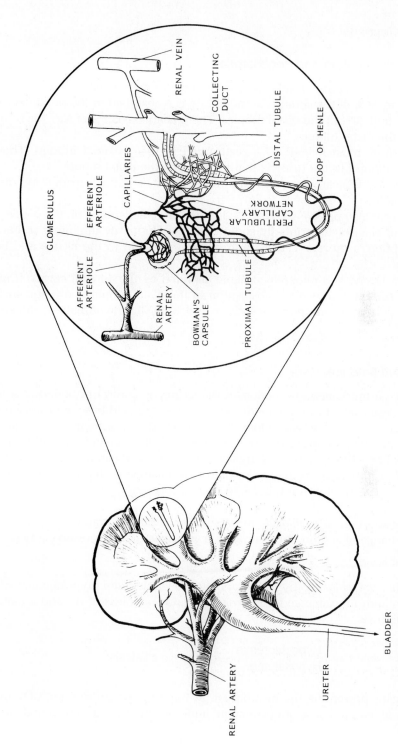

FIG 18–1. Basic structure of the kidney, with a detailed view of the nephron.

Electrolyte Filtration and Reabsorption

The following important ions are filtered and exchanged in the tubules:
Sodium: 80% of the sodium in the filtrate is reabsorbed in the proximal tubules, and 20% in the distal tubules. There is an exchange of Na^+ for H^+ or
K^+ in the distal tubules.
Potassium: most filtered K^+ is reabsorbed in the proximal tubules. Then
what is found in the urine is that secreted by the distal tubule.
Chloride and Bicarbonate: are passively reabsorbed in the proximal and distal tubules.

Water is also passively reabsorbed or excreted, depending on the concentration of electrolyte, primarily sodium, in the filtrate. By inhibiting sodium
reabsorption, a diuretic causes more water to remain in the filtrate and be
excreted.

Aldosterone is a mineralocorticoid secreted by the adrenal cortex; it increases sodium and water reabsorption in the distal tubule. A diuretic such
as spironolactone can increase sodium and water loss by inhibiting aldosterone.

Acid-Base Balance

Since a fundamental function of the kidney is control of buffering substances, especially bicarbonate, diuretics may cause acid-base imbalances to
occur as they increase water loss. Figure 18−2 gives a schema of hydrogen
and bicarbonate pathways that regulate pH. The filtration and reabsorbtion of
Na^+, Cl^-, and HCO_3^- have already been described and can be seen in Figure
18−2. The important exchange for acid-base balance is that of sodium. Sodium is reabsorbed in the tubules by several means:

- Reabsorption with *chloride* to preserve electrical neutrality
- Exchange of sodium for hydrogen or *potassium*, again preserving neutrality

Either *low chloride* (hypochloremia) or *low potassium* (hypokalemia) will
force sodium to exchange for hydrogen, producing a loss of H^+ and a metabolic alkalosis.

$$\left.\begin{array}{l} \text{Hypochloremia} \\ \text{Hypokalemia} \end{array}\right\} \rightarrow \text{metabolic alkalosis}$$

Finally, preventing the bicarbonate in the *filtrate* from forming CO_2 and
water will lead to a loss of bicarbonate buffer in the urine and metabolic acidosis.

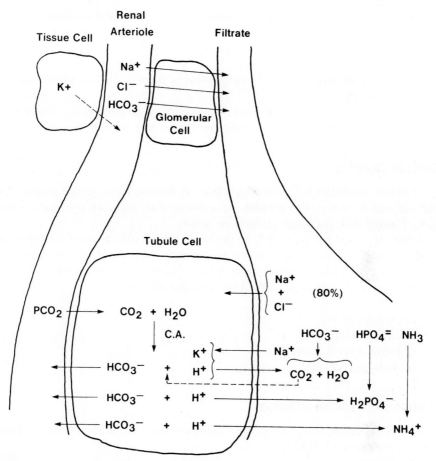

FIG 18–2. Renal regulation of acid-base. Basic mechanisms for kidney retention of bicarbonate with hydrogen ion buffering. Sodium exchange with chloride and for hydrogen is also indicated. C.A., carbonic anhydrase.

DIURETIC GROUPS

On the basis of the nephron function described, drugs could increase water loss by either increasing the glomerular rate of filtration or by inhibiting the reabsorption of water in the tubules. Diuretics can inhibit water reabsorption by the following mechanisms:

- Inhibition of sodium reabsorption, which lowers osmotic reabsorption of water
- Increasing the osmotic concentration in the filtrate directly, thus carrying off more water

- Antagonism of aldosterone to inhibit sodium and water reabsorption
- Inhibition of carbonic anhydrase, which decreases the amount of hydrogen available for sodium reabsorption

The mode of action for each major class of diuretic will be identified and explained briefly.

The major clinical uses of diuretics include congestive heart failure with edema, and hypertension, previously mentioned in Chapter 17.

Osmotic Diuretics

Osmotic diuretics are substances that are filtered through the glomerulus but *not* reabsorbed in the tubules. As a result, they carry an osmotic equivalent of water with them for urinary excretion.

They are used intravenously to decrease intraocular or cerebral pressure, to decrease circulatory volume, and to prevent acute renal failure caused by decreased glomerular filtration in trauma or cardiovascular surgery.

Examples of osmotic diuretics include the following:

Urea (Ureaphil)
Mannitol (Osmitrol)
Glycerin (Glyrol, Osmoglyn)
Isosorbide (Ismotic)

Carbonic Anhydrase Inhibitors

The enzyme carbonic anhydrase catalyzes the conversion of CO_2 and water to carbonic acid, H_2CO_3:

$$CO_2 + H_2O \overset{\text{C.A.}}{\rightleftharpoons} H_2CO_3 \rightleftharpoons H^+ + HCO_3^-$$

The ionic dissociation of H_2CO_3 is not enzyme dependent. The reaction is reversible. From Figure 18–2, it is seen that CO_2 dissociates in the tubule cell to form free hydrogen. Inhibition of carbonic anhydrase prevents or slows this reaction. With lack of hydrogen ions, sodium is not reabsorbed. There is an increased excretion of Na^+, K^+, HCO_3^-, and water.

Such agents may increase tissue levels of CO_2 and can cause *metabolic acidosis* by loss of bicarbonate in the filtrate. If HCO_3 does not combine with H^+ under the action of carbonic anhydrase, it will not be reabsorbed as CO_2 and will be excreted in the urine.

Carbonic anhydrase inhibitors are rarely used as diuretics today, but they can be used to reduce intraocular pressure in treating glaucoma. The most commonly seen agent in this group is acetazolamide, which is a sulfonamide.

Examples of carbonic anhydrase inhibitors are as follows:

Acetazolamide (Diamox)
Dichlorphenamide (Daranide)
Methazolamide (Neptazane)

Thiazide Diuretics

The thiazide group of diuretics is also termed *benzothiadiazide* or *thiadiazide.* They resulted from research on carbonic anhydrase inhibitors and are also derivatives of the sulfonamide structural family. The mode of action by which these agents increase diuresis is inhibition of sodium and chloride reabsorption in the distal tubule, with a corresponding loss of water.

There is also a depletion of potassium, which can lead to *metabolic alkalosis* as more hydrogen ions must exchange for the sodium that *is* reabsorbed. This can be seen in Figure 18–2.

The thiazide diuretics have largely replaced the older mercurial diuretics and acid-forming salts, both of which groups are identified subsequently. Thiazide derivatives are potent and convenient agents given orally for diuresis in congestive heart failure and hypertension. Their exact mechanism in hypertension is unknown. After initial therapy, cardiac output normalizes, but peripheral vascular resistance remains lowered. Chlorothiazide was the prototype agent in this group, and the numerous analogues listed below all have the same basic pharmacological action as chlorothiazide. Agents in this group, with representative trade names, include:

Chlorothiazide (Diuril)
Hydrochlorothiazide (Esidrix)
Bendroflumethiazide (Naturetin)
Chlorthalidone (Hygroton)
Cyclothiazide (Anhydron)
Polythiazide (Renese)
Quinethazone (Hydromox)
Benzthiazide (Exna, Hydrex)
Methyclothiazide (Enduron)
Hydroflumethiazide (Diucardin)
Trichlormethiazide (Metahydrin)
Metolazone (Diulo)
Indapamide (Lozol)

Loop Diuretics

The loop diuretics are extremely potent and have been termed *high-ceiling diuretics.* They exhibit a peak diuretic effect greater than that of other agents. They act by inhibiting the reabsorption of sodium and chloride in the proximal and distal tubules, as well as in the loop of Henle. Their potency is due to this pervasive action.

Because of their mode of action, the high-ceiling diuretics may lead to a chloride loss and a resulting hypochloremia, which can cause *metabolic alkalosis.* This has been explained previously in discussing acid-base regulation by the kidney. There can, additionally, be a loss of potassium (hypokalemia), which can likewise lead to metabolic alkalosis.

These agents are used when greater diuresis is needed, especially to relieve edema in congestive heart failure, hepatic cirrhosis, and renal disease.

Examples of loop diuretics are as follows:

Furosemide (Lasix)
Ethacrynic acid (Edecrin)
Bumetanide (Bumex)

Potassium-Sparing Diuretics

Normally, potassium is reabsorbed throughout the proximal tubule and the ascending loop of Henle, along with sodium. Diuretics that interfere with sodium reabsorption at these sites (thiazides, loop diuretics) also cause a loss of potassium, leading to metabolic alkalosis, as previously discussed. Potassium is usually secreted into the urine in the distal tubule. Instead of acting to prevent potassium (and sodium) reabsorption in the proximal tubule or ascending loop, potassium-sparing diuretics block sodium reabsorption in the *distal* tubule, which actually decreases the loss of potassium at this site where it would normally exchange for the sodium. Potassium is then saved, or spared. Three agents act in this fashion: spironolactone, amiloride, and triamterene. Spironolactone has a mode of action different from the other two agents, and so they are discussed separately.

Spironolactone (Aldactone)

Aldosterone has been identified as a steroid hormone (a mineralocorticoid) that functions to increase the rate of sodium reabsorption in the tubules. Spironolactone is a competitive antagonist for aldosterone receptor sites. This leads to increased sodium and chloride excretion, along with water.

Spironolactone is used for edema resistant to other drugs, with hypersecretion of aldosterone, and as adjunct therapy in treating hypertension.

Amiloride (Midamor) and Triamterene (Dyrenium)

These two agents act by inhibiting sodium reabsorption in the distal tubule. They are not aldosterone antagonists.

There is a saving of potassium by these two agents when other diuretic groups are used. Their major use is to enhance other diuretics and counteract potassium loss.

Other Diuretic Groups

There are three classes, or groups, or diuretics that are now considered obsolete and have been replaced by the thiazide, loop, and potassium-sparing diuretics. These groups are:

- Acid-forming salts such as ammonium chloride (NH_4Cl)
- Mercurial diuretics such as mercaptomerin (Thiomerin) and meralluride (Mercuhydrin)
- Xanthines such as theophylline

Acid-forming salts caused diuresis by contributing chloride (Cl^-) to the tubules, which combined with sodium for excretion, with a corresponding loss of water. Since ammonium chloride also contributed hydrogen ions, *metabolic acidosis* was produced; once the kidneys compensated to balance the pH, such agents lost their diuretic effect. The hydrogen was exchanged for sodium and buffered in the filtrate by ammonia (NH_3) and chloride, one of the buffering mechanisms stated when reviewing the acid-base regulation by the kidney.

The **mercurial diuretics** inhibited the active reabsorption of sodium by the tubules to increase sodium and water loss. The mercurial group could induce a *hypochloremic alkalosis* by their effect on chloride.

The **xanthines** are not usually used as primary diuretics. However, since theophylline has a diuretic effect by increasing sodium and chloride excretion and is often used with asthmatic patients as a bronchodilator, its potential for causing dehydration should be noted. It is often difficult to achieve adequate hydration of patients with chronic obstructive pulmonary disease who are already drinking tea, beer, and cola, all of which cause water loss. A further dehydrating side effect with a xanthine bronchodilator can cause decreased water for the formation of respiratory mucus, with increased mucous viscosity. Correct and adequate fluid intake should be prescribed for patients requiring theophylline for maintenance therapy.

BIBLIOGRAPHY

Haughey EJ Jr, Sica FM: Diuretics: how safe can you make them? Nursing 77 7(2):34, 1977.

Hutcheon DE, Mehta D, Romano A: Diuretic action of furosemide, Arch Intern Med 115:542, 1965.

Modell W, Schild HO, Wilson A: The Kidneys. In Applied Pharmacology, Philadelphia, 1976, WB Saunders Co.

Ram CVS: Diuretics in the treatment of hypertension, Hosp Formul 16:741, 1981.

Romankiewicz JA: Loop diuretics. I. J Pract Nurs 32:9, May 1982.

Diuretics: II. J Pract Nurs 32:11, June 1982.

Thiazides: III. J Pract Nurs 32:7, July/Aug 1982.

19

Aerosolized Drug Delivery in Neonates and Children

Chapter 19 reviews the delivery of inhaled aerosol drugs in infants and children. The following specific topics are discussed:

- Factors affecting drug therapy in young subjects
- Methods of calculating pediatric doses
- Pediatric doses of aerosolized drugs
- Methods of administering aerosol drugs to infants and children

FACTORS AFFECTING DRUG THERAPY IN THE YOUNG

A detailed discussion of neonatal and pediatric respiratory pharmacology requiring a review of physiologic and pathologic conditions common to this age level is well beyond the scope of the text. The intent of this chapter is to provide a working overview of and practical guidelines for respiratory drug therapy in neonates and children.

Two general factors that affect drug therapy are *size* and *age*. There is a direct relationship between body weight (size) and mass of drug: The greater the mass of drug in relation to body size, the greater the effect to be expected. Age, however, adds other factors that can cancel a drug's effect (such as lack of receptors) or produce a toxic effect (lack of enzymes to break down a drug). This is the basis for the pediatrician's maxim that neonates and children are not simply small adults. By using the three phases of drug action outlined in Chapter 1 (pharmaceutical, pharmacokinetic, and pharmacodynamic), some of these important differences can be highlighted. Although not exhaustive, the factors cited serve to point out the important difference between neonatal/pediatric and adult drug therapy. The following definitions are usual in the literature:

Premature Neonate: <36 weeks gestational age.

Neonate: first month of postnatal life.

Infant: 1 to 12 months.

Child: 1 to 12 years.

Adolescent: 12 to 18 years.

Adult: >18 years.

General reviews of pediatric pharmacology can be found in Kelly (1987), MacLeod and Radde (1985), and Mirkin (1978). A detailed review of the literature on aerosolized drug delivery in infants and children is given in Rau (1991).

Pharmaceutical Factors

Dosage form and route of administration must be tailored to the age level. Infants cannot take pills, tablets, or capsules, and liquids taken orally may not be swallowed. Instant regurgitation, spitting, and drooling are common with babies. Liquids can be given with a small medicine cup, dropper, or plastic syringe without the needle. Injection may be reliable depending on the size of the child, but children have an adultlike fear of needles. Parenterally administered dosage volumes for infants and neonates may result in errors because there are no small syringes below 1.0 ml with minimal dead space. Topical administration is more practical at all ages. Aerosols can be given to infants, as well as children, and will be discussed separately in a subsequent section.

Pharmacokinetic Factors

Neonates and children differ dramatically from adults in the absorption, distribution, metabolism, and elimination of drugs. Total body water as a percentage of weight is 85% in the premature neonate, 70% in the full-term infant, 65% in the child, and 60% in the adult. Extracellular fluid as a percentage of weight is 50% in the premature neonate, and 40%, 25%, and 15% in the infant, child, and adult respectively. These factors affect the distribution of water-soluble drugs. Hepatic oxidation and glucoronide conjugation are deficient in the newborn. Maturation of these liver enzyme systems may take 1 month to 1 year. For example, the half-life of theophylline is 14 to 58 hours in premature neonates, but 3.5 to 8 hours in adults. Chloramphenicol, useful in treating *Haemophilus influenzae* cannot be metabolized in the newborn, and the unconjugated form cannot be adequately excreted in the urine, causing accumulation and toxicity ("gray baby syndrome"). Glomerular filtration rate and tubular function are immature in the neonate, requiring approximately 6 months to develop fully. Decreased renal clearance reduces the ability of neonates to excrete drug metabolites in urine, requiring dosage adjustments of many drugs.

Pharmacodynamic Factors

Infants and children often respond differently than adults when a drug does combine with its target receptors. For example, central nervous system stimulants such as amphetamine or methylphenidate (Ritalin) *increase* attention span and *decrease* outbreaks of disruptive behavior in so-called hyperactive children. This is the opposite of what would be expected. It is theorized that the central nervous system is not fully developed in infants and children. Of importance for respiratory care is the question of whether infants less than 1 year old possess bronchial beta receptors or sufficient bronchiolar smooth muscle to respond to sympathomimetic bronchodilators (Lenney and Milner, 1978). If infants did lack bronchial beta receptors, then a bronchodilating response would not be expected, nor detected. Actually, recent research has indicated the presence of β_2 receptors at birth, and airway response to beta agonists has been found (Rau, 1991).

CALCULATING PEDIATRIC DOSES

Because of the factors noted, infants and children require different doses of drugs than adults. Clinical trials of drugs are not usually conducted in children, so pediatric doses may be established by the manufacturer. The following sources should be consulted to determine if there is a recommended and established pediatric dose:

Physicians' Desk Reference (PDR)
Pediatric Dosage Handbook (American Pharmaceutical Association)
Manual of Pediatric Therapeutics (Little, Brown & Co)
The Harriet Lane Handbook (Mosby-Year Book, Inc)

Practitioners should always check the product information sheet in each drug package before administration.

There are several rules used to estimate a pediatric dose if established doses are not given. These rules give fractions of the adult dose based on the child's age (Fried's rule, Young's rule), weight (Clark's rule), and body surface area (BSA rule). Each rule is defined below:

Fried's Rule (infants under 1 year):

$$\text{Infant dose} = \frac{\text{infant age (months)}}{150 \text{ months}} \times \text{adult dose}$$

For a child of 12.5 years (= 150 months), the full adult dose would be given, which is the usual practice.

Young's Rule (1 to 12 years):

$$\text{Child dose} = \frac{\text{child age (years)}}{\text{child age} + 12 \text{ years}} \times \text{adult dose}$$

Clark's Rule

$$\text{Child dose} = \frac{\text{child weight (lb)}}{150 \text{ lb}} \times \text{adult dose}$$

In similar fashion to Fried's rule, Clark's rule assumes a 150-lb (70-kg) "child" is an adult, and the full adult dose would be given.

BSA Rule (body surface area):

$$\text{Child dose} = \frac{\text{child BSA} \times \text{m}^2}{1.73 \text{ m}^2} \times \text{adult dose}$$

The BSA rule is considered to be the most accurate method of estimating a pediatric dose. Body surface area must be obtained from nomograms using the child's height and weight.

Because so many variables can affect drug action in neonates and children, it is absolutely necessary to monitor these patients for side effects or adverse reaction, especially with initial dosing.

TABLE 19–1.

Aerosolized Bronchoactive Drugs

Drug	Delivery Device*	Dosage
Sympathomimetic (adrenergic) bronchodilators		
Racemic epinephrine	Nebulizer	0.05 ml/kg of 2.25% solution p.r.n. but not more frequently than q.2hr; maximum single dose, 0.5 ml
Isoproterenol	MDI	1-2 puffs q.3hr to q.4hr
	Nebulizer	0.25 ml of 1:200 solution t.i.d. or q.i.d. or 0.01 ml/kg; maximum, 0.5 ml q.4hr p.r.n.
Isoetharine	Nebulizer	0.25-0.5 ml of 1% solution q.4hr p.r.n.
Metaproterenol	Nebulizer	0.2-0.3 ml of 5% solution q.4hr to q.6hr
	MDI	1-3 puffs q.3hr to q.4hr up to 12 puffs/day
Terbutaline	MDI	2 puffs q.4hr to q.6hr
Albuterol	MDI	1-2 puffs q.4hr to q.6hr
	Nebulizer	0.01-0.03 ml/kg of 0.5% solution; maximum, 0.5 ml t.i.d. or q.i.d.
	DPI	Children ≥ 4 yr, 200 μg (1 caps.) q.4-6hr
Bitolterol†	—	—
Pirbuterol†	—	—

Parasympatholytic (anticholinergic) bronchodilators		
Atropine sulfate	Nebulizer	0.05 mg/kg diluted in saline; minimum, 0.25 mg; maximum, 1 mg
Ipratropium	MDI	Usual dose, 2 puffs q.i.d.; no specific pediatric dosages given
Mucolytic		
Acetylcysteine‡	Nebulizer	3-5 ml of 10% or 20% solution t.i.d. or q.i.d. by face mask, mouthpiece, or endotracheal tube adapter
Corticosteroids		
Dexamethasone sodium phosphate	MDI	2 puffs t.i.d. or q.i.d.; maximum, 8 puffs/day
Beclomethasone	MDI	Children 6-12 yr, 1-2 puffs t.i.d. or q.i.d.; maximum, 10 puffs/day
Flunisolide	MDI	Children 6-15 yr, 2 puffs b.i.d.; safety and efficacy not established for children under age 6 yr
Triamcinolone	MDI	Children 6-12 yr, 1-2 puffs t.i.d. or q.i.d.; maximum, 12 puffs/day; no dose established for children under age 6 yr
Antiasthmatic		
Cromolyn sodium	MDI	Children ≥ 5 yr, 2 puffs q.i.d.
	Nebulizer	Children > 2 yr, 20 mg (1 amp.) q.i.d.
	DPI	Children > 5 yr, 20 mg (1 cap.) q.i.d.
Nedocromil sodium	MDI	No dose established for children under age 12 yr
Antiinfective		
Ribavirin	SPAG nebulizer	6 g/300 ml (2%) 12-18 hr/day for 3-7 days
Pentamidine	Respirgard II nebulizer	Children ≥ 5 yr, 300 mg q.mo; (limited by child's ability to use nebulizer)

*MDI, metered-dose inhaler; DPI, dry-powder inhaler; SPAG, small-particle aerosol generator.
†No pediatric dose established.
‡The 10% solution is less irritating to the airway. Larger volumes up to 300 ml have been used for nebulization in tents or croupettes. The amount used is the volume that maintains a heavy mist for the desired treatment period.

PEDIATRIC DOSES OF AEROSOLIZED DRUGS

Table 19–1 lists bronchoactive drugs and recommendations for dosages by aerosol. While pediatric doses are given for some drugs, many aerosols are not approved by the Food and Drug Administration for use in children under 12. The doses given are taken from the manufacturer's literature and from the *Harriet Lane Handbook* previously cited. Dosage guidelines for aerosolized drugs used in both maintenance therapy of childhood asthma and treatment of acute episodes are given in Chapters 7 and 8 of the National Asthma Education Program report (1991). In addition to those sources, the following articles have reported doses to be used with pediatric practice: Alderson and Warren (1984), Canny and Levison (1988), Davis et al. (1990), Kelly (1987), and Tabachnik and Levison (1981).

Burgess and Chernick (1982) also provide a chapter on pediatric pharmacology in their text. Since new research may revise such doses, it is strongly urged that neonatal/pediatric practitioners consult current product literature and the research literature in neonatal and pediatric respiratory care for updated recommendations concerning these drugs.

The amount of diluent, such as normal saline, to be added to the doses in Table 19–1 is based on the volume fill requirements of the nebulizers used. Recall from Chapter 2 that most small-reservoir nebulizers operate efficiently with 3 to 5 ml volumes. For example, if the dose of the drug gives 0.5 ml, then 2 to 3 ml of normal saline is needed for mechanically efficient nebulization. This is not to *dilute* the dosage (see Chapter 3) since the same amount of the drug (0.5 ml) is in the total mixture. The volume is simply expanded.

It should also be pointed out that actual *neonatal aerosol* dosages used in clinical practice often differ from the schedules given in the previously cited sources. For aerosolized bronchodilators, it is often the case that an adult dose will be given to a neonate. For example, 0.25 ml of 1% isoetharine has been used in an infant. Similarly, an entire ampule of cromolyn sodium has been nebulized for an infant with bronchopulmonary dysplasia. The safe use of such doses may be due to immature development of smooth muscle and receptors, which is normal for babies and which would require a higher dose for the effect needed. As always, close monitoring of infants for either the desired effect or adverse side effects is needed.

PEDIATRIC AEROSOL ADMINISTRATION

The numerous variables in aerosol delivery of medication were discussed in Chapter 2, and those considerations apply to pediatric and infant use, with the added factor of the age variable in young patients. Yet aerosols *can* be given successfully to pediatric subjects and are the logical delivery method for treating the lung and airways. The following summarizes the general guidelines on age requirements for use of different methods to administer aerosolized drugs to infants and children.* These are averages, and individual children may differ in their ability to use different aerosol devices.

*From Rau JL. Delivery of aerosolized drugs to neonatal and pediatric patients, Respir Care 36:514, 1991. Used with permission.

Delivery Device	Minimum Age
Small-volume nebulizer	Neonate
MDI	7 yr
With spacer	3 yr
With spacer and mask	Infant
With endotracheal tube	Neonate
DPI	3-4 yr

Metered-Dose Inhaler

Pressurized MDI canisters are popular, convenient to use, and deliver well-controlled doses of a drug. The experience of clinicians has shown that children over age 6 years can learn to use an MDI correctly, and those 4 to 6 years of age can easily use an MDI with a spacer device such as the InspirEase (Key Pharmaceuticals, Inc). As with adults, approximately 10% of the total dose reaches the lung. Although an open-mouth technique has been advocated when using an MDI *without* a spacer device, one study has shown no advantage in bronchodilator response with the mouth open as opposed to a closed mouth (Unzcitig et al., 1983). Holding an MDI in front of an open mouth does add a degree of difficulty for adults and children alike.

Dry-Powder Inhalers

Cromolyn sodium and albuterol are available in a DPI formulation in the United States. However, this technique is being investigated for other drugs. Current dry-powder systems require high inspiratory flow rates of 60 to 120 L/min for efficient capsule dispersion, and this may not be possible with children under 4 or 5 years of age. Newer dry-powder systems have been developed that are effective with lower flow rates and may be released in the future.

Jet Nebulizers

The usual method of nebulization for drug delivery is the small-reservoir, gas-powered jet, although ultrasonic nebulizers have been used. Young children and infants can use pediatric face masks held in place by parents or clinicians while the patient is cuddled. Treatment times may need to be shortened with young children, depending on the degree of cooperation, and this will affect the delivered dose.

Aerosol Delivery with Face Masks or Endotracheal Tubes

Both MDI and nebulizer aerosol generators can be interfaced to young patients either by using face masks or, in the case of more critical support, through endotracheal tubes (ETTs). Data have begun to accumulate on both of these methods of aerosol delivery.

Face Mask Delivery

Delivery of an aerosol drug with a face mask was evaluated with cromolyn sodium by Salmon and co-workers (1990). They quantitated the amount of aerosol drug reaching the lungs, based on urinary excretion, for nebulizer and face mask and for MDI with spacer and face mask, in infants between 9 and 36 months of age. Adults inhaling nebulized solution with nasal breathing, by using a facemask, were included for comparison. The following amounts of lung deposition were estimated:

- Infants
  Nebulizer and face mask, 0.76%
  MDI with spacer and face mask, 0.30%
- Adults
  Nebulizer and face mask, 1.5%

Kraemer and associates (1991) found the administration of aerosolized albuterol by using an MDI with a spacer and mask to be substantially better than placebo in wheezy infants.

Another study by Lowenthal and Kattan (1992) compared face masks versus mouthpieces for delivering aerosolized albuterol from nebulizers to asthmatic patients between the ages of 6 and 19 years. There was no substantial difference in pulmonary function improvement by either method, although they noted a greater incidence of tremor in the face mask group.

Endotracheal Tube Delivery

Delivery of aerosol through an ETT was described previously in Chapter 2. Both MDI and nebulizer systems have been used with ETTs, and in addition ultrasonic nebulizers and special-purpose nebulizers, such as the Ultravent used in nuclear medicine, have been investigated for this purpose. Table 19–2 summarizes some of the results of data accumulating on delivery of aerosolized drugs to the lung through an ETT in neonatal populations. The studies cited included both in vivo and in vitro methodologies, lung models and animal models, and different drugs such as cromolyn sodium, albuterol, and budesonide (a corticosteroid). A variety of measurement methods were used. Full details can be found in the referenced articles.

SUMMARY

The present chapter has a limited scope of presentation. The general context of pediatric drug therapy is outlined, with the primary focus on aerosol

TABLE 19-2.

Amount of Aerosolized Drug Delivered to the Lung Through a Neonatal Endotracheal Tube

Delivery Device*	ETT Size (mm)	Percentage Delivered	Reference
SVN	3.0	8.5	Ahrens
SVN	3.5	0.02-0.68	Arnon
MDI-Aerovent		3.62	
MDI-Aerochamber		14.20	
SVN	—	0.28	Banks
SVN	2.5	2.11	Benson
	3.0	2.0	
	3.5	2.14	
SVN	3.5	0.69	Cameron
MDI + spacer	2.5	1.8	Everard
	3.0	1.54	
SVN	3.0	0.19-1.9	Flavin
USN	3.5	1.3	Grigg
MDI-Aerochamber		1.72	
SVN	3.0	0.97-1.78	Rau

*SVN, Small-volume nebulizer; USN, ultrasonic nebulizer.

delivery. For dosages of drugs given orally or parenterally, the following sources can be consulted: product literature; *Drug Facts and Comparisons* (Lippincott); and the *Harriet Lane Handbook*. A good presentation of pharmacotherapy in bronchopulmonary dysplasia is found in Blanchard et al. (1987), which discusses all of the bronchoactive drugs. Zaritsky (1987) provides a discussion of cardiopulmonary resuscitation (CPR) in children, in the context of which, dosages of CPR drugs are provided.

BIBLIOGRAPHY

Ahrens RC et al: The delivery of therapeutic aerosols through endotracheal tubes, Pediatr Pulmonol 2:19, 1986.

Alderson SH, Warren RH: Pediatric aerosol therapy guidelines, Clin Pediatr 23:553, 1984.

Arnon S et al: Delivery of micronized budesonide suspension by metered dose inhaler and jet nebulizer into a neonatal ventilator circuit, Pediatr Pulmonol 13:172, 1992.

Banks JL et al: Pulmonary aerosol deposition in the mechanically ventilated newborn piglet, Pediatr Res 27:295, 1990 (abstract).

Benson JM et al: The impact of changing ventilator parameters on availability of nebulized drugs in an in vitro neonatal lung system, Drug Intell Clin Pharmacol 25:272, 1991.

Blanchard PW, Brown TM, Coates AL: Pharmacotherapy in bronchopulmonary dysplasia, Clin Perinatol 14:881, 1987.

Burgess WR, Chernick V: Pharmacology. In Respiratory therapy in newborn infants and children, New York, 1982, Thieme-Stratton, Inc.

Canny GJ, Levison H: Ann Allergy 60:12, 1988.

Cameron D, Clay M, Silverman M: Evaluation of nebulizers for use in neonatal ventilator circuits, Crit Care Med 18:866, 1990.

Davis JM, Sinkin RA, Aranda JV: Drug therapy for bronchopulmonary dysplasia, Pediatr Pulmonol 8:117, 1990.

Everard ML et al: New aerosol delivery system for neonatal ventilator circuits, Arch Dis Child 67:826, 1992.

Flavin M et al: Aerosol delivery to the rabbit lung with an infant ventilator, Pediatr Pulmonol 2:35, 1986.

Greene MG, editor: The Harriet Lane Handbook, ed 12, Chicago, 1990, Mosby-Year Book.

Grigg J et al: Delivery of therapeutic aerosols to intubated babies, Arch Dis Child 67:25, 1992.

Kelly HW: Pharmacotherapy of pediatric lung disease: differences between children and adults, Clin Chest Med 8:681, 1987.

Kraemer R et al: Short-term effect of albuterol, delivered via a new auxiliary device, in wheezy infants, Am Rev Respir Dis 144:347, 1991.

Lenney W, Milner AD: At what age do bronchodilator drugs work? Arch Dis Child 53:532, 1978.

Lowenthal D, Kattan M: Facemasks versus mouthpieces for aerosol treatment of asthmatic children, Pediatr Pulmonol 14:192, 1992.

MacLeod SM, Radde IC: Textbook of pediatric clinical pharmacology, Littleton, Mass, 1985, PSG Publishing Co.

Mirkin BL: Clinical pharmacology and therapeutics: a pediatric perspective, Chicago, 1978, Year Book Medical Publishers, Inc.

National Asthma Education Program: Guidelines for the diagnosis and management of asthma. Bethesda, Md, 1991, U.S. Department of Health and Human Services, National Institutes of Health.

Rau JL Jr: Delivery of aerosolized drugs to neonatal and pediatric patients, Respir Care 36:514, 1991.

Rau JL Jr, Harwood RJ: Comparison of nebulizer delivery methods through a neonatal endotracheal tube: a bench study. Respir Care 37:1233, 1992.

Salmon B, Wilson NM, Silverman M: How much aerosol reaches the lungs of wheezy infants and toddlers? Arch Dis Child 65:401, 1990.

Tabachnik E, Levison H: Infantile bronchial asthma, J Allergy Clin Immunol 67:339, 1981.

Unzcitig JC, Richards W, Church PA: Administration of metered-dose inhalers: Comparison of open- and closed-mouth techniques in childhood asthmatics. Ann Allergy 51:571, 1983.

Zaritsky A: Cardiopulmonary resuscitation in children, Clin Chest Med 8:561, 1987.

Appendix A

Apothecary, Avoirdupois, and Household Units

Units of measurement in the apothecary and avoirdupois systems are not consistent, as with the metric system. The units also have characteristic symbols, which are listed in Table 1–1 (Abbreviations and Prescriptions). In the tables below, the units are spelled out, for easy recognition.

Several conventions apply if apothecary measure is used.

1. If the abbreviation or symbol for a unit is used, then the amount *follows* the symbol and is written in small Roman numerals.

   Example:
   2 grains is gr. ii
   6 drams is 3 vi

2. Fractions are written as fractions, with the order as given in 1 above. The exception to this rule is use of $\overline{ss}$ instead of ½.

   Example:
   ½ ounce is oz. $\overline{ss}$
   ¼ grain is gr. ¼

3. The following rules apply to the use of Roman numerals:

   i, I = 1
   v, V = 5
   x, X = 10
      L = 50
      C = 100
      D = 500
      M = 1,000

   Reading from left to right, *add* amounts placing largest numerals to left.
   Example: 27 is XXVII
   If a smaller numeral is before (to the left of) a larger numeral, *subtract* the smaller from the larger.
   Example: 29 is XXIX
   Use the shortest form of a number when more than one is possible.
   Example: LLIV   CIV =   104
               XIIII   XIV =   14

The apothecary weight and fluid (volume) measures are given in the following tables.

Apothecary's weight
20 grains = 1 scruple
3 scruples = 1 dram
8 drams = 1 ounce
12 ounces = 1 pound

Apothecary's fluid measures
60 minims = 1 fluid dram
8 fluid drams = 1 fluid ounce
16 fluid ounces = 1 pint
2 pints = 1 quart
4 quarts = 1 gallon

THE AVOIRDUPOIS SYSTEM

The avoirdupois system contains only *weight measurement,* not *volume.* The avoirdupois system uses the same terms as found in the apothecary system of weight; however, the grain is the only unit identical in both systems. There are 12 ounces per pound apothecary and 16 ounces per pound avoirdupois. Therefore 1 pound apothecary is 5,760 grains, while 1 pound avoirdupois is 7,000 grains.

Avoirdupois weight
437 ½ grains = 1 ounce
16 ounces = 1 pound
7,000 grains = 1 pound

In addition to the three systems of measure noted, there exists a set of household measures, which are included in the list of equivalents.

Intersystem Conversions

All drugs manufactured today in America should have metric units for dosage strengths and amounts. All orders for drugs should similarly use metric units. However, a list of approximate equivalents is given to aid in conversion from one system to another, including household measures. It is stressed that this set of equivalents is only *approximate* and has been considered to be helpful clinically. Slightly different sets of equivalents can be found in different texts. For accurate drug administration, drug orders should always employ the units in which the drug is supplied by the manufacturer.

Approximate Equivalents

Metric:

1 milligram	= 0.015 grain = 1/65 grain
1 gram	= 15 grains
1 kilogram	= 2.2 pounds (avdp)
1 milliliter	= 16 minims or 16 drops (gtts)

Apothecary:

1 grain	= 65 milligrams
1 ounce (apoth)	= 31.1 grams
1 fl. oz. (apoth)	= 29.57 milliliters
1 pint	= 473.2 milliliters = approx. 500 ml
1 quart	= 986.4 milliliters = approx. 1,000 ml
1 minim	= 1 drop (gtt). = .062 milliliters

Avoirdupois:

1 pound	= 454 grams
1 ounce	= 28.3 grams

Household equivalents:

1 teaspoon	= 5 milliliters
1 tablespoon	= 15 milliliters
1 cup	= 240 milliliters

Several examples are provided to illustrate the apothecary and avoirdupois systems and conversions with the metric system.

1. How many milliliters are equivalent to 8 minims?
   equivalence: 16 minims = 1 milliliter
   1 ml/16 minims × 8 minims = 0.5 ml

2. 1/150 grain equals how many milligrams (approximately)?
   equivalence: 1 grain = 65 milligrams
   1/150 grain × 65 mg/grain = 0.43 mg = 0.4 mg

3. How many milliliters are contained in 4 drops?
   equivalence: 16 drops = 1 milliliter
   1 ml/16 drops × 4 drops = 0.25 ml

4. If Tempra liquid contains 120 mg per teaspoon, how much active ingredient is contained in 2.5 ml?
   equivalence: 1 teaspoon = 5 ml

$$\frac{120 \text{ mg}}{5 \text{ ml}} = \frac{X \text{ mg}}{2.5 \text{ ml}}$$

$$X = 60 \text{ mg}$$

5. 8 fluid ounces apothecary equals how many milliters?
   equivalence: 1 fluid ounce = 29.57 ml
   29.57 ml/l fl. oz. × 8 fl. oz. = 236.6 ml = 240 ml

6. How many kilograms in 135 pounds (avdp)?
   equivalence: 1 kg = 2.2 pounds
   1 kg/2.2 pounds × 135 pounds = 61 kg

Arithmetic Related to Drug Calculations

ARITHMETIC SELF-TEST

1. Change to whole numbers or to mixed numbers.
   a. $\dfrac{24}{12}$ = _____
   b. $\dfrac{9}{4}$ = _____
   c. $\dfrac{100}{25}$ = _____
   d. $\dfrac{16}{3}$ = _____
   e. $\dfrac{500}{25}$ = _____
   f. $\dfrac{67}{15}$ = _____

2. Add the following fractions.
   a. ⅕,½, ⅟ = _____
   b. ⅙,⅜, ¾ = _____
   c. 2¾, 4⅛, 5½ = _____

3. Subtract the following fractions and mixed numbers.
   a. ⅔ − ½ = _____
   b. ⅘ − ⅓ = _____
   c. 4½ − 2⅓ = _____
   d. 10¼ − 6⅜ = _____

4. Write as a decimal.
   a. forty-five and five tenths = _____
   b. thirty-five and three hundredths = _____
   c. two and five ten thousandths = _____
   d. one hundred sixty and three thousandths = _____

5. Add the following decimals.
   a. 0.05, 0.010, 0.156 = _____
   b. 1.005, 20.1, 400.5 = _____
   c. 0.004, 42.015, 1004.05 = _____

6. Subtract the following decimals.
   a. 12.05 − 10.50 = _____
   b. 9.00 − 5.50 = _____
   c. 125.50 − 100.60 = _____
   d. 95.05 − 5.25 = _____

7. Multiply the following.
   a. 525 × 0.51 = _____
   b. 550.10 × 0.05 = _____
   c. 594.99 × 0.99 = _____
   d. 841.08 × 0.08 = _____

8. Divide the following.
   a. $\frac{3}{5} \div \frac{3}{10}$ = _____
   b. $\frac{4}{8} \div \frac{1}{16}$ = _____
   c. 14.25 ÷ 3.5 = _____
   d. 150.25 ÷ 0.25 = _____

9. Change the following fractions to decimals.
   a. $\frac{7}{10}$ = _____
   b. $5\frac{1}{4}$ = _____

10. Solve the following proportions.
    a. 1 : 2 :: X : 15
    b. 30 : 45 :: 35 : X
    c. $\frac{3}{4} = \frac{1}{X}$
    d. $\frac{17}{22} = \frac{34}{X}$
    e. X : 60 :: 3 : 12

11. Change the following to percents.
    a. $\frac{1}{2}$ = _____
    b. 0.007 = _____
    c. $\frac{3}{4}$ = _____
    d. 0.05 = _____

12. What is:
    a. 5% of 75 = _____
    b. 0.5% of 500 = _____

    c. 6% of 400 = _____

    d. 0.7% of 750 = _____

13. Metric conversions:

    a. 2 milligrams = _____ grams

    b. 10 milliliters = _____ liters

    c. 0.0025 grams = _____ milligrams

    d. 200 micrograms = _____ milligrams

Answer key—Self-Test

1. a. 2
  b. 2¼
  c. 4
  d. 5⅓
  e. 20
  f. 4⁷⁄₁₅

2. a. ¹⁹⁄₂₀
  b. ³¹⁄₂₄
  c. ⁹⁹⁄₈

3. a. ⅙
  b. ⁷⁄₁₅
  c. ¹³⁄₆
  d. ³¹⁄₈

4. a. 45.5
  b. 35.03
  c. 2.0005
  d. 160.003

5. a. 0.216
  b. 421.605
  c. 1046.069

6. a. 1.55
  b. 3.50
  c. 24.90
  d. 89.90

7. a. 267.75
  b. 27.505
  c. 589.0401
  d. 67.2864

8. a. ³⁰⁄₁₅ = 2
  b. ⁶⁴⁄₈ = 8
  c. 4.07
  d. 601

9. a. 0.7
  b. 5.25

10. a. 7.5
    b. 52.5
    c. ⅓ or 1⅓
    d. 44
    e. 15
11. a. 50%
    b. 0.7%
    c. 75%
    d. 5%
12. a. 3.75
    b. 2.5
    c. 24
    d. 5.25
13. a. 0.002 g
    b. 0.010 L
    c. 2.5 mg
    d. 0.2 mg

REVIEW AND SUMMARY OF ARITHMETIC

I. Fractions

Definition: A fraction is a portion of a whole.
Terms:
  Numerator: upper number of fraction, which is the dividend.
  Denominator: lower number of fraction, the divisor.
    Example: 2 _____ numerator

    3____denominator
  Least Common Denominator (L.C.D.): for a group of fractions, the *small-est* number that all of the denominators will divide into evenly.
    Example: ½, ⅓ L.C.D. = 6; ½ = ³⁄₆, ⅓ = ²⁄₆
  Proper Fraction: numerator is *less than* denominator.
    Example: ⅕
  Improper Fraction: numerator is *greater than* denominator.
    Example: 5⁄4
  Complex Fraction: a fraction whose numerator, or denominator, or both, are fractions.

    Example: $\dfrac{½}{3}$, $\dfrac{½}{⅔}$

  Mixed Number: a whole number and a fraction.
    Example: 1⅔

Reducing Fractions:

Rule: to reduce fractions, find a number that divides evenly into both numerator and denominator.

Exercise I–1: Reduce the following fractions:

a. $\dfrac{6}{24} =$

b. $\dfrac{9}{27} =$

c. $\dfrac{1}{3} =$

d. $\dfrac{2}{8} =$

e. $\dfrac{2}{4} =$

f. $\dfrac{4}{16} =$

g. $\dfrac{2}{7} =$

h. $\dfrac{3}{4} =$

i. $\dfrac{9}{16} =$

j. $\dfrac{4}{24} =$

Exercise I–2: Find the least common denominator:

a. $\dfrac{3}{4}, \dfrac{1}{6}, \dfrac{1}{2}$: L.C.D. =

b. $\dfrac{1}{18}, \dfrac{1}{9}, \dfrac{3}{18}$: L.C.D. =

c. $\dfrac{3}{4}, \dfrac{3}{12}, \dfrac{4}{9}$: L.C.D. =

d. $\dfrac{3}{20}, \dfrac{1}{9}, \dfrac{3}{18}$: L.C.D. =

e. $\dfrac{7}{20}, \dfrac{5}{8}$: L.C.D. =

f. $\dfrac{1}{24}, \dfrac{3}{12}, \dfrac{1}{4}$: L.C.D. =

g. $\dfrac{1}{24}, \dfrac{5}{6}, \dfrac{1}{48}$: L.C.D. =

h. $\dfrac{9}{27}, \dfrac{2}{3}, \dfrac{1}{8}$: L.C.D. =

i. $\dfrac{6}{13}, \dfrac{1}{26}, \dfrac{5}{6}$: L.C.D. =

j. $\dfrac{6}{18}, \dfrac{3}{6}, \dfrac{1}{2}$: L.C.D. =

Mixed Numbers and Improper Fractions:

Rules:

Mixed Numbers to Improper Fractions:
1. Multiply the whole number by the fraction's denominator.
2. Add this product to the numerator.
3. The denominator stays the same.

Example: $1\frac{2}{3} = \dfrac{3+2}{3} = \frac{5}{3}$

Improper Fractions to Mixed Numbers:
1. Divide the denominator into the numerator.
2. Write the remainder as a fraction, with the original denominator.

Exercise I–3: Change to mixed numbers and improper fractions:

a. $1\frac{1}{4}$ =

b. $1\frac{2}{3}$ =

c. $4\frac{1}{8}$ =

d. $1\frac{1}{6}$ =

e. $3\frac{2}{5}$ =

f. $4\frac{2}{3}$ =

g. $13\frac{1}{2}$ =

h. $7\frac{7}{8}$ =

i. $1\frac{3}{7}$ =

j. $2\frac{1}{6}$ =

k. $\frac{42}{7}$ =

l. $\frac{56}{8}$ =

m. $\frac{9}{6}$ =

n. $\frac{8}{7}$ =

o. $\frac{19}{5}$ =

p. $\frac{43}{12}$ =

q. $\frac{13}{3}$ =

r. $\frac{16}{4}$ =

s. $\frac{7}{2}$ =

t. $\frac{16}{7}$ =

Addition:

Rule: find a common denominator, then add the numerators together. Reduce improper fractions to mixed numbers. Reduce fractions whenever possible after adding.

Exercise I–4: Add the following fractions and reduce improper fractions to mixed numbers:

a. $\dfrac{3}{4} + \dfrac{1}{4}$ =

b. $\dfrac{2}{3} + \dfrac{1}{3}$ =

c. $\dfrac{3}{4} + \dfrac{1}{2} =$

d. $\dfrac{1}{2} + \dfrac{4}{6} =$

e. $\dfrac{2}{3} + \dfrac{3}{4} =$

f. $\dfrac{1}{2} + \dfrac{7}{12} =$

g. $\dfrac{3}{4} + \dfrac{1}{8} =$

h. $\dfrac{2}{7} + \dfrac{1}{8} =$

i. $\dfrac{5}{6} + \dfrac{1}{7} =$

j. $\dfrac{6}{8} + \dfrac{2}{4} =$

Multiplication/Division of Fractions:

Rules:

Multiplication:

1. Change any mixed numbers to improper fractions.
2. Cancel whenever possible.
3. Multiply remaining numerators to get final numerator and remaining denominators to get denominator.

   Example: $1\frac{3}{5} \times \frac{2}{8} = ?$

   $\frac{8}{5} \times \frac{2}{8} = \frac{2}{5}$

Division:

Rules:

1. Follow Rule 1 for multiplication.
2. Invert the divisor (fraction after division sign) and then multiply. Follow rules of multiplication.

Exercise I–5: Multiply or divide these fractions:

a. $\frac{1}{2} \times \frac{3}{4} =$

b. $2\frac{1}{7} \times \frac{3}{21} =$

c. $\frac{6}{18} \times 1\frac{3}{6} =$

d. $\frac{1}{2} \times \frac{3}{8} =$

e. $\frac{3}{8} \times 4\frac{1}{2} =$

f. $\frac{4}{12} \times \frac{1}{3} =$

g. $\frac{3}{16} \times 2 =$

h. $\frac{12}{24} \times \frac{3}{4} =$

i. $\frac{1}{2} \div \frac{3}{16} =$

j. $\frac{1}{2} \div 1\frac{1}{6} =$

k. $4\frac{1}{2} \div \frac{1}{2} =$

   l. $6 \div \frac{2}{3} =$
m. $2\frac{1}{4} \div \frac{1}{8} =$
n. $\frac{2}{3} \div \frac{1}{3} =$
o. $\frac{1}{2} \div 3 =$

II. Decimals

Decimals are based on tens and multiples or fractions of ten. Reading decimals is as follows:

```
t t h t u   •   t h t t
e h u e n       e u h e
n o n n i       n n o n
  u d s t       t d u
t s r   s       h r s t
h a e           s e a h
o n d           d n o
u d s           t d u
s s             h t s
a               s h a
n                 s n
d                 d
s                 t
                  h
                  s
```

Example: 0.29 is twenty-nine hundredths
             1.2 is one and two-tenths

Addition/Subtraction:

Rule: line up all decimals in a column, with the decimal points of all numbers in the same line.

   Example: 0.04
             +1.3
           ————
           1.34

Exercise II–1: Add or subtract:

   a. $27.1 + 3.007 =$
   b. $127 + 0.1 =$
   c. $3.4 + 1 =$
   d. $6.9 + 1.745 =$
   e. $10.9 + 0.0075 =$
   f. $27.9 - 0.3 =$
   g. $375.4 - 1.7542 =$
   h. $10 - 0.001 =$
   i. $9.5 - 0.3 =$
   j. $675.2 - 3 =$

Multiplication:
Rules:
1. Multiply as with whole numbers.
2. Count off the *total* number of decimal places in the figures multiplied from the right (to left) in your answer.

Example: $0.23 \times 1.01 = 0.2323$

Exercise II–2: Multiply:

a. $3.1 \times 1.75 =$
b. $10 \times 0.1 =$
c. $6.97 \times 1.34 =$
d. $6 \times 0.003 =$
e. $125 \times 1.0 =$
f. $10 \times 0.9 =$
g. $3.10 \times 2 =$
h. $3.3 \times 11 =$
i. $4.6 \times 2.3 =$
j. $5.91 \times 3.1 =$

Division:
Rule: convert the divisor to a whole number (no decimals in it) if necessary, and move the decimal place in the dividend the same number of places to the *right*.

Example: $0.18 \div 1.3$ becomes
$$1.8 \div 13$$

Exercise II–3: Divide:

a. $10.3 \div 14.13 =$
b. $193 \div 0.2 =$
c. $0.13 \div 15.1 =$
d. $12{,}400 \div 0.19 =$
e. $87.6 \div 93.45 =$
f. $1 \div 16 =$
g. $1 \div 375 =$
h. $2.478 \div 2.43$
i. $76.648 \div 0.04 =$
j. $3.0 \div 2.0 =$

III. Proportions

Proportions are commonly expressed in two formats: as fractions: $\frac{1}{2} = \frac{2}{4}$ as proportional terms:

$1 : 2 :: 2 : 4$

extreme : means :: means : extreme

To solve:

As fractions, cross multiply the numerators with opposite denominator;

As proportions, multiply the extremes, which will then equal the result of multiplying the means.

In the example above, this is:

$1 \times 4 = 2 \times 2$

If any one of the means or extremes is unknown, it can be called X and then solved for:

$1 \times 4 = 2 \times X$

$2X = 4$

$X = \frac{4}{2} = 2$

Exercise III–1: Solve the proportions or fractions:

a. $1 : 3 :: X : 5$

b. $0.02 : X :: 101 : 43$

c. $X : 55 :: 0.75 : 4.5$

d. $\dfrac{12.2}{X} = \dfrac{1.1}{150}$

e. $\dfrac{X - 3}{5} = \dfrac{8}{10}$

f. $\dfrac{X}{46} = \dfrac{0.002}{0.47}$

g. $\dfrac{0.13}{1.8} = \dfrac{9}{X}$

h. $\dfrac{7}{13} = \dfrac{X}{65}$

i. $1 : 4 :: X : 35$

j. $1.5 : 2.35 :: 5 : X$

IV. Percentages

Definition: percentage means parts per hundred. 25% is 25 parts per hundred.

In decimals, this would be 0.25 or twenty-five hundreths

In fractions: $\dfrac{25}{100}$

To express a percent as a decimal: *divide* by a hundred, which is to move the decimal 2 places toward the *left*.

Example: $15.5\% = 0.155$

To express a decimal as a percent: *multiply* by a hundred, which is to move the decimal 2 places toward the *right*.

Example: $0.364 = 36.4\%$

(For a fraction, divide the denominator into the numerator to obtain a decimal.)

Exercise IV–1: Express as a decimal:
a. 47% =
b. 0.2% =
c. 50% =
d. 150% =
e. 15% =
f. 36% =
g. 0.1% =
h. 0.005% =

Exercise IV–2: Express as a percentage:
a. 0.5 =
b. 0.125 =
c. 0.56 =
d. 0.3 =
e. 0.95 =
f. $\frac{1}{200}$ =
g. $\frac{1}{50}$ =
h. $\frac{1}{1000}$ =
i. $\frac{1}{100}$ =

V. Metric Conversions

Since the metric system of weight and volume is based on powers of 10, conversion of units within the metric system can be accomplished by shifting decimal places to the right or left.

To substitute smaller units for larger units (e.g., milligrams for grams), move the decimal to the *right*.

Example: 0.5 grams = 500 milligrams Since 1 gram = 1000 milligrams, multiply by 10^3.

To use larger units for smaller units (e.g., grams for milligrams), move the decimal to the *left*.

Example: 250 milligrams = 0.25 grams
1 milligram = $\frac{1}{1000}$ gram, multiply by 10^{-3}

Exercise V–1: Perform the following conversions:
a. 125 ml = _____ L
b. 100 mg = _____ g
c. 10 mg = _____ g
d. 0.002 g = _____ mg
e. 0.4 L = _____ ml
f. 0.002 L = _____ ml
g. 12 mg = _____ g
h. 12 mg = _____ kg
i. 12 mg = _____ μg
j. 1.2 g = _____ μg

k. 1 cc = _____ ml
l. 0.0025 g = _____ mg
m. 370 µg = _____ mg
n. 90 µg = _____ mg

Answer key: Arithmetic review

I–1: a. ¼
  b. ⅓
  c. ⅓
  d. ¼
  e. ½
  f. ¼
  g. ²⁄₇
  h. ¾
  i. ⁹⁄₁₆
  j. ⅙
I–2: a. 12
  b. 18
  c. 36
  d. 180
  e. 40
  f. 24
  g. 48
  h. 216
  i. 78
  j. 18
I–3: a. ⁵⁄₄
  b. ⁵⁄₃
  c. ³³⁄₈
  d. ¹⁰⁄₆
  e. ¹⁷⁄₅
  f. ¹⁴⁄₃
  g. ²⁷⁄₂
  h. ⁶³⁄₈
  i. ¹⁰⁄₇
  j. ¹³⁄₆
  k. 6
  l. 7
  m. 1½
  n. 1⅐
  o. 3⅘
  p. 3⁷⁄₁₂

      q. $4\frac{1}{3}$

      r. 4

      s. $3\frac{1}{2}$

      t. $2\frac{2}{7}$

I–4: a. $\frac{4}{4} = 1$

      b. $\frac{3}{3} = 1$

      c. $\frac{5}{4} = 1\frac{1}{4}$

      d. $\frac{7}{6} = 1\frac{1}{6}$

      e. $\frac{17}{12} = 1\frac{5}{12}$

      f. $\frac{13}{12} = 1\frac{1}{12}$

      g. $\frac{7}{8}$

      h. $\frac{23}{56}$

      i. $\frac{41}{42}$

      j. $\frac{10}{8} = 1\frac{2}{8} = 1\frac{1}{4}$

I–5: a. $\frac{3}{8}$

      b. $\frac{45}{147}$

      c. $\frac{1}{2}$

      d. $\frac{3}{16}$

      e. $\frac{27}{16}$

      f. $\frac{4}{36} = \frac{1}{9}$

      g. $\frac{6}{16}$

      h. $\frac{3}{8}$

      i. $\frac{8}{3} = 2\frac{2}{3}$

      j. $\frac{3}{7}$

      k. $\frac{9}{1} = 9$

      l. 9

     m. 18

     n. 2

     o. $\frac{1}{6}$

II–1: a. 30.107

      b. 127.1

      c. 4.4

      d. 8.645

      e. 10.9075

      f. 27.6

      g. 373.6458

      h. 9.999

      i. 9.2

      j. 672.2

II–2: a. 5.425

      b. 1.0

      c. 9.3398

      d. 0.018

     e. 125
     f. 9.0
     g. 6.20
     h. 36.3
     i. 10.58
     j. 18.321

II–3: a. 0.72894
     b. 965.0
     c. 0.00860
     d. 65,263.157
     e. 0.93739
     f. 0.0625
     g. 0.00266
     h. 1.01975
     i. 1,916.20
     j. 1.5

III–1: a. $X = 1.667$
     b. $X = 0.0085$
     c. $X = 9.167$
     d. $X = 1663.636$
     e. $X = 7$
     f. $X = 0.196$
     g. $X = 124.615$
     h. $X = 35$
     i. $X = 8.75$
     j. $X = 7.83$

IV–1: a. 0.47
     b. 0.002
     c. 0.5
     d. 1.50
     e. 0.15
     f. 0.36
     g. 0.001
     h. 0.00005

IV–2: a. 50%
     b. 12.5%
     c. 56%
     d. 30%
     e. 95%
     f. $0.005 = 0.5\%$
     g. $0.02 = 2\%$
     h. $0.001 = 0.1\%$
     i. $0.01 = 1\%$

V−1:   a. 0.125 L
    b. 0.1 g
    c. 0.01 g
    d. 2 mg
    e. 400 ml
    f. 2 ml
    g. 0.012 g
    h. 0.000012 kg
    i. 12,000 μg
    j. 1,200,000 μg
    k. 1 ml
    l. 2.5 mg
    m. 0.37 mg
    n. 0.09 mg

Appendix C

Drug Preparation for Nebulization

Solutions for nebulization often require the drawing up and mixing of a small amount of active drug with a larger amount of diluent, to achieve a total volume suitable for nebulizer efficiency. This volume is 2.5 to 4.0 ml. If only one agent is needed and the dose gives the required volume, no mixing is needed, and either a single syringe or a unit-dose preparation can be used. Commercial unit-dose preparations of solutions for nebulization minimize the chance for error and maximize convenience. For example, the usual dose of 0.5 ml of 0.5% albuterol for nebulization is currently available as a premixed 3-ml solution of 0.083% strength. The premixed unit dose contains the same 2.5 mg of active albuterol as the 0.5 ml of the 0.5% solution and is ready for nebulization with no additional diluent (volume). Unit-dose preparations can be expensive and lack flexibility for dosage adjustments. In the event that a unit-dose preparation cannot be used, the following guidelines are offered for preparing nebulized drugs.

Measuring Medications. Use one separate syringe for each drug agent or diluent, with tuberculin syringes for measuring potent bronchodilators or drugs with small, critical amounts. Add the measured drug or drugs, and diluent if needed, to a 3-ml syringe through the needle adapter on the syringe barrel; this 3-ml syringe will be the delivery vehicle for an actual unit dose. After filling the delivery syringe or other suitable delivery container, it can be capped and labeled with the medication name, dose, date, patient's name, and location. A convenient label is the press-apply type of strip. This gives a unit-dose container, and as a method of drug measurement, can be employed within a fully developed unit-dose drug preparation system or by individual staff. The procedure is more efficient with one person drawing up a number of unit syringes from the individual drug agents, rather than many staff members each drawing up a few doses. One medication technician would also better utilize a well-established work space for preparing medications. An aseptic, established work space for medication preparation, with all suitable supplies, is a must for efficient operation.

Clarifying Physician Orders. Check the physician's order for accuracy and communicate to physicians the drugs available for aerosol use and suggested strengths and dosages. This can be accomplished through the medical director or memoranda to the hospital's medical board.

Manufacturers' Specifications. Check and follow all recommendations concerning drug use. Valuable information is contained in drug literature inserts.

Basic Methodology. A review of procedures should check for sound methods in all aspects of medication preparation. This includes basic hand washing, asepsis of the medication area and storage area, labeling of drug doses, dating opened medications and discarding expired drugs, needle storage, and the overall process of drug distribution between the physician's order and actual administration of the drug to the patient. This process should be examined for streamlined efficiency and accuracy.

Drug Interactions

In this appendix, drug-drug interactions with respiratory care drugs are noted. Each class of drug is given and those drugs or groups with interaction are listed.

Drug-drug interaction: Modification of the effect of one drug by another.

The following source provides detailed listings of drug-drug interactions for all drugs, not just those used in respiratory care:

Drug Interaction Facts, available from JB Lippincott, Facts and Comparisons Division.

I. Sympathomimetic bronchodilators.
   A. Effects antagonized by beta-blocking agents (e.g. propranolol).
   B. Antagonize the effect of some antihypertensive agents such as guanethidine or propranolol.
   C. Effect is increased by tricyclic antidepressants and some antihistamines.
   D. Have additive effects with each other and with anticholinergic and xanthine bronchodilators.
   E. May necessitate increased doses of insulin or oral hypoglycemic agents.
   F. Effect may be enhanced by corticosteroids.
II. Anticholinergic bronchodilators.
   A. Additive effects with sympathomimetic bronchodilators.
   B. No adverse effects have been noted for ipratropium (Atrovent) used concomitantly with methylxanthines, steroids, or cromolyn sodium.
III. Xanthine bronchodilators.
   A. Effect decreased by
      1. Cigarette and marijuana smoking.
      2. Phenobarbital.
      3. Aminoglutethimide (adrenal steroid inhibitor).
      4. Beta-adrenergic blocking agents.
   B. Effect increased by
      1. Cimetidine (Tagamet).
      2. Erythromycin.
      3. Influenza virus vaccine.

      4. Oral contraceptives.

      5. Troleandomycin.

      6. Clindamycin.

      7. Lincomycin.

      8. Possibly corticosteroids.

  C. Decreases the effect of

      1. Phenytoin (Dilantin).

      2. Lithium.

      3. Nondepolarizing muscle relaxants.

IV. Mucolytic (acetylcysteine).

  A. Incompatible when mixed in solution with

      1. Amphotericin B.

      2. Chlortetracycline.

      3. Tetracycline.

      4. Erythromycin.

      5. Oxytetracycline.

      6. Sodium ampicillin.

      7. Iodized oil USP.

      8. Chymotrypsin.

      9. Trypsin.

     10. Hydrogen peroxide.

  B. Reactive with iron, copper, and rubber.

V. Corticosteroids.

  A. Increased effect with erythromycin.

  B. May enhance response to beta-adrenergic bronchodilators.

  C. Have increased clearance with barbiturates, phenytoin, rifampin, and possibly ephedrine.

  D. Decrease the effect of acetyl salicylic acid, coumarin anticoagulants, and isoniazid.

  E. May decrease potassium levels with amphotericin B or potassium-depleting diuretics.

  F. May increase insulin and hypoglycemic agent requirements.

  G. Can increase reaction to attenuated-virus vaccines by enhanced virus replication.

VI. Cromolyn sodium.

  A. Animal studies have shown adverse fetal effects in high parenteral doses (40 to 300 times human dose) when given with high doses of isoproterenol.

VII. Neuromuscular blocking agents.

  A. Curare preparations.

      1. Effect intensified by aminoglycoside antibiotics, bacitracin, polymyxin B, tetracyclines, and potassium depletion due to diuretics.

      2. Effect antagonized by acetylcholine, anticholinesterases, and potassium.

B. Pancuronium bromide.
  1. Effect intensified by quinidine, the aminoglycoside antibiotics, clindamycin, lincomycin, and bacitracin.
  2. Effect antagonized by acetylcholine, anticholinesterases, theophylline, and potassium.
C. Atracurium.
  1. Effect intensified by the aminoglycoside antibiotics, bacitracin, capreomycin, polymyxin B, clindamycin and lincomycin, lithium, verapamil, procainamide, and quinidine.
  2. Effect reduced by theophylline and phenytoin.
D. Vecuronium.
  1. Effect intensified and prolonged with the following antibiotics: aminoglycosides, tetracyclines, bacitracin, polymyxin B, and colistin.
E. Succinylcholine.
  1. Enhanced or prolonged effect with acetylcholine, anticholinesterases (neostigmine), some nonpenicillin antibiotics, beta-adrenergic blockers, quinidine, procainamide, lidocaine, lithium, and furosemide.

Index